General Veterinary Pathology and Oncology

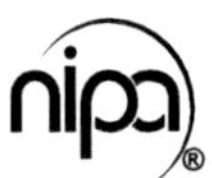

NIPA® GENX ELECTRONIC RESOURCES & SOLUTIONS P. LTD.
New Delhi-110 034

About the Authors

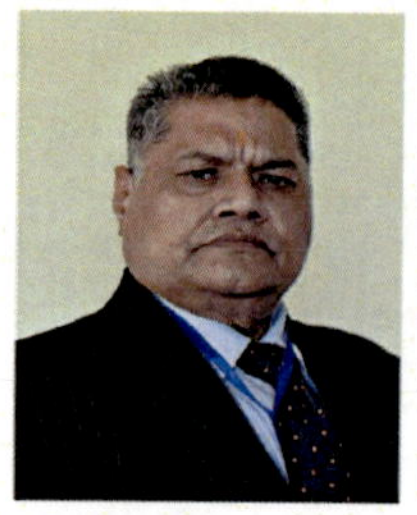

Prof RS Chauhan – Cowpathy Man, MVSc, PhD, FNAVS FSIIP, FIAVP, Diplomat ICVP, PDCR, ACPPM, OCTT MBA EX- Director ICAR-IVRI, JD CADRAD, Director IBT National Fellow, Advisor WHO. Member, Animal Welfare Board of India; Member, CPCSEA (Govt. of India); Chairman Scientific Advisory Committee, ICMR-NARFBR.

Born on September 10th, 1958 in a farmer's family, Dr. Chauhan completed his Bachelors (80.3%) with honours, Master (85.8%) and Doctoral degree (90.0%) in Veterinary Sciences with specialization in veterinary pathology from G.B. Pant University of Agric. & Tech., Pantnagar. He served the country in various capacities including Assistant Professor/ADIO (1983-96), Associate Professor (1996-1999), National Fellow (1999-2004) and Joint Director (CADRAD), IVRI, Izatnagar(2004-2009), Director & Vice-Chancellor(2009), ICAR-IVRI and Campus Director, IBT, Patwadangar (2009-2013). During his tenure as academician and scientist, he has written 112 books including 35 manuals and 1 monograph very popular among the students world over. He contributed 99 chapters in different books and published 235 research and 59 review papers. Besides, he participated in International / National Conferences and presented 178 papers. He is life member of 15 scientific bodies and has been in several executive committee such as Chairman, Panch Gavya Professionals' Club; President, Cow Therapy Society; Secretary-General, Society for Immunology and Immunopathology; Vice President, Indian Society of Veterinary Educators; Zonal Secretary, Indian Association of Veterinary Pathologists and Joint Secretary, Indian Virology Society, President, Dr. J.L. Vegad Foundation, Expert Member Research Group, Committee for Certification of Pathologists, Vice-President, IAVP; Registrar, ICVP, etc.

Based on his contributions and scientific achievements, he has been awarded with several prizes, medals and honours including Best Young Scientist Award (1992), IAAVR Award (1996), National Fellow Award (1999), Fellow NAVS (2000), Fellow SIIP (2001), K.S. Nair Memorial Award (1999), Vigyan Bharti Award (2000), Dr. C.M. Singh Trust Award (2002), Dr. Rajendra Prasad Award (2002), Shri Ramlal Agrawal National Award (2000), Best Paper Award SIIP (2003), Best Paper Award IAVA (2001, 2002, 2003), Best Teacher Award (2004) by GBPUAT, Fellow, IAVP (2006), Gopal Gaurav (2007), Bharat Excellence Award (2007), Diplomat, ICVP (2008), Intas-ISVE Best Veterinary Scientist Award (2008), Best Academician Award (2012), Moropant Pingle Go Sewa National Award (2015), Outstanding Scientist Award (2019), Research Excellence Award (2020), Indo

Asian-Claude Bourgelat Distinguished Innovative Scientist Award-2020 in Animal Immunopathology and MAN OF COWPATHY at GADVASU Ludhiana etc. in recognition of his research and teaching endeavor. He has been inducted in many national and international scientific/advisory committees and boards including Member, WHO/IPCS Committee on Environmental Health Criteria. Dr. Chauhan added many new including Enterotoxaemia, Pyometra, ETEC infection in camels, isolated camel pox virus, developed rapid diagnostic test DIA for the first time in India. He reported role of cell mediated immunity in rotavirus infection in calves. His pioneer work includes immunopathology due to pesticides, heavy metals, mycotoxins and nanoparticles. Dr. Chauhan developed a new method using MTT dye for detection of CMI response. He has scientifically validated Panchgavya and named it as "Cowpathy".

He have been recognized internationally as visiting Professor, University of Wageningen and Advisor, WHO. Dr. Chauhan guided more than 50 scholars for their Masters and Doctoral research; most of them are placed as Professors, Scientists, Officers in Indian Army, banks and industry in India and abroad. At present he is working as Head Veterinary Pathology, Chairman Scientific Advisory Committee ICMR-NARFBR, Member AWBI and CPCSEA (Govt of India). Prof Chauhan superannuated on 30th June 2024 after distinguish service of 41.5 years and still contributing to the profession through lectures, writings and research and particularly developing literature/ books for the benefit of students and young generation.

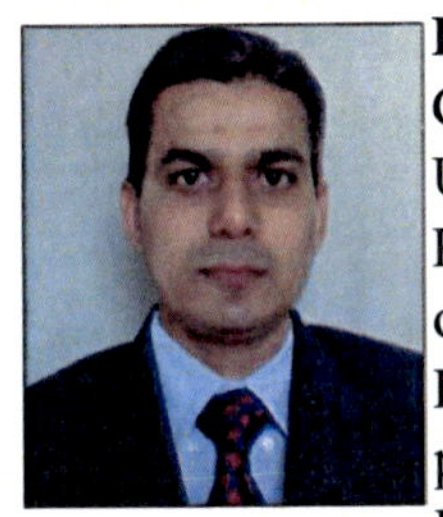

Dr. Desh Deepak Singh is Veterinary Graduate and Post Graduate in Veterinary Pathology from Govind Ballabh Pant University of Agriculture and Technology (GBPUA&T), Pantnagar (Uttarakhand) India in 2001 and 2003. He is awarded outstanding student award by GBPUA&T, Pantnagar in 2003. He visited Istanbul, Turkey to present research paper in world poultry congress-2004. He joined as Assistant Professor, Department of Veterinary Pathology, College of Veterinary Sciences & Animal Husbandry, Acharya Narendra Dev University of Agriculture & Technology (ANDUA&T), Kumarganj, Ayodhya, Uttar Pradesh in 2004. He completed his Ph.D. as in-service candidate from Uttar Pradesh Pandit Deen Dayal Upadhyay Pashu Chikitsha Vigyan Vishwavidyalaya Evam Go Anusandhan Sansthan (DUVASU), Mathura-281001, Uttar Pradesh, India in 2017 and promoted to Associate Professor in 2017 in ANDUA&T, Kumarganj, Ayodhya. Dr Singh was selected as Professor, Veterinary Pathology, DUVASU, Mathura in 2023 and presently working as Professor & Head, Veterinary Pathology, DUVASU, Mathura. He is having more than 20 years' experience of teaching Under Graduate

(UG) and Post Graduate (PG) courses of Veterinary Pathology along with vast experience of disease diagnosis, research and extension. He has published more than 48 research papers in referred journals, 08 review articles, 10 book chapters, 53 technical/popular articles, 04 laboratory manuals for Under Graduate students, 02 manuals for Veterinary Officers and 01 book. He is awarded Young Scientist award by Society of Immunology and Immunopathology, Prakash best poster award, best paper presentation award by Indian Society of Veterinary Anatomy, best poster award by UP chapter of Indian Society of Veterinary Surgery and best paper award in National Conference held at ANDUA&T, Kumarganj, Ayodhya.

General Veterinary Pathology and Oncology

R.S. Chauhan
M.V.Sc., Ph.D. (Path.), FNAVS, FSIIP, FIAVP, PDCR, OCTT, ACPPM, MBA
(Ex- Advisor WHO, Ex- Director IVRI, Ex-JDCADRAD, Ex-Director IBT, Ex-National Fellow ICAR)
Member Animal Welfare Board of India (Govt. of India)
Member, CCSEA (Govt of India)
Chairman, SAC, ICMR-NARFBR
Ex-Professor and Head, Department of Veterinary Pathology
GB Pant University of Agriculture & Technology Pantnagar - 263 145
Uttarakhand, India

Desh Deepak Singh
M.V.Sc., Ph.D.
Professor & Head
Department of Veterinary Pathology
Uttar Pradesh Pandit Deen Dayal Upadhyay Pashu Chikitsha Vigyan Vishwavidyalaya Evam Go Anusandhan Sansthan (DUVASU), Mathura-281001
Uttar Pradesh, India

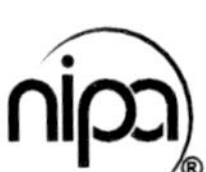

NIPA® GENX ELECTRONIC RESOURCES & SOLUTIONS P. LTD.
New Delhi-110 034

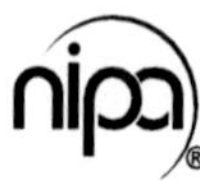

**NIPA® GENX ELECTRONIC
RESOURCES & SOLUTIONS P. LTD.**

101,103, Vikas Surya Plaza, CU Block
L.S.C.Market, Pitam Pura, New Delhi-110 034
Ph : +91 11 4386 0225, 9717133558, 9540816132
E-mail: newindiapublishingagency@gmail.com
Website: www. niparesources.com

Print ISBN: 978-93-58877-19-9

ebook ISBN: 978-93-58877-75-5

NIPA® also publishes books in a variety of electronic formats. Some content that appears in print may not be available in electronic books, and vice versa

Composed and Designed by NIPA®.

Preface

Veterinary Pathology is an important discipline of Veterinary Sciences which makes a bridge in between the basic and clinical sciences. The knowledge of Veterinary Pathology makes the veterinarian a perfect diagnostician particularly when his patient (animal) can't speak his/her illness to the doctor. Keeping the need of study of Veterinary Pathology to become a good Veterinary doctor, book "General Veterinary Pathology and Oncology" is written for the use of teachers, students and field veterinarians. The complexity of the subject was presented in a simplified way particularly keeping the view of Indian geo-climatic conditions and animal population. However, students of Veterinary Science desire a compact text of General Veterinary Pathology and Oncology covering the VCI new syllabus of Pathology which can be utilized during their study and examinations particularly competitive examinations. Hence, this text book is prepared as a text material to all those who want to study Pathology at undergraduate and postgraduate level and is interested in any kind of competitive examination or interview. It covers all the topics of Veterinary General Veterinary Pathology like etiology, disturbances in circulation, cell metabolism, growth and pigment metabolism besides inflammation, immunity and immunopathology. Animal cancers are discussed in detail with their occurrence in India, carcinogenesis, staging and grading, diagnosis and prognosis. The text is described in a very simple format including definition, etiology, clinical manifestations, macroscopic and microscopic features and diagnosis and only salient features are mentioned avoiding detailed text.

Hope this book "Veterinary General Pathology and Oncology" will find a place in the young fraternity of Veterinary Science. The help rendered by our colleagues and students in preparation and designing of this book is duly acknowledged. Readers' comments are welcome to further improve the book.

R.S. Chauhan
D.D. Singh

Contents

1

Introduction

Definitions

Pathology

Pathology is the study of the anatomical, chemical and physiological alterations from normal as a result of disease in animals. It is a key subject because it forms a vital bridge between preclinical sciences (Anatomy, Physiology, Biochemistry) and clinical branches of Medicine and Surgery (Fig.1.1). Pathology is derived from the Greek word pathos = disease, logos = study. It has many branches, which are defined as under:

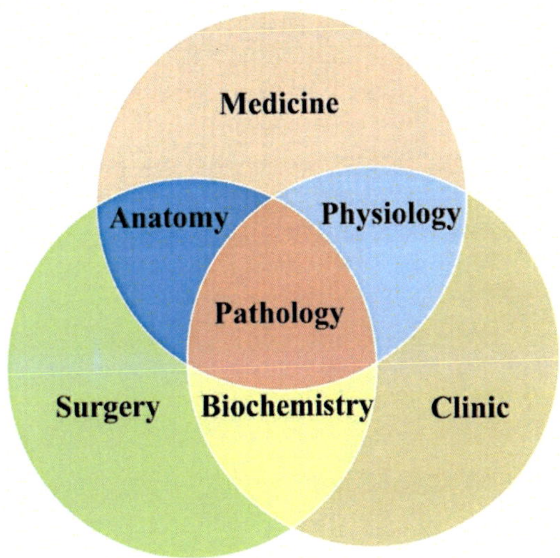

Fig. 1.1: Pathology- Relationship with other disciplines

General Pathology

General Pathology concerns with basic alterations of tissues as a result of disease. e.g. fatty changes, thrombosis, amyloidosis, embolism, necrosis (Fig. 1.2).

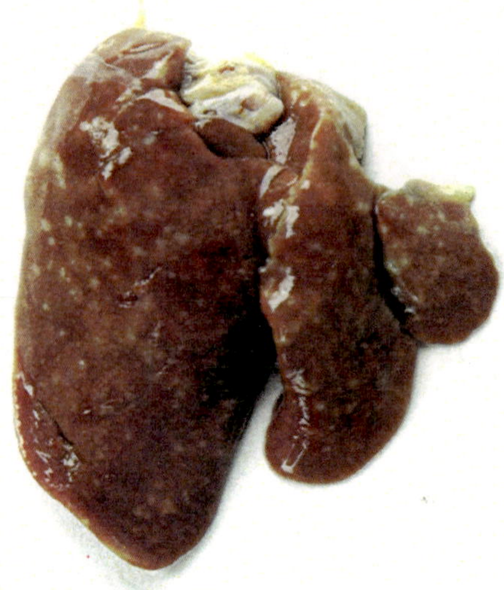

Fig. 1.2: Necrosis in liver

Systemic Pathology

Systemic Pathology deals with alterations in tissues/organs of a particular system. e.g. respiratory system, genital system etc. (Fig. 1.3).

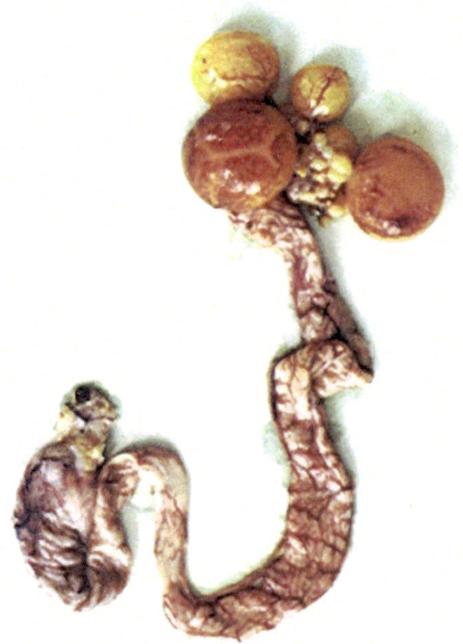

Fig.1.3: Female genital system of poultry

Specific Pathology

Specific Pathology is the application of the basic alterations learned in general pathology to various specific diseases. It involves whole body or a part of body. e.g. tuberculosis, rinderpest.

Experimental Pathology

Experimental Pathology concerns with the production of lesion through experimental methods. e.g. Rotavirus calves enteritis/ diarrhoea in calves (Fig. 1.4).

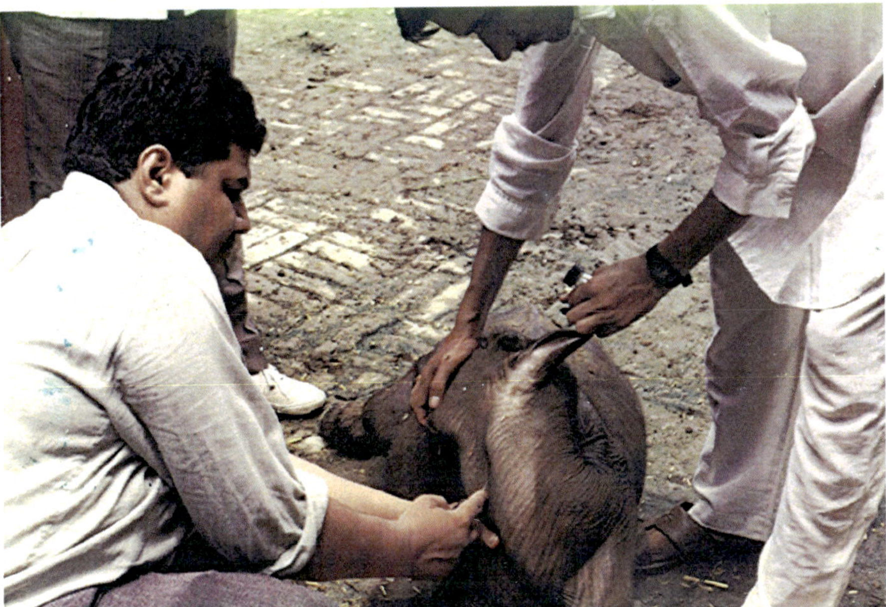

Fig. 1.4: Experimental Pathology

Clinical Pathology

Clinical Pathology includes certain laboratory methods which help in making the diagnosis using an excretions/secretions/blood/skin scrapings/ biopsy etc. e.g. urine examination, blood examination (Fig. 1.5).

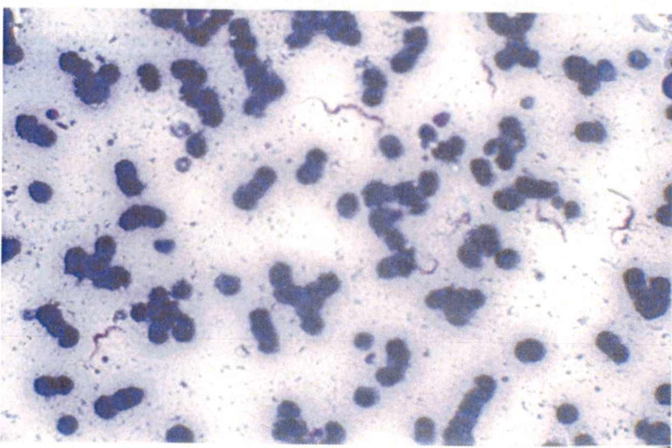

Fig.1.5: Examination of blood for protozoan parasites

Post-mortem Pathology

Post-mortem Pathology is examination of an animal after death. Also known as Necropsy or Autopsy. It forms the base for study of pathology (Fig. 1.6).

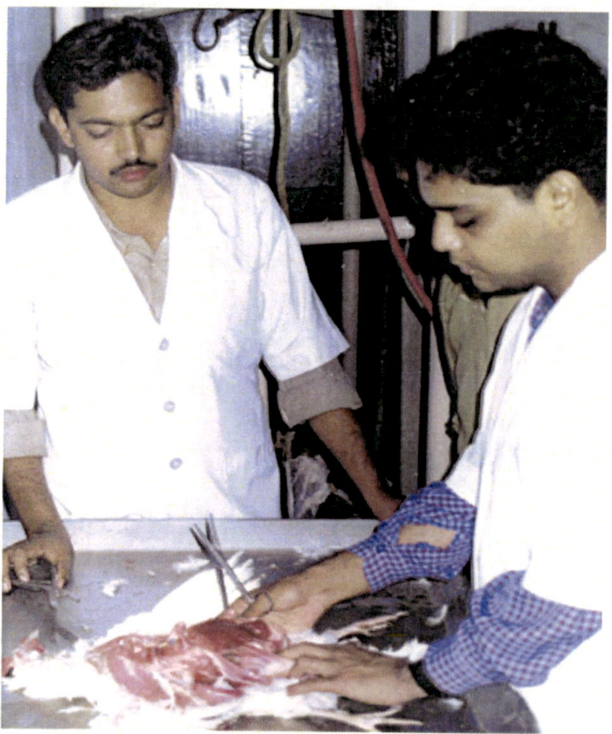

Fig. 1.6: Post-mortem examination of poultry

Microscopic Pathology

Microscopic Pathology deals with examination of cells/tissues/organs using microscope. It is also known as histopathology/cellular pathology. e.g. microscopy, electron microscopy (Figs. 1.7 & 1.8).

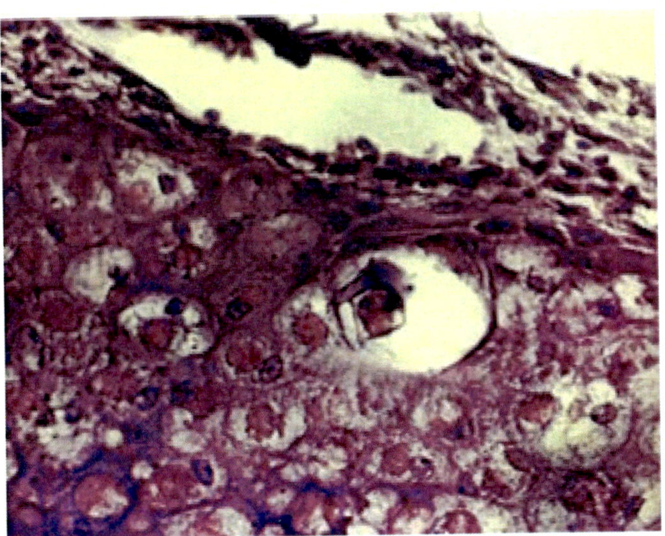

Fig. 1.7: Histopathology of skin showing inclusion bodies.

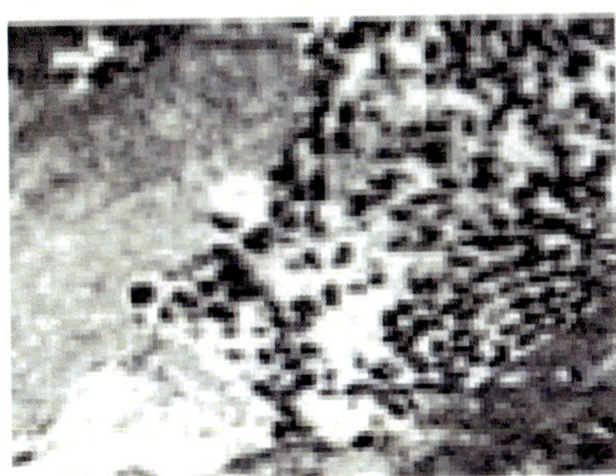

Fig. 1.8: Electron micro photograph showing poxvirus in cytoplasm of a cell

Humoral Pathology

Humoral Pathology is the study of alterations in fluids like antibodies in serum (Fig. 1.9).

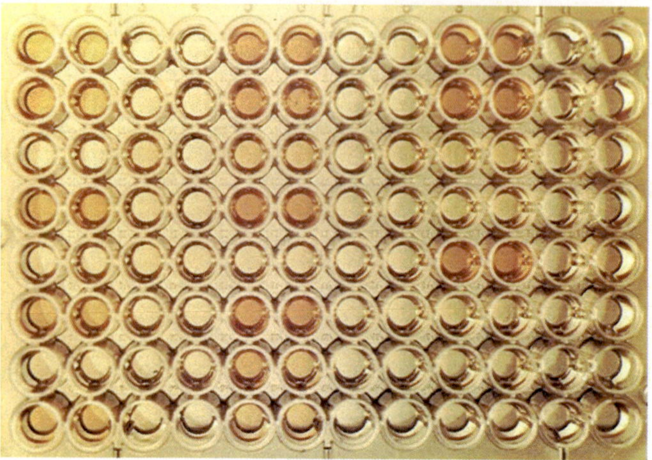

Fig. 1.9: A calf showing diarrhoea

Chemical Pathology

Chemical Pathology is the study of chemical alterations of body fluids/tissues. e.g. enzymes in tissue.

Physiological Pathology

Physiological Pathology deals with alteration in the functions of organ/system. It is also known as Pathophysiology. e.g. indigestion, diarrhoea, miscarriage (Fig. 1.10).

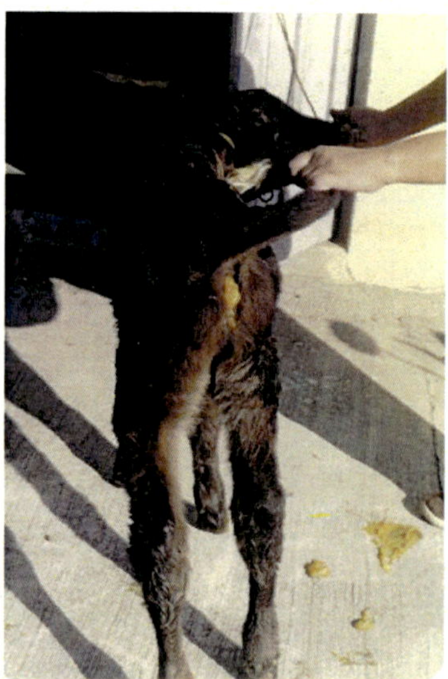

Fig. 1.10: Humoral Pathology- Detection of antibodies in serum.

Nutritional Pathology

Nutritional Pathology is the study of diseases due to deficiency or excess of nutrients. e.g. Vit.-A deficiency induced nutritional roup, rickets due to calcium deficiency (Fig. 1.11).

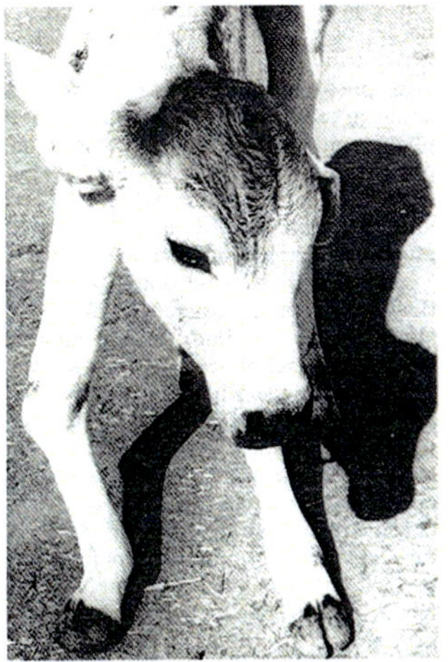

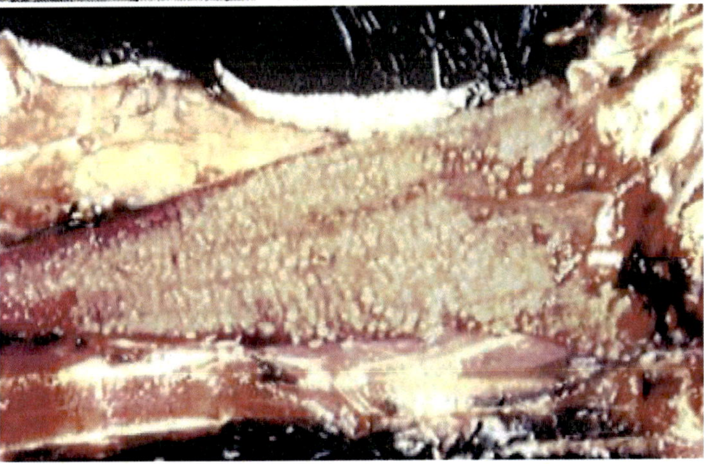

Fig. 1.11: Nutritional Pathology- Above: Rickets in a calf, Below: Nutritional roup due to vitamin A deficiency in poultry

Comparative Pathology

Comparative Pathology is the study of diseases of animals with a comparative study in human beings and other animals. e.g. zoonotic diseases such as tuberculosis (Fig. 1.12).

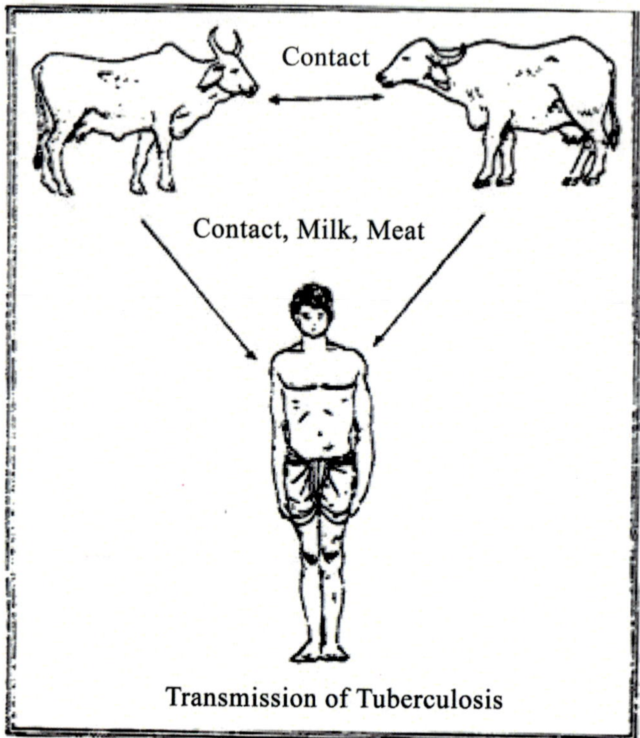

Fig. 1.12: Comparative Pathology- Diseases from animals to man

Oncology

Oncology is the study of cancer/tumor/neoplasms (Fig. 1.13).

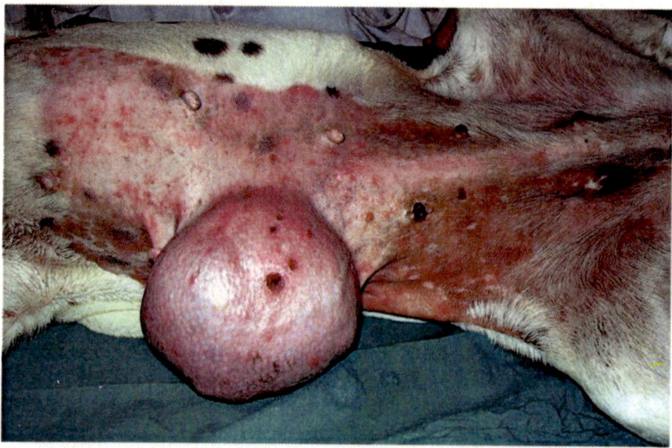

Fig. 1.13: Oncology- Mammary gland cancer in a bitch.

Immunopathology

Immunopathology deals with the study of diseases mediated by immune reactions. It includes Immunodeficiency diseases, autoimmunity and hypersensitivity reactions (Fig. 1.14).

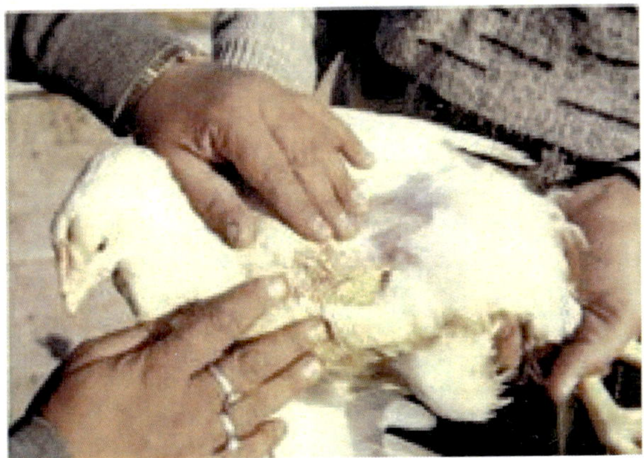

Fig. 1.14: Immunopathology-DTH reaction

Cytopathology

Cytopathology is the study of cells shed off from the lesions for diagnosis (Fig. 1.15).

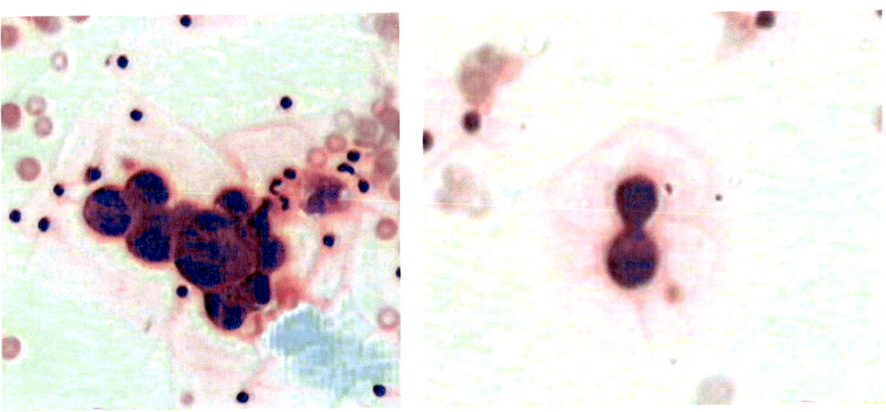

Fig. 1.15: Cytopathology

Health

Health is a state of an individual living in complete harmony with his environment/surroundings (Fig. 1.16).

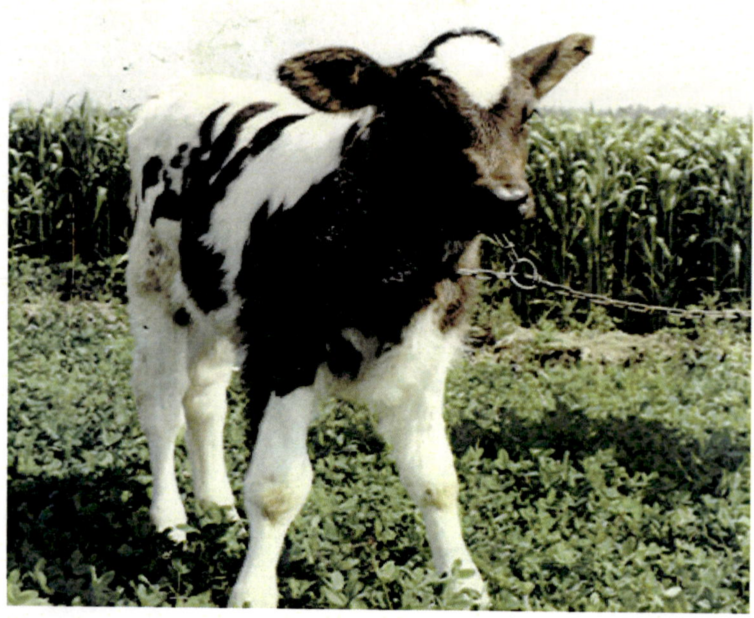

Fig. 1.16: A heathy calf

Disease

Disease is a condition in which an individual shows an anatomical, chemical or physiological deviation from the normal. (Discomfort with environment & body) (Fig. 1.17).

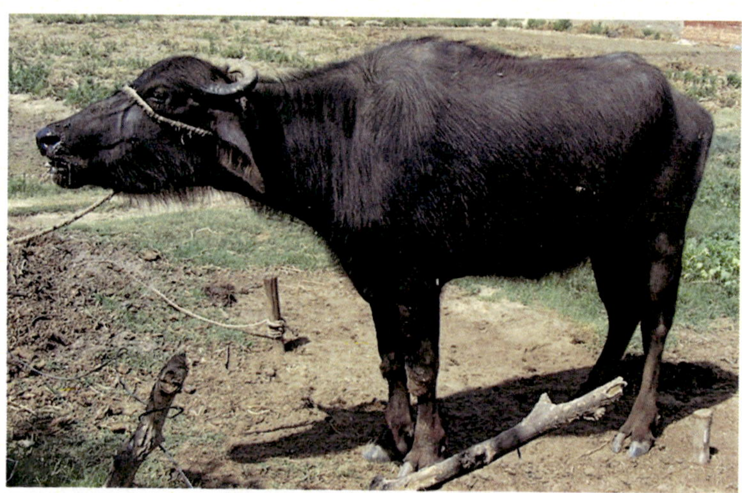

Fig. 1.17: Disease in a buffalo- dysnoea

Illness

Illness is the reaction of an individual to disease in the form of illness.

Forensic Pathology

Forensic Pathology includes careful examination and recording of pathological lesions in case of veterolegal cases.

Homeostasis

Homeostasis is the mechanism by which body keeps equilibrium between health and disease. e.g. Adaptation to an altered environment.

Toxopathology

Toxopathology or Toxic Pathology deals with the study of tissue/organ alterations due to toxins/poisons (Fig.1.18).

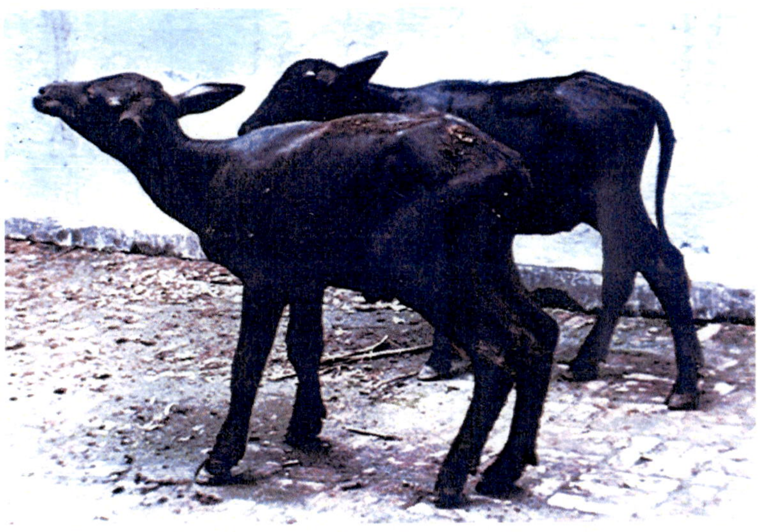

Fig. 1.18: Toxopathology- Strychnine poisoning in buffalo calves

Etiology

Etiology is the study of causation of disease (Fig. 1.19).

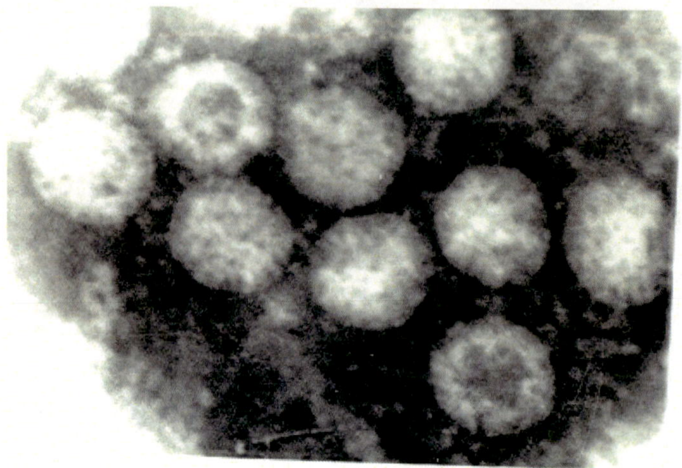

Fig. 1.19: Etiology-Rotavirus cause of diarrhoea in calves

Diagnosis

Diagnosis is an art of precisely knowing the cause of a particular disease (Dia= thorough, gnosis= knowledge) (Fig 1.20).

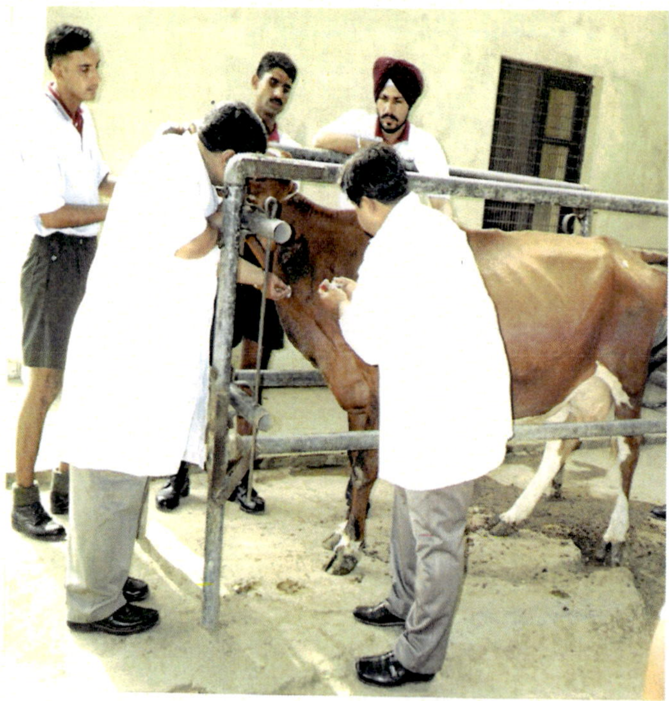

Fig. 1.20: Diagnosis of disease in animals- Tuberculin uesting

Symptoms

Any subjective evidence of disease of animal characterized by an indication of altered bodily or mental state as told by owner (complaints of the patients).

Signs

Indication of the existence of something, any objective evidence of disease perceptible to veterinarian (observations of the clinicians).

Syndrome

A combination of symptoms caused by altered physiological process.

Lesion

Lesion is a pathological alteration in structure/ function that can be detectable (Fig. 1.21).

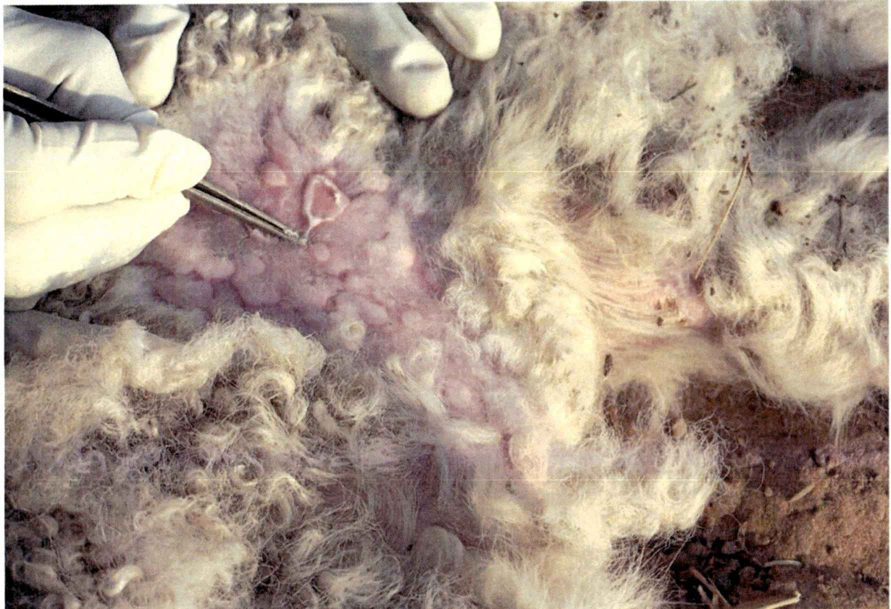

Fig.1.21: Skin of a sheep showing pock lesions.

Pathogenesis

Pathogenesis is the progressive development of a disease process. It starts with the entry of causal agent in body and ends either with recovery or death. It is the mechanism by which the lesions are produced in body.

Incubation period

Incubation period is the time that elapses between the action of a cause and manifestation of disease.

Course of disease

Course of disease is the duration for which the disease process remains till fate either in the form of recovery or death.

Prognosis

Prognosis is an estimate by a clinician of probable severity/outcome of disease.

Morbidity rate

Morbidity rate is the percentage/proportion of affected animals out of total population in a particular disease outbreak. e.g. out of 100 animals 20 are suffering from diarrhoea, the morbidity rate of diarrhoea will be 20%.

Mortality rate

Mortality rate is the percentage/proportion of animals out of total population died due to disease in a particular disease outbreak. e.g. if in a population of 100 animals, 20 fall sick and 5 died, the mortality rate will be 5%.

Case fatality rate

Case fatality rate is the percentage/proportions of animals died among the affected animals. If in a population of 100 animals, 20 fall sick and 5 die,. the case fatality rate will be 25%.

Biopsy

Biopsy is the examination of tissues received from living animals.

Infection

Infection is the invasion of the tissues of the body by pathogenic organisms resulting in the development of a disease process (Fig. 1.22).

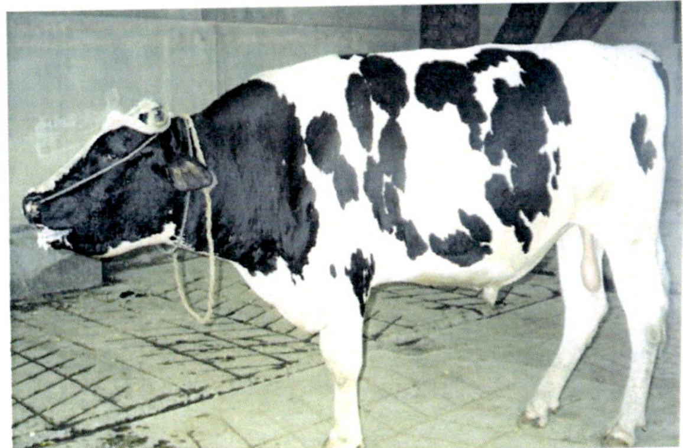

Fig. 1.22: Bull showing illness due to infection of *Pasteurella multocida.*

Infestation

Infestation is the superficial attack of any parasite/organism on the surface of body (Fig. 1.23).

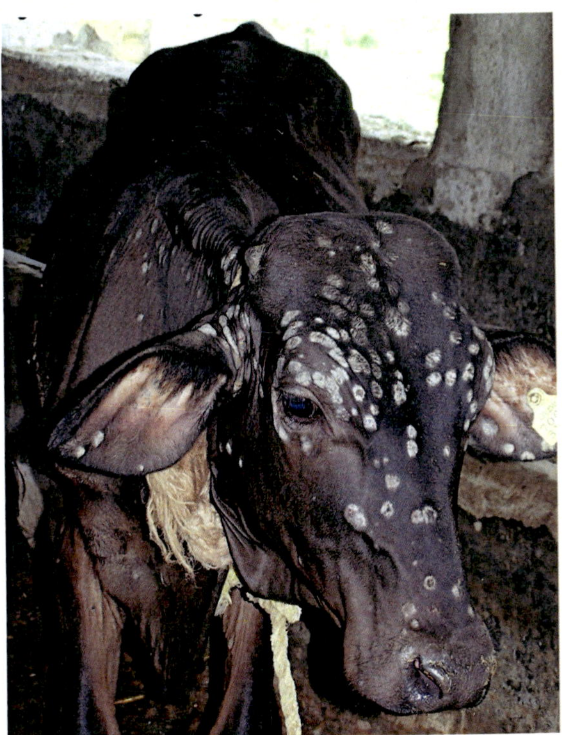

Fig.1.23: Infestation of demodectic mange in cattle

Pathogenicity

Pathogenicity is the capability of an organism for producing a disease.

Virulence

Virulence is the degree of invasiveness of pathogenic organism.

Historical Milestones

2500-1500 BC	Shalihotra (Indian)	• First known veterinarian of the world • Wrote Haya Ayurved/ Ashwa- Ayurved in Sanskrit, 8 volumes on equine medicine with diagnosis, treatment, effect of planetary forces and evils on health
	Muni Palkapya (Indian)	• Wrote a treatise on elephants — Gaj Ayurved
2100 BC	Hammurabi	• Conduct of Veterinary Practitioners, "Laws of Hammurabi"
1000 BC	Krishna (Indian) Nakul (4th Pandav) (Indian) Sahdev(5th Pandav) (Indian)	• Mathura is known for best cattle production/ milk production
		• Wrote Ashwa- Chikitsa, a book on equine medicine.
		• He is considered as an expert of equine management
		• Expert in cattle rearing and disease management.
800 BC	Charak (Indian)	• Wrote Charak Sanhita with details of cause of diseases and impact of environment.
500 BC	Jeevak (Indian)	• Described the pathology of brain.
460-375 BC	Hippocrates (Greece)	• Physician, studied malaria, pneumonia , also known as "Father of Medicine"
384-323 BC	Aristotle (Greece)	• Humoral theory of disease • Father of Zoology • Originator of Modern Anatomy & Physiology
300 BC	Chandra Gupta Maurya period	• In Kautilya, Arthshashtra description on "Animal Husbandry and Veterinary Sciences", rules on animal ethics and jurisprudence
	Samrat Ashok	• First Veterinary Hospital established for treatment of animal diseases • Prevention of cruelty on animals advertised through writings on walls.

53 BC-37 AD	Cornelius Celsus (Rome)	• Wrote 8 volumes of pathology (1st special pathology) • Cardinal signs of inflammation (redness, swelling, heat and pain)
131-206 AD	Claudius Galen (Rome)	• Meat inspection • 5th cardinal sign of inflammation "Loss of function"
450-500 AD	Renatus Vegetius (Rome)	• Father of Veterinary Medicine • Disregard divine pleasure • Disease of animals' influence on man
600 AD	Madhav	• Described pathology of diarrhoea, dysentery, icterus, tuberculosis and various toxic conditions.
980-1037 AD	Avicenna	• Cause of disease are minute organism • Spreads through air, food, water.
1497 AD-1558 AD	Jean Fernel	• Compiled the information of his time First to attempt to codify the knowledge of Pathology.
1564 AD-1642 AD	Galileo Galilei	• Developed single microscope
1578-1657 AD	William Harvey	• Blood vascular system and its impact on pathology
1617 AD-1619 AD	Drebbel	• Developed double lens microscope
1617-1680 AD	Solleysel (French)	• Book on Le Parfact Marechal
1632 AD-1723 AD	Antony van	• Saw microbes first
	Leeuwen-hoek	• Book — Little animals
1682-1771 AD	G.B. Morgagni (Italian)	• Conducted 700 autopsies • Began modern pathology • Book The seats and causes of disease
1712-1779 AD	Bourgelat, C (French)	• New knowledge of equine medicine
1728- 1793 AD	John Hunter (English)	• First experimental pathologist
1753-1793 AD	Saint Bel (French)	• Teacher at Alfort established Vet School in England 1791 and in 1793 died due to glanders.
1762 AD	Bourgelat, C (French)	• 1st Veterinary school established — Ecole Veterinaire • Nationale'd Alfort
1771-1802 AD	Bichat (French)	• Father of pathological anatomy • Foundation for the study of histology • Father of histology
1801-1858 AD	Mueller. J. (German)	• Cellular pathologist, known for his work "The fine structure and form of morbid tumors"

1804-1878 AD	Carl Rokitanskey (German)	• Supreme descriptive pathologist
1818-1865 AD	Semmelwiss (Hungarian)	• Surgery/autopsy • Started hospital sanitation
1821-1902 AD	R. Virchow (German)	• Journal Virchow's Archives • Great work on cellular pathology, "Father of modern Pathology"
1822-1895 AD	Louis Pasteur (French)	• Bacteria cause of disease
1839-1884 AD	J. Cohnheim (German)	• Originator of modern experimental pathology • Detected leucocytes at the site of inflammation • His work forms the basis for the pathology of Inflammation • Introduced frozen sections
1843-1890 AD	R. Koch (German)	• Koch's postulates • Identified Tuberculosis, Staphylococcus and Vibrio as cause of disease
1850-1934 AD	W.H. Welch (U.S.A)	• Professor Pathology • Started pathology in USA.
1869 AD	Bruck Muller (USA)	• Textbook of pathological anatomy of domestic and zoo animals.
1883-1962 AD	G.N. Papanicolaou	• Father of exfoliative cytology
1884 AD	E. Metchnikoff	• Phagocytosis (microphages/macrophages)
1884-1955 AD	Robert Feulgen (German)	• Founder of Histochemistry
1885-1979 AD	William Boyd (Canadian)	• Author of Textbook of Pathology
1889 AD		• Establishment of Imperial Bacteriological Laboratory at Mukteshwar (Now IVRI)
1905-1993 AD	L. Ackerman (American)	• Authority on interpretation of frozen sections.
1913 AD	India	• Imperial Bacteriological Laboratory (now IVRI) established at new campus at Izatnagar- Bareilly
1924 AD	India	• The Publication of Indian Veterinary Journal started
1926 AD	E. Joest	• Wrote 5 volumes of Veterinary Pathology

1931 AD	India	• The publication of Indian Journal of Veterinary Sciences and Animal Husbandry (Presently Indian Journal of Animal Sciences) started
1933 AD	Ruska and Lorries	• First developed electronmicroscope.
1936 AD	Bittner	• Milk transmission of cancer
1938 AD	R.A. Runnels	• Wrote book on "Animal Pathology".
1953 AD	Watson and Crick	• Structure of DNA
1968 AD	G.A. Sastry (India)	• Author of Veterinary Pathology textbook.
1973 AD		• The Publication of Indian Veterinary Medical Journal started from Lucknow
1976 AD		• The publication of Indian Journal of Veterinary Pathology started from Izatnagar
1983 AD		• Indian Association of Veterinary Pathologist established.
1989 AD		• Veterinary Council of India established • Dr. C.M. Singh became 1st President of VCI • 1st Veterinary and Animal Sciences University established in Madras (now Chennai).
1998 AD		• Establishment of " Society for Immunology and Immunopathology" at Pantnagar.
		• Publication of "Journal of Immunology and Immunopathology" started from Pantnagar

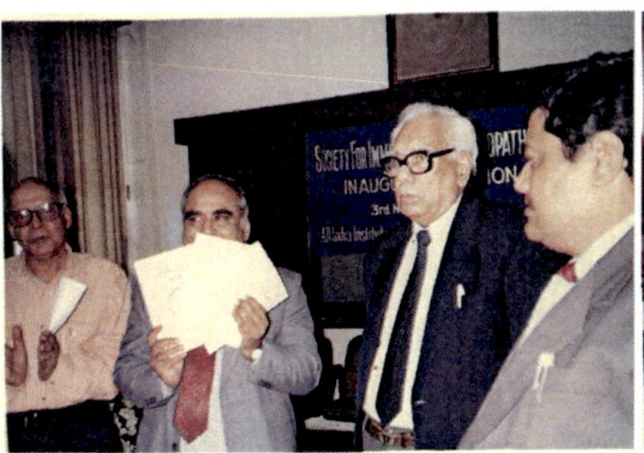
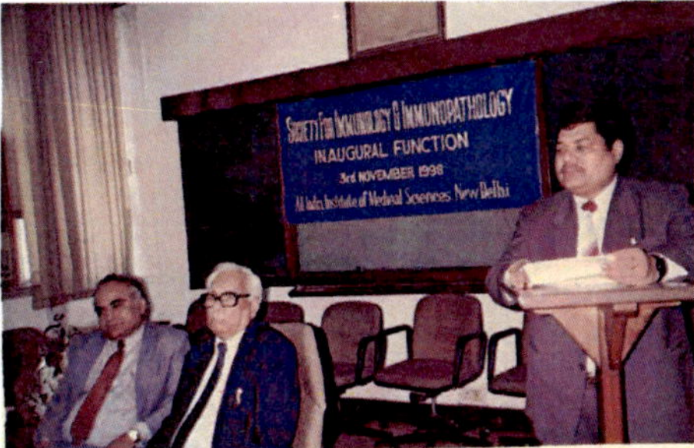

From left to right: Dr. Ramesh Kumar, Professor, Microbiology, AIIMS; Dr. N.K. Ganguly, Director General Indian Council of Medical Research; Dr. C.M. Singh, Former Director, IVRI and President VCI; Dr. R.S. Chauhan, National Fellow, at inaugural function of Society for Immunology and

Immunopathology.

2008 AD Silver Jubilee Annual Conference of IAVP and International Symposium on "Quality Assurance in Pathology and Disease Diagnosis" and Satellite Seminar on "Descriptive Gross and Microscopic Veterinary Pathology in Necropsy, Biopsy and Certification Examination during November 10-12, 2008 at IVRI, Izatnagar (UP). Establishment of Indian College of Veterinary Pathology (ICVP). Ist batch of 22 certified Chartered member and Diplomat ICVP passed out including Drs. AT Rao, MC Prasad, B Murali Manohar, C Balachandran, AK Srivastava, TV Anil Kumar, M Krishna Nair, VK Gupta, BN Tripathi, RS Chauhan, R Somvanshi, P Dwivedi, AK Sharma, JL Vegad, PP Gupta, RNS Gowda, MV Joshi, Lal Krishna, NK Sood, Syed SYH Qadri, Rajendra singh and VM Shingtagiri.

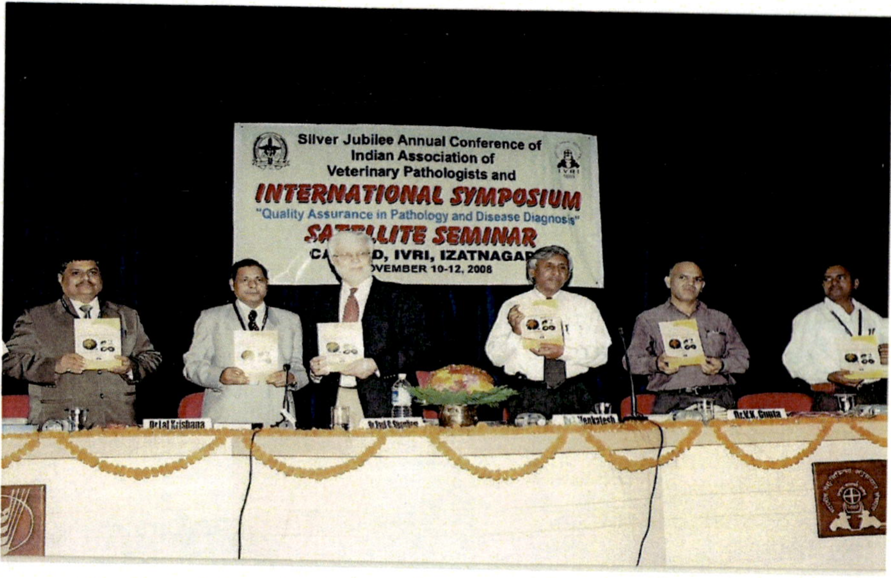

(Photo: From left to right) Drs. RS Chauhan, Chairman Silver Jubilee Conference IAVP; Lal Krishna, President IAVP; Paul C Stroberg, President ACVP; Venktesh; V K Gupta, Secretary General IAVP and Rajendra Singh, Organising Secretary in inaugural function of silver jubilee annual conference of Indian Association of Veterinary Pathologists)

2

Etiology

Etiology

Etiology is the study of cause of disease. It gives precise causal diagnosis of any disease. Broadly, the cause of diseases can be divided into two

a. Intrinsic causes.

b. Extrinsic causes.

Intrinsic Causes

Those causes which determine the type of disease present within an individual over which he has no control. These causes are further divided into following subgroups:

Genus

Specific diseases occur in a particular genus or species of animals. e.g. Hog cholera in pigs, Canine distemper in dogs

Breed/Race

Diseases do occur in particular breed of animals such as: dairy cattle are more prone for mastitis. Brain tumors are common in Bull dog/ Boxer.

Family

Genetic relationship plays a role in occurrence of diseases in animals. e.g. some chickens have resistance to leucosis; hernia in pigs due to weak abdominal wall.

Age

Age of animal may also influence the occurrence of diseases such as:

- At young age diarrhoea/pneumonia (Fig. 2.1).

- Old age tumor
- Canine distemper – Young dogs
- Strangles – Young horse
- Prostatic hyperplasia – Old dogs
- Coccidiosis – Young chickens

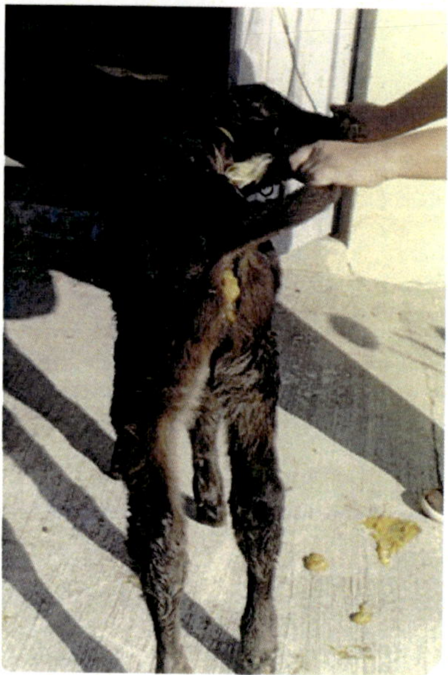

Fig. 2.1: A calf showing diarrhoea

Sex

Reproductive disorders are more common in females

- Milk fever, mastitis and metritis in females.
- Nephritis is more common in male dogs than female, but Bovine nephritis is more common in females.

Colour

Colour may also play role in occurrence of diseases. e.g. squamous cell carcinoma in white coat colour cattle, melanosarcoma in grey and white horses

Idiosyncracy

An unusual reaction of body to some substances such as

- Drug reaction: Small dose of drug may produce reaction.
- Individual variations.

Genetic Disorders

Aberration in Chromosomes

- A large number of chromosomal aberrations are removed due to death of gamete or zygote which is termed as "species cleansing effect". However, some aberrations persist and are expressed in phenotype leading to illness.

- **Aberration in number**
  - Chromosomes are in pairs (2n). When number of chromosomes are other than (n) or (2n). It is known as heteroploidy.

(a) Heteroploidy

The number of chromosomes are other than (n) or (2n). When abnormal number is exact multiplies of the haploid set due to errors in mitosis. The polar body may fail to be extruded from ovum leaving diploid set to be fertilized by sperm (n) i.e. 2n + n = 3n (Triploid zygote). When abnormal number is not the exact multiplies of haploid set. It may have specific chromosome in triple number (trisomy) or in single number (monosomy).

(b) Duplication and deficiencies

- Duplication or deficiency may occur in a section of chromosome and total number of chromosomes remains same.
- Translocation is the rearrangement of a part of chromosome in two non-homologous chromosomes. It may be reciprocal or non-reciprocal. Absence of a piece of chromosome is known as deletion.

(c) Mosaicism

- In mosaicism, there is more than one population of cells in body; each population differs in their chromosomes/ genes due to error during development.
- May be due to chromosomal non-disjunction there is, e.g. XXY in some cells, XY in other cells.

(d) Chimerism

- In this, one type of cells are acquired in utero from a twin e.g. Bovine twin, 1 male and 1 female, with joint placenta. The blood cells of male may go in female counterpart. Then the female will have two types of cell population, one of its own and another acquired from twin. Similarly, male may also have XX leucocytes in its blood. Such chimeric bulls are sterile.

2. Abnormalities in sex chromosomes

(a) Klinefelters syndrome

- Males have sex chromatin i.e. XXY = 47(2n) in man.
- In some cells, different number of chromosomes i.e. XX, XXY, XXXY, XXYY.
- It is recognized in adolescence by small testes, tall body, and low sexual characters, mostly infertile.
- May occur in sheep, cattle and horse.

(b) Tortoiseshell male cat

- Male cat has small testes, lack of libido and absence of spermatozoa in testes with 3n chromosomes (XXY).

(c) Turner's syndrome

- Mare are with XO karyotype having gonadal dysgenesis and such animals are sterile and do not have sex chromatin.
- In mice XO karyotype is normal.

(d) Intersexes

- In this condition ambiguity occurs in genitalia or the secondary sex characters are present for both the sexes including male and female.
- Hermaphrodites have male and female genitalia while pseudohermaphrodites have external genitalia of one sex and gonads of opposite sex.

(e) Freemartinism

- In bovine twins, one male with (XY) and one female (XX) karyotype but they share placental circulation so cells of embryo establish in other co-twin.

(f) Testicular feminization

- The animal has female genitalia as external and internal organs but in place of ovaries, there are testes. It occurs due to single gene defect and makes tissues unresponsive to androgenic hormones.

3. Abnormalities in autosomal chromosomes

(a) ***Down's syndrome/ Mongolism***

- It occurs as a result of trisomy, number of a particular chromosome increases leaving 2n, as 61 in bovines, 77 in dogs and 47 in man e.g. bovine lymphosarcoma occurs in animals with 2n=61. Male dog with 2n= 77 are prone to lymphoma.

(b) ***Sterility in hybrids***

Q. Donkey has 2n=62 and horse has 2n=64. Their cross mule has 2n=63.

R. Cause of sterility in mules is not known, may be due to uneven number of chromosomes.

4. Abnormalities in genes

- Lethal genes are those genes which are responsible for death of zygote.
- Sublethal genes
- X-linked or sex linked: Diseases transmitted by heterozygous carrier females only to male offsprings who are homozygous for X-chromosome.

Anomalies

Anomaly is a developmental abnormality that occurs in any organ/tissue. It may be due to genetic disorder and may affect the zygote itself within a few days after fertilization or may occur during any stage of pregnancy. It may be classified as under:

1. Imperfect development

(a) ***Agenesis***

Agenesis is incomplete development of an organ or mostly it is associated with absence of any organ.

Acrania is absence of cranium.

Anencephalia is absence of brain.

Hemicrania is absence of half of head. Agnathia is absence of lower jaw.

Anophthalmia is absence of one or both eyes. Abrachia is absence of fore limbs.

Abrachiocephalia is absence of forelimbs and head.

Adactylia is absence of digits.

Atresia is absence of normal opening e.g. Atresia ani is absence of anus opening.

(b) *Fissures*

Fissures are a cleft or narrow opening in an organ on the median line of head, thorax and abdomen.

- Cranioschisis is a cleft in skull.
- Chelioschisis is a cleft in lips also known as harelip.
- Palatoschisis is a cleft in palates; also known as cleft palate.
- Rachischisis is a cleft in spinal column.
- Schistothorax is a fissure in thorax.
- Schistosomus is a fissure in abdomen.

(c) *Fusion*

Fusion is joining of paired organs.

- Cyclopia is fusion of eyes.
- Renarcuatus is fusion of kidneys; also known as horseshoe kidneys.

2. Excess of development

1. Congenital hypertrophy of any organ.
2. Increase in the number of any organ or part /tissue.
3. Polyotia is increased number of ears.

Polyodontia is increased number of teeth. Polymelia is increased number of limbs. Polydactylia is increased number of digits.

Polymastia is increased number of mammary gland.

Polythelia is increased number of teats.

3. Displacement during development

(a) *Displacement of organ*

1. Dextrocardia is the transposition of heart into right side instead of left side of thoracic cavity.
2. Ectopia cordis is the displacement of heart into neck.

(b) *Displacement of tissues*

1. Teratoma is a tumor arising due to some embryonic defect and composed of two or more types of tissues. In this at least two tissues should be of origin.
2. Dermoid cyst is a mass containing skin, hair, feathers or teeth depending on the species and often arranged as cyst. It mostly occurs in the subcutaneous tissues.

Monster

Monster is a disturbance of development in several organs and causes distortion of the foetus e.g. Duplication of all or most of the organs (Fig. 2.2 and 2.3).

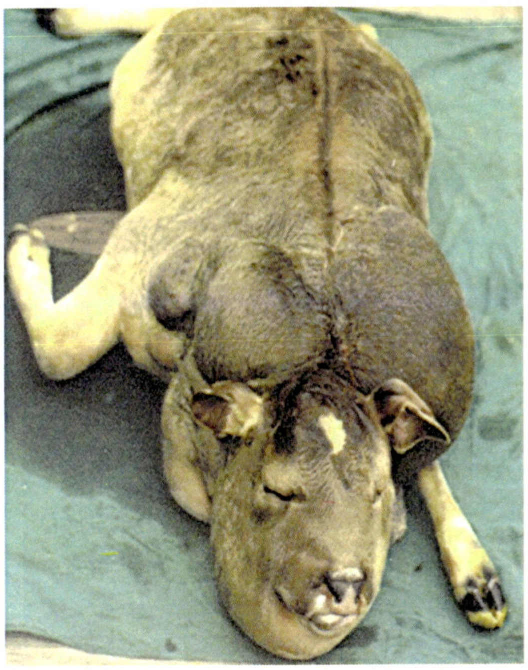

Fig. 2.2: Monster- duplication of most of the organs- incomplete twining.

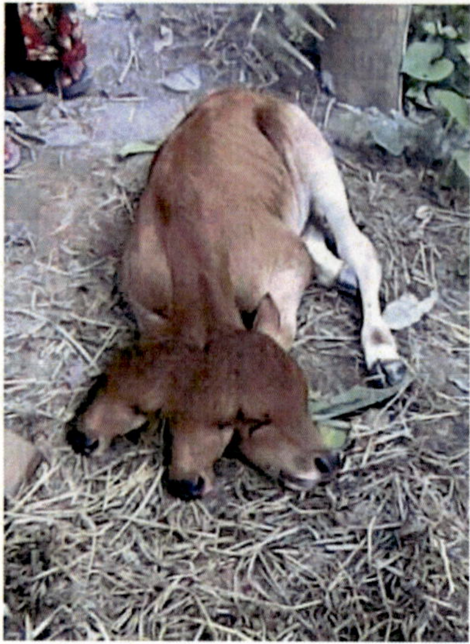

Fig. 2.3: Monster- Tricephely

- Monsters develop from a single ovum; these are the product of incomplete twinning.
- Monsters are classified as under:

1. Separate twins

One twin is well developed while another is malformed and lacks the heart, lungs or trunk, head, limbs.

2. United twins

These twins are united with symmetrical development and are further classified as

(a) ***Anterior twinning***

Anterior portion of foetus is having double structures while posterior remains as single.

- Pyopagus is a monster twin united in the pelvic region with the bodies side by side.
- Ischiopagus is a monster twin united in the pelvic region with the bodies at more than a right angle.
- Dicephalus is a monster having two separate heads, neck, thorax, and trunk.

- Diprosopus is a monster having double organs in cephalic region without complete separation of heads and with double face.

(b) *Posterior twinning*

When in monsters, the anterior portion remains single and posterior parts become double.

- Craniopagus is a monster having separate brain with separate bodies arranged at an acute angle.
- Cephalothoracopagus is the monster having united head and thorax.
- Dipygus is the monster having double posterior extremities and posterior parts of body.

(c) *Almost complete twining*

In some monster, twins have complete development with joining in thorax and abdomen.

- Thoracopagus is a monsters united in thorax region.
- Prosopothoracopagus is the monster twin united at thorax, head, neck and abdomen.
- Rachipagus is the monster in which thoracic and lumber portion of vertebral column are united in twin.

Extrinsic Causes

Some etiological factors which are present in the outside environment may cause/influence the occurrence of disease. These are also known as exciting cause/acquired cause. Majority of causes of diseases fall under this group which are further classified as physical, chemical, biological and nutritional causes.

Physical Causes

Trauma

Traumatic injury occurs due to any force or energy applied on body of animal e.g. during control / restraining, shipping or transport of animal.

Contusions/Bruises

Contusions or bruises arise from rupture of blood vessel with disintegration of extravassated blood (Fig. 2.4).

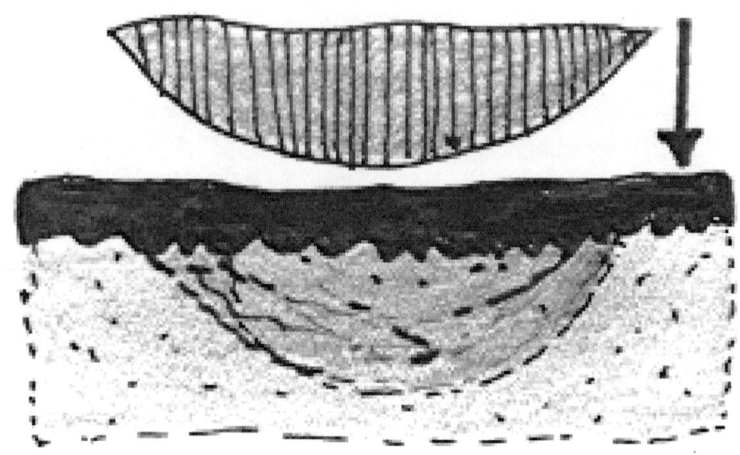

Fig. 2.4: Contusions

Abrasions

Abrasions are circumscribed areas where epithelium has been removed by injury and it may indicate the direction of force (Fig. 2.5).

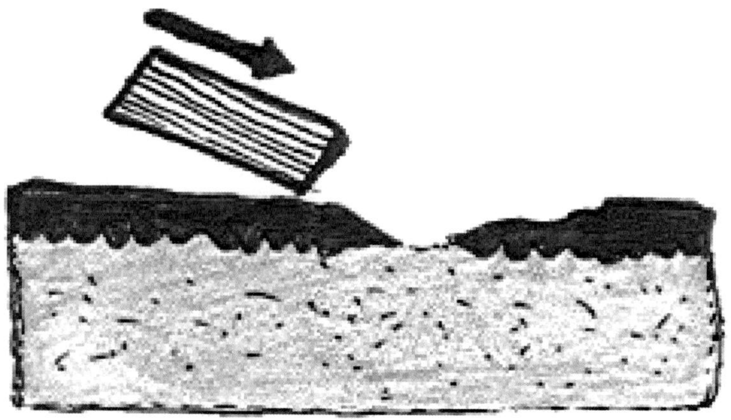

Fig. 2.5: Abrasion

Erosions

Partial loss of surface epithelium on skin or mucosal surface is termed as erosion (Fig. 2.6).

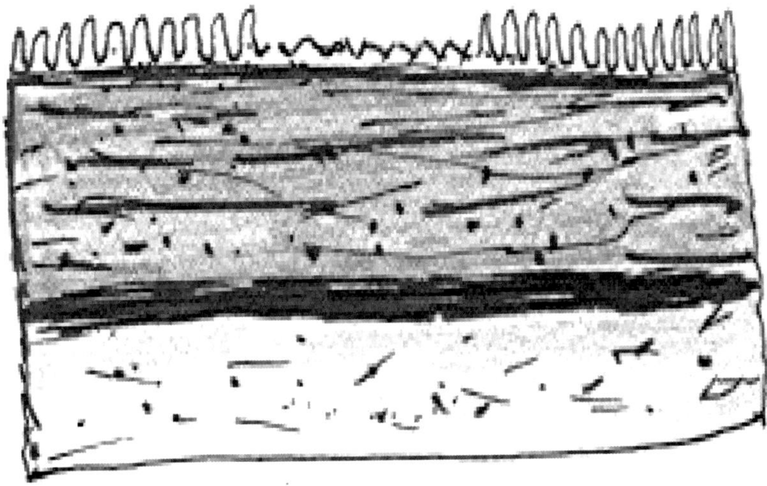

Fig. 2.6: Erosion

Incised wounds/cuts

Incised wounds are produced by sharp-edged instrument. They are longer than deep (Fig. 2.7).

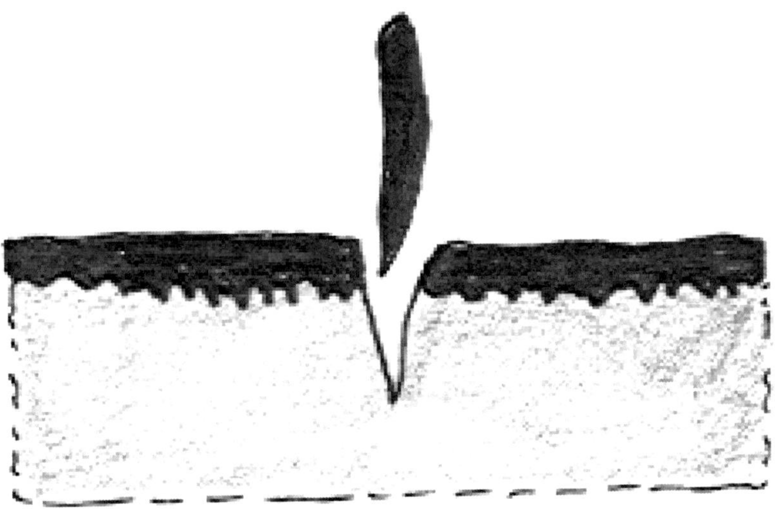

Fig. 2.7: Incised wound/ cut

Stab wound

Stab wounds are deeper than longer produced by sharp edged instrument.

Laceration

Severance of tissue by excessive stretching and is common over bony surfaces or are produced by cut through a dull instrument (Fig. 2.8).

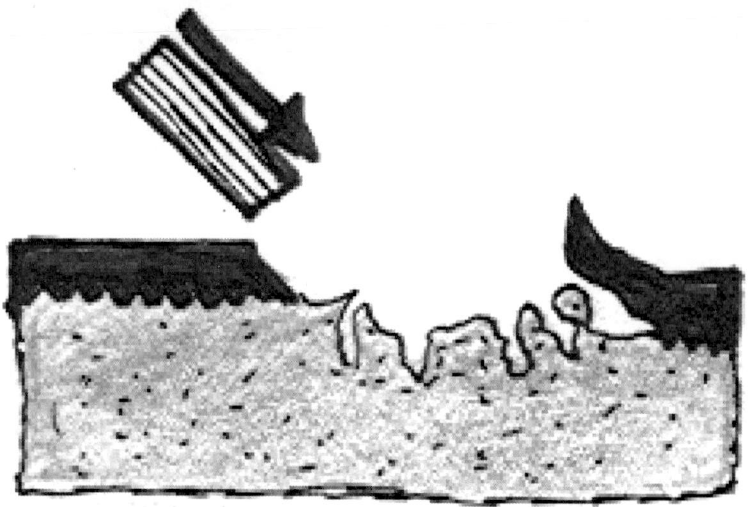

Fig. 2.8: Laceration

Compression

Compression injury is produced as a result of force applied slowly e.g. during parturition.

Blast injury

Force of compression waves against surfaces followed by a wave of reduced pressure. It can rupture muscles/viscera.

Bullet wound

Hitting at 90° by firearms to produce uniform margins of abrasion. Exit wounds are irregular and lacerated.

Electrical Injury

High voltage current induces tetanic spasms of respiratory muscles and hits the respiratory centre of brain. It also produces flash burns. Lightning causes cyanotic carcass, post-mortem bloat, congestion of viscera, tiny haemorrhage and skin damage.

Temperature

Burns

1st degree burns

There is only congestion and injury to the superficial layers of epidermis e.g. sun burn on hairless parts or white skinned animal.

2nd degree burns

Epidermis is destroyed; hair follicles remain intact and provide a nidus for healing of epithelium.

3rd degree burns

Epidermis and dermis both are destroyed leading to fluid loss, local tissue destruction, laryngeal and pulmonary oedema, renal failure, shock and sepsis. Till 20 hrs of burn, the burn surface remains sterile then bacterial contamination occurs. After 72 hrs millions of bacteria enter in the affected tissue. Bacteria such as Staphylococci, Streptococci and *Pseudomonas aeruginosa* invade the deeper layers of skin and cause sepsis. There is a state of immunosuppression in severe burns leading to impaired phagocytosis by neutrophils (Fig. 2.9).

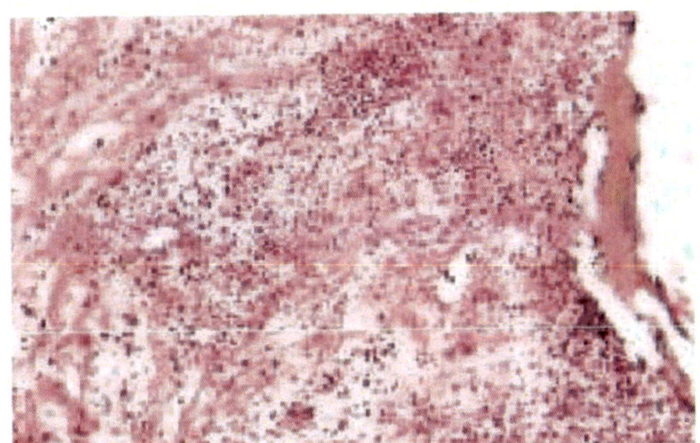

Fig. 2.9: Photomicrograph of third degree burn injury in skin

Hyperthermia

Hyperthermia means increased body temperature due to high environmental temperature e.g. pets in hot environment without water. Hyperthermia leads to increased respiration (hyperpnoea), rapid heart beat (tachycardia), and degeneration in myocardium, renal tubules and brain.

Hypothermia

Hypothermia means decreased body temperature and includes freeze induced necrosis of tissues at extremities

Radiation Injury

Radiation as a result of exposure to X-rays, Gamma rays or ultra violet (UV) rays leads to cell swelling, vacuolation of endoplasmic reticulum, swelling of mitochondria, nuclear swelling and chromosomal damage resulting in mutation. The impact of radiation is more on dividing cells of ovary, sperm, lymphocytes, bone marrow tissue and intestinal epithelium. It is characterized by vomiting, leucopenia, bone marrow atrophy, anemia, oedema, lymphoid tissue and epithelial necrosis.

Biological Causes

Virus

Viruses are smallest organisms, which have only one type of nucleic acid DNA or RNA in their core covered by protein capsid (Fig. 2.10 and 2.11).

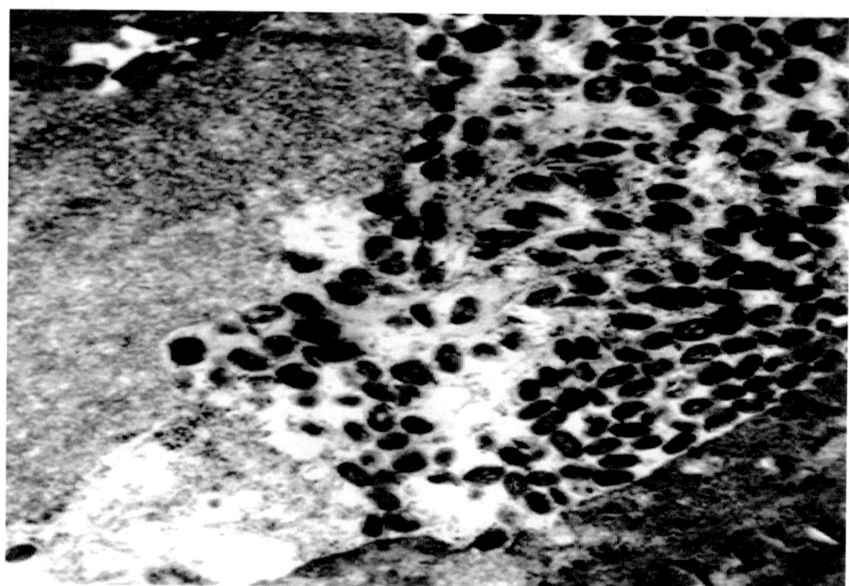

Fig. 2.10: DNA virus- Pox virus as seen in electron microscope

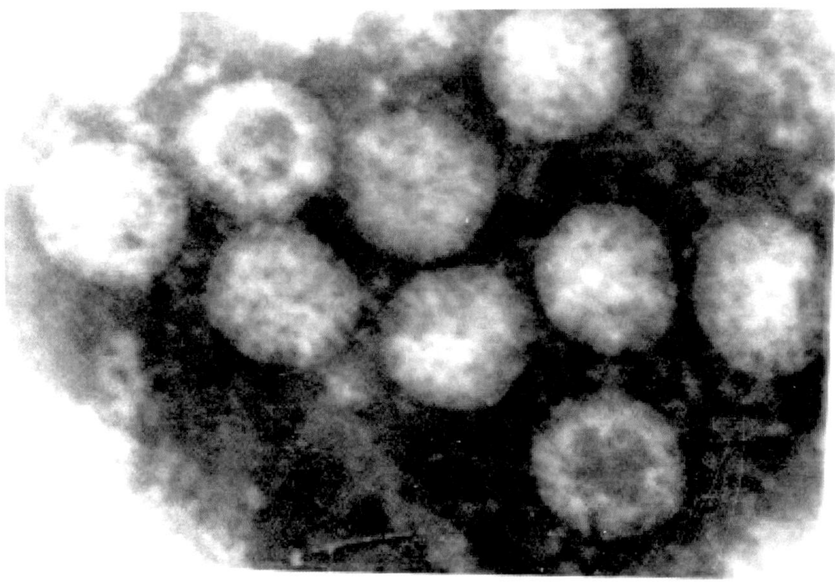

Fig. 2.11: RNA virus- Rotavirus as seen in electron microscope

Subviral agents

- Prion proteins are infectious proteins without any nucleic acid. e.g. Bovine spongiform encephalopathy.
- Viroids have only nucleic acid without proteins. They do not cause any disease in animals. However, They are associated with plant diseases.

Rickettsia

Coxiella burnetti causes Q-fever

Mycoplasma

Mycoplasma mycoides is responsible for pneumonia, joint ailments and genital disorders

Chlamydia

Chlamydia trachomatis, *C. psittaci* cause abortions, pneumonia, and eye ailments.

Spirochaete

Leptospira sp. causes abortion, icterus.

Borrelia anserina causes fowl spirochetosis in chickens (Fig. 2.12).

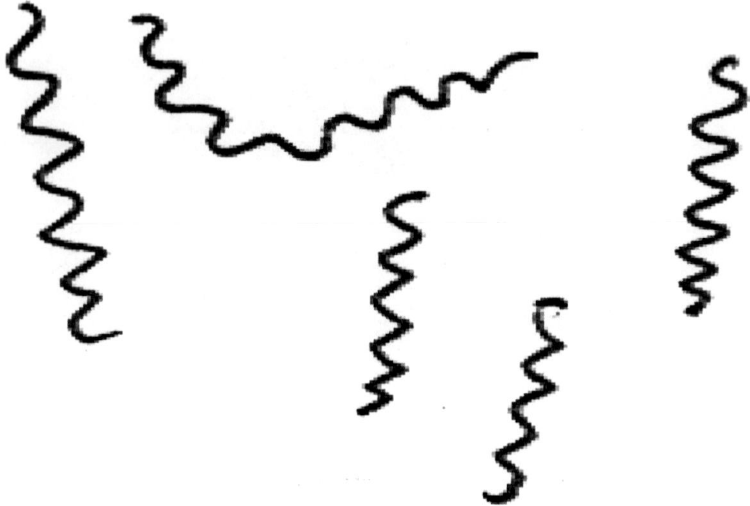

Fig. 2.12: Spirochete

Viruses of Veterinary Importance with their classification

(International Committee on taxonomy of viruses, 2005)

DNA Viruses (Fig. 2.10)

S. No.	Family	Genus	Virus species	Disease
Group I - ds DNA viruses (Double stranded DNA virus)				
1.	Adenoviridae	Aviadenovirus Atadenovirus Mastadenovirus	Fowl adenovirus Ovine adenovirus A Canine adenovirus 1	IBH, EDS, HPS in birds Pneumonia in Sheep ICH in Dog
2.	Herpesviridae	Alphaherpes virus	Herpes suis	Pseudorabies in pigs
			Bovine herpes virus – 1 (BHV-1)	IBR, IPV in cattle
			Equine herpes virus – 1 (EHV-1)	Equine viral abortion
			Equine herpes virus – 4 (EHV-4)	Rhinopneumonitis in equines
			Equine herpes virus – 3 (EHV-3)	Coital exanthema
			Avian herpes virus type-1 (AHV-1)	ILT in birds
		Betaherpes virus	Porcine cytomegalo virus	Inclusion body rhinitis in pigs

S. No.	Family	Genus	Virus species	Disease
		Gammaherpes virus	Malignant catarrhal fever virus	MCF in cattle
			Marek's disease virus	Marek's disease in birds
3.	Papillomaviridae	Papillomavirus	Bovine papillomavirus Canine oral papillomavirus Rabbit papillomavirus	Cutaneous papilloma in cattle Oral papilloma in dogs Cutaneous papilloma in rabbits
4.	Poxviridae	Orthopox virus	Vaccinia virus, Cowpox virus, Buffalopox virus, Monkeypox virus, Rabbitpox virus Camelpox virus	Pox in animals
		Avipox virus	Fowlpox virus, Pigeonpox virus, Turkeypox virus, Canarypox virus	Fowl pox, Pigeon pox, Turkeypox, Canarypox
		Capripox virus	Sheeppox virus, Goatpox virus	Sheep pox, Goat pox
		Leporipox virus	Myxoma virus	Myxomatosis in Rabbits
		Suipox virus	Swinepox virus	Swine pox
		Parapox virus	Orfpox virus	Orf in sheep
Group II - ss DNA viruses (Single stranded DNA virus)				
1.	Circoviridae	Circovirus	Porcine circovirus	-
		Gyrovirus	Chicken anemia virus	Chicken infectious anemia
2.	Parvoviridae	Parvovirus	Murine minute virus	
		Bocavirus	Bovine parvovirus	Diarrhoea in cattle
			Canine parvovirus	Enteritis, myocarditis in dogs
			Porcine parvovirus	Infertility, fetal death in pigs

RNA Viruses (Fig. 2.11)

S. No.	Family	Genus	Virus species	Disease
Group III - ds RNA virus (Double stranded RNA virus)				
1.	Birnaviridae	Avibirnavirus	IBD virus	IBD in birds
		Aquabirnavirus	Infectious pancreatic necrotic virus	Infectious pancreatic necrosis
2.	Reoviridae	Orthoreovirus	Mammalian orthoreo virus	Pneumoenteritis in calves
		Orbivirus	Blue tongue virus	Blue tongue in sheep
		Rotavirus	Rotavirus	Diarrhoea in neonates
Group IV - (+ve) ss RNA virus (Positive single stranded RNA or M RNA like)				
1.	Arteriviridae	Arterivirus	Equine arteritis virus	Equine viral arteritis
2.	Coronaviridae	Coronavirus	Infectious bronchitis virus	Infectious bronchitis in birds
			Bovine coronavirus	Diarrhoea in calves
3.	Astroviridae	Avastrovirus	Turkey astrovirus	-
4.	Calciviridae	Vesivirus	Swine vesicular exanthema virus	Vesicular exanthema in pigs
		Lagovirus	Rabbit haemorrhagic disease virus	Haemmorhagic disease in rabbit
		Norovirus	Norwalk virus	-
5.	Flaviviridae	Flavirus	Yellow fever virus	Yellow fever in man
		Hepacivirus	Hepatitis C virus	Hepatitis in man
		Pestivirus	BVD virus, CSF virus	BVD, CSF
6.	Picornaviridae	Enterovirus	Poliovirus	Polio in man
		Rhinovirus	Rhinovirus	Rhinitis
		Hepatovirus	Hepatitis A virus	Hepatitis
		Cardiovirus	Encephalomyocarditis virus	Encephalomyocarditis
		Aphthovirus	FMD virus	FMD
		Erbovirus	Equine rhinitis B virus	Respiratory disease in equines

S. No.	Family	Genus	Virus species	Disease
7.	Togaviridae	Alphavirus	Equine Encephalomyelitis virus	Equine encephalomyelitis
		Rubivirus	Rubellavirus	
Group V – (-ve) ss RNA virus (Negative single stranded RNA)				
1.	Paramyxoviridae	Paramyxovirus	Parainfluenza virus 1 (PI-1)- Pigs, Parainfluenza virus 2 (PI-2)- Dogs, Parainfluenza virus 3 (PI-3)- Cattle	Respiratory diseases in pigs Kennel cough in dogs Respiratory disease in cattle
		Avulavirus	Ranikhet disease virus	Ranikhet disease in birds
		Morbillivirus	Canine Distemper virus Rinderpest virus PPR virus	CD in dogs RP- in animals PPR – sheep, goat
2.	Bornaviridae	Borna disease virus	Borna disease virus	Borna disease in sheep
3.	Filoviridae	Ebolavirus	-	-
		Filovirus	-	-
4.	Rhabdoviridae	Vesiculovirus	Vesicular stomatitis virus	Vesicular stomatitis in bovines
		Lyssavirus	Rabies virus	Rabies
		Ephemerovirus	Ephemeral fever virus	Ephemeral fever in animals
5.	Bunyaviridae	Hantavirus	Hantaanvirus	Hantavirus pulmonary syndrome, Korean haemorragic fever
		Phlebovirus	Nairobi sheep disease virus, Rift valley fever virus, Akabana disease virus	Nairobi Sheep disease, RVF Akabana disease
6.	Orthomyxoviridae	Influenza virus A Influenza virus B Influenza virus C	Influenza virus A Influenza virus B Influenza virus C	Influenza in animals

S. No.	Family	Genus	Virus species	Disease
Group VI ss RNA-RT virus (Single stranded RNA virus with reverse transcriptase)				
1.	Retroviridae	Alpharetrovirus	Avian leucosis virus	ALC in birds
		Betaretrovirus	Mouse mammary tumour virus	Cancer in mice
		Gammaretrovirus	Murine leukemia virus	Leukemia in mice
			Feline leukemia virus	Leukemia in cats
		Deltaretrovirus	Bovine leukemia virus	Bovine leukemia
		Lentivirus	Bovine immunodeficiency virus	Bovine immunodeficiency syndrome
			Feline immunodeficiency virus	Feline immunodeficiency syndrome
Group VII ds DNA-RT virus (Double stranded DNA virus with reverse transcriptase)				
1.	Hepadnaviridae	Orthohepadnavirus	Hepatitis B virus	Hepatitis
		Avihepadna virus	Duck hepatitis B virus	Duck hepatitis

Bacteria

Bacteria are classified as Gram positive and Gram negative on the basis of Gram's staining. Gram positive bacteria include *Staphylococci, Streptococci, Corynebacterium, Listeria, Bacillus Clostridia*. Gram negative bacteria are *Escherichia coli, Salmonella, Proteus, Klebsiella, Pasteurella, Pseudomonas, Brucella, Yersinia, Campylobactor* etc. Besides, there are certain organisms stained with Zeihl Neelson stain and are known as acid fast bacilli e.g. *Mycobacterium tuberculosis* and *M. paratuberculosis* (Fig. 2.13).

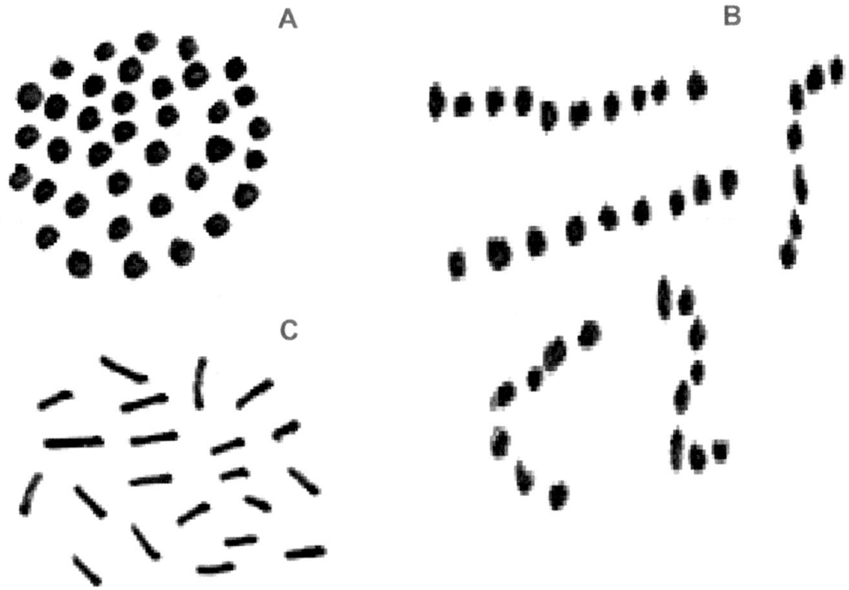

Fig. 2.13: Bacteria- Cocci in bunches (A), in chains (B) and rods (C).

Fungi

Fungi pathogenic for animals mostly belong to fungi imperfecti. e.g. Histoplasmosis.

Fungi cause three type of disease – Mycosis e.g. Actinomycosis; Allergic disease e.g. Ringworm; Mycotoxicosis e.g. Aflatoxicosis (Fig. 2.14 A&B).

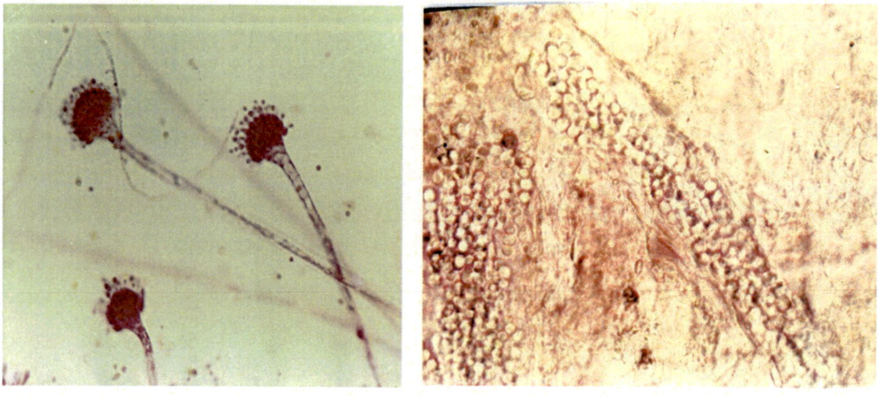

A B

Fig. 2.14: Fungus- *Aspergillus* spp **(A)** and *Trichophyton* spp **(B)**.

Parasites

Parasites are classified mainly in 3 groups:

Protozoan parasites

Trypanosoma evansi, Theileria annulata, Babesia bigemina, Toxoplasma gondii, Eimeria Spp. (Fig. 2.15).

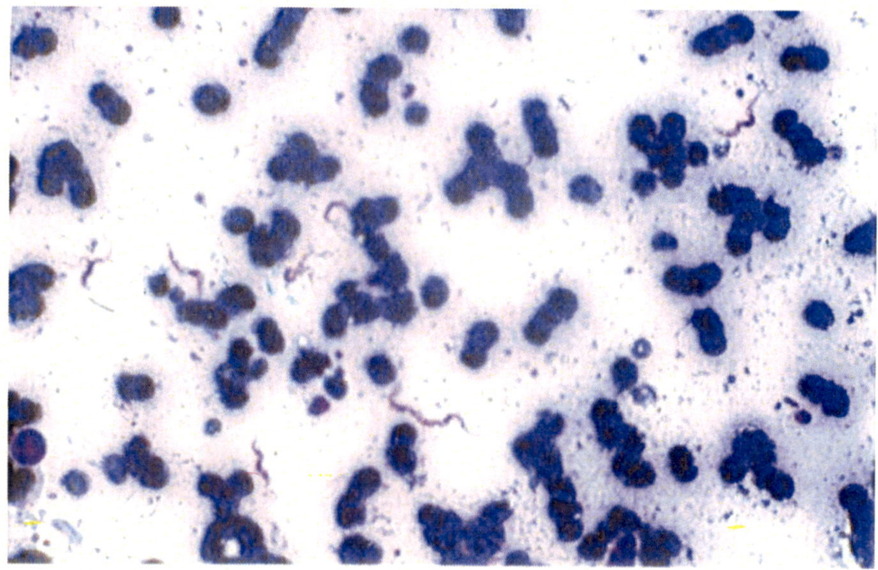

Fig. 2.15: Protozoan parasite *Trypanosoma evansi*

Helminths

Nematodes – Roundworms e.g. Ascaris. Trematod – Flat worms e.g. Liver fluke (Fig.2.16).

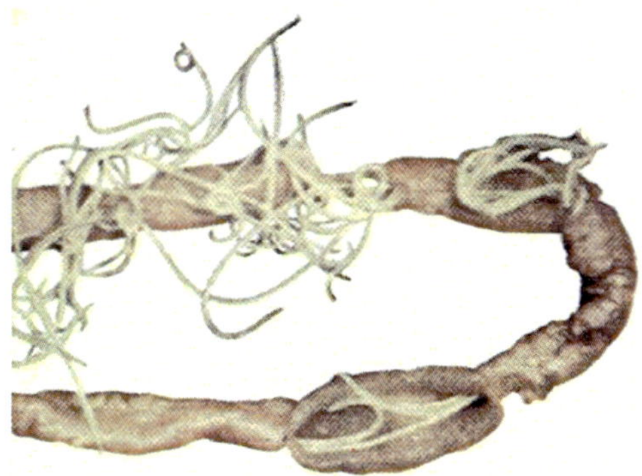

Fig. 2.16: Parasite Round worms

Cestodes – Tapeworms e.g *Taenia* spp. (Fig. 2.17).

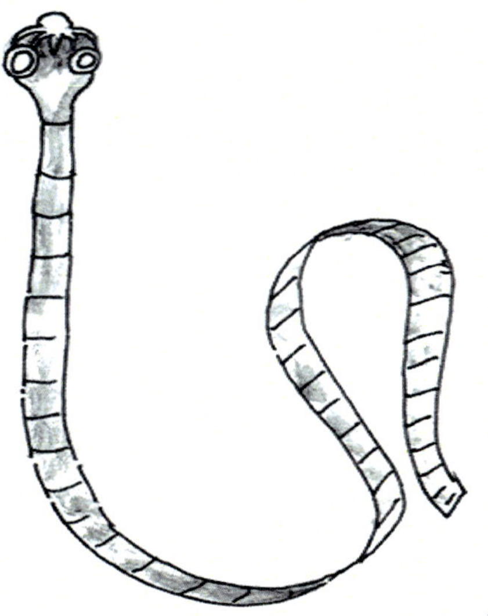

Fig. 2.17: Parasite Tape worm

Arthropods

Ticks, Mites, Flies, Lice (Figs. 2.18 and 2.19).

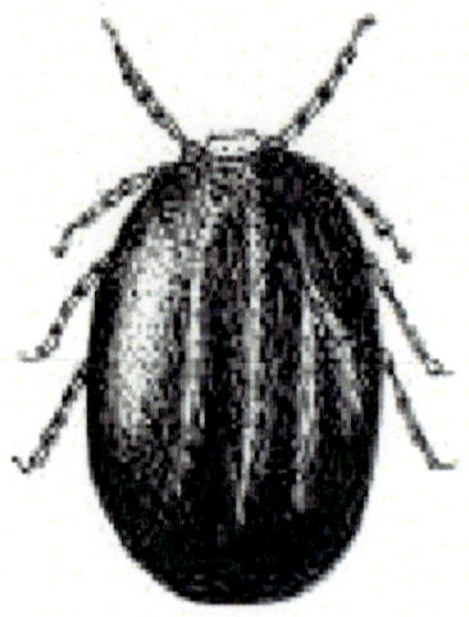

Fig. 2.18: Parasite-Tick

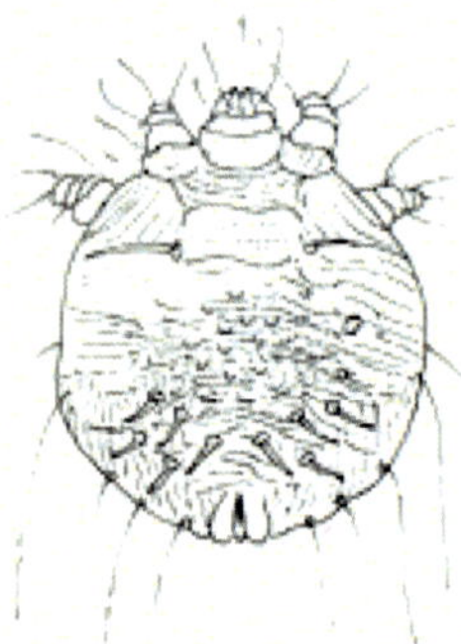

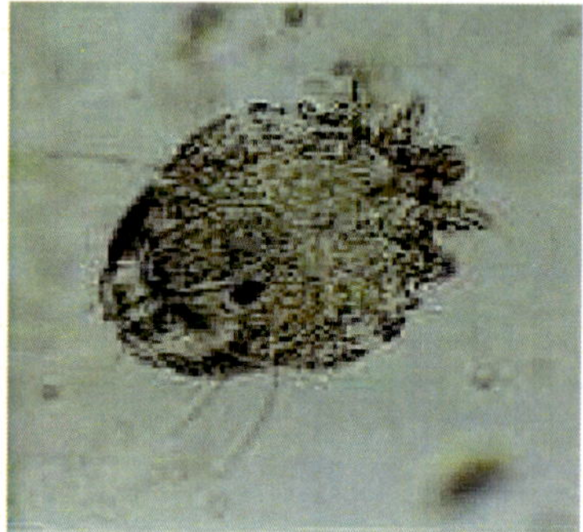

Fig. 2.19: Parasite-Mite

Transmission

Biological agents are transmitted from one animal to another through horizontal or vertical transmission.

Horizontal Transmission

Horizontal transmission of biological causes occurs through direct contact or indirectly via animal or inanimate (fomites) objects. It is also known as lateral transmission as it occurs in a population from one to another. Various methods of horizontal transmission are as under:

Ingestion

Food, water, faecal-oral route e.g. Salmonellosis, Johne's disease, Rotavirus infection.

Inhalation

Air-borne infections, droplet infection e.g. R.P., FMD, Tuberculosis.

Contact

Fungal infection, Bacterial dermatitis, Flu, Brucellosis, Rabies through bite.

Inoculation

Introduction of infection in body through puncture either mechanically through needles or by arthropods such as by ticks. Ticks transmit diseases through transovarian (one generation to next generation) or transstadial (through developmental stages) transmission.

Iatrogenic

Transmission of infection during surgical procedures or caused by doctor, through dirty instrument and contaminated preparations.

Coitus

Through sexual contact of animals, biological agents spread from one to another animals. e.g. Campylobacteriosis, Trichomonosis.

Vertical Transmission

Vertical transmission occurs from one generation to another generation in ovo/ in utero or through milk. These include:

Hereditary

Infection/disease carried in the genome of either parent e.g. Retrovirus

Congenital

Diseases acquired either in utero/in ovo

- Infection in ovary/ ovum (Germinative transmission) e.g. ALC in chickens, lymphoid leukemia in mice, Salmonellosis in poultry.
- Infection through placenta. e.g. Feline panleukopenia virus (Transmission to embryo)

- Ascending infection from lower genital canal to amnion / placenta e.g. Staphylococci.
- Infection at parturition: Infection from lower genital tract during birth. e.g. Herpex simplex virus.

Maintenance of Infection

Biological agents face difficulty of survival at both places – in environment and in host. Two types of hazards which create problem to agent are:

Internal hazards e.g. Host's immune system External hazards e.g. Desiccation, UV light Agents try to maintain themselves by adopting following maintenance strategies

- Avoidance of a stage in the external environment.
- Resistant forms e.g. Anthrax spores.
- Rapidly in-rapidly out strategy e.g. Viruses of respiratory tract.
- Persistence within the host e.g. *Mycobacterium tuberculosis*, Slow viral diseases.
- Extension of host range.
- Infection in more than one host e.g. Foot and mouth disease.

Chemical Causes

Biological Toxins

Snake venom

Snake venom has phospholipase A_2 which causes lytic action on membranes of RBC and platelets. The presence of hyaluronidase, phosphodiesterase and peptidase in snake venom are responsible for oedema, erythema, haemolytic anemia, swelling of facial/laryngeal tissues, haemoglobinurea, cardiac irregularities, fall in blood pressure, shock and neurotoxicity.

Microbial toxins

Microbial toxins are those toxins/poisons that are produced by microbial agents particularly by bacteria and fungi.

Bacterial toxins

Bacterial toxins include structural proteins (endotoxins) and soluble peptides/

secretary toxins (exotoxins). Endotoxins are present in cell wall of Gram-negative bacteria and are found to be responsible for septicemia and shock. Exotoxins are secreted by bacteria outside their cell wall and are responsible for protein lysis and damage to cell membrane. e.g. Clostridium toxins suppress metabolism of cell. Most potent clostridial toxins are botulinum and tetanus, which are the cause of hemolysis and are powerful neurotoxin. Besides, Clostridium chauvei toxins are responsible for black leg disease in cattle.

Fungal Toxins (Mycotoxins)

There are several fungi known for production of toxins. Such toxins are known as mycotoxins and they are mostly found in food/ feed items, which cause disease in animals through ingestion.

Aflatoxins

Aflatoxins are produced by several species of fungi including mainly Aspergillus flavus, A. parasiticus and Penicillium puberlum. These aflatoxins are classified as B_1, B_2, G_1, G_2, M_1, M_2, B_2a, G_2a and aspertoxin. Aflatoxins are produced in moist environment in grounded animal/poultry feed on optimum temperature and are more common in tropical countries where storage conditions are poor and provide suitable environment for the growth of fungi. These toxins are known to cause immunosuppression, formation of malignant neoplasms and hepatopathy.

Ergot

Ergot is produced by *Claviceps purpura* in grains which causes blackish discoloration. It produces gangrene by chronic vasoconstriction, ischemia and capillary endothelium degeneration. It is also associated with summer syndrome in cattle characterized by gangrene of extremities.

Fusarium toxins

Fusarium toxins are produced by *Fusarium tricinctum* in paddy straw, which are found to cause gangrene in extremities. Zearalenone toxin is the cause of ovarian abnormality in sow.

Ochratoxins

Ochratoxins are produced by *Aspergillus ochraceous* and *A. viridicatum* fungi in grounded feed on optimum temperature and moisture and are found to cause renal tubular necrosis in chickens and pigs.

Plant toxins

Over 700 plants are known to produce toxin. e.g. Braken fern which causes haematuria and encephalomalacia. Strychnine from *Strychnos nuxvomica* is highly toxic and causes death in animals with nervous signs. It is used for dog killing in public health operations to control rabies (Fig. 2.20). HCN is found in sorghum which is known to cause clonic convulsions and death in animals characterized by haemorrhage in mucous membranes.

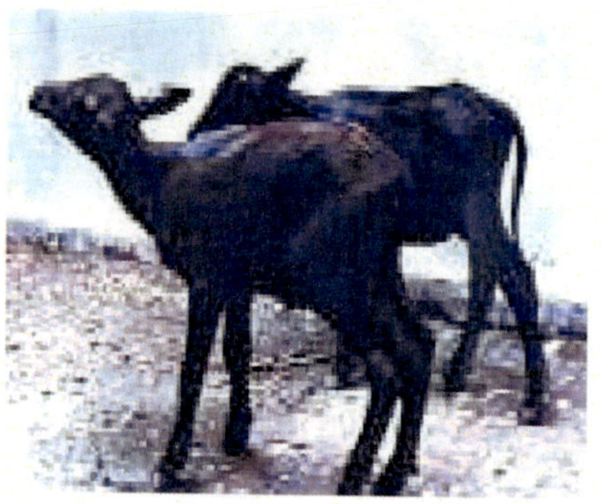

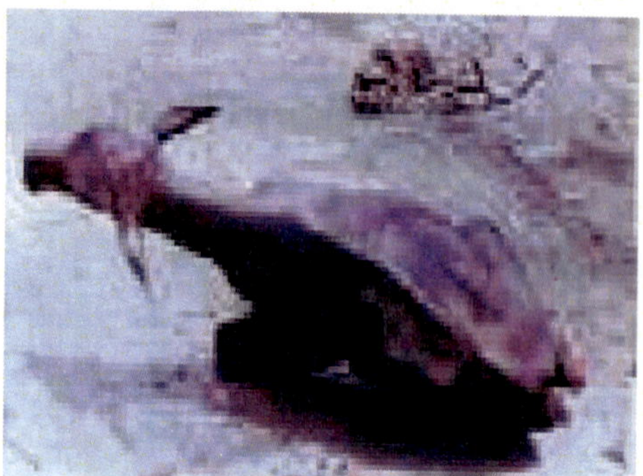

Fig. 2.20: Plant toxin- Strychnine poisoning

Drug toxicity

- *Antibiotics*: Cause direct toxicity by destroying gut microflora. Oxytetracyline, sulfonamides are nephrotoxic. Neomycin and Lincomycin cause Malabsorption diarrhoea and immunosuppression.
- *Anti-inflammatory drugs*, like acetaminophen causes hepatic necrosis, icterus and hemolytic anemia.
- *Anticoccidiostate drug*: Monensin is responsible for necrosis of cardiac and skeletal muscles.
- *Trace elements*: There are various trace elements, excess of which may cause poisoning in animals. e.g. Selenium poisoning "Blind staggers" or "Alkali Disease" in cattle characterized by chronic debilitating disease. It also causes encephalomalacia in pigs.

Environmental pollutants

Environment is polluted due to presence of unwanted materials in food, water, air and surroundings of animals, particularly by agrochemicals including pesticides and fertilizers. The environmental pollutants exert their direct or indirect effect on the animal health and production. The main pollutants are:

- Heavy metals such as mercury, lead, cadmium are found in industrial waste, automobile and generator smoke, soil, water and also as contaminants of pesticides and fertilizers. They are responsible for damage in kidneys, immune system and neuropathy. They are also associated with immune complex mediated glomerulonephritis.
- Sulphur dioxide is produced by automobiles, industries and generators. It is responsible for loss of cilia in bronchiolar epithelium.
- Hydrogen sulphide is produced by animal's decay and in various industries. It inhibits mitochondrial cytochrome oxidase leading to death.
- Pesticides are agrochemicals used in various agricultural, animal husbandry and public health operations. They are classified as insecticides, herbicides, weedicides and rodenticides. Chemically, insecticides are grouped mainly as organochlorine organophosphates, carbamates and synthetic pyrethroids. Acute poisoning of pesticides causes death in animals after nervous clinical signs of short duration. Chronic toxicity is characterized by immunosuppression, nephropathy, neuropathy, hypersensitivity and autoimmunity in animals (Fig. 2.21).

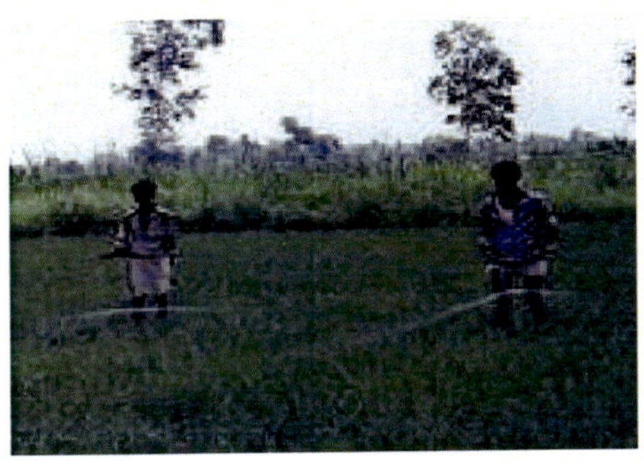

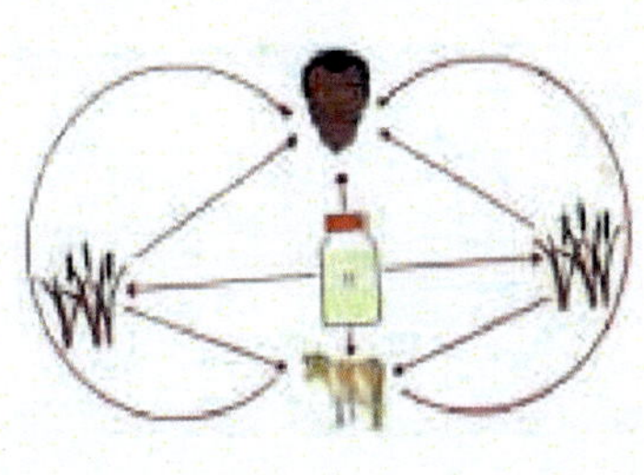

Fig. 2.21: Pesticide toxicity

Nutritional Causes

Malnutrition causes disease in animals either due to deficiency or excess of nutrients. It is very difficult to diagnose the nutritional causes and sometimes it is not possible to find a precise cause as in case of infectious disease because functions of one nutrient can be compensated by another in cell metabolism. Experimental production of nutritional deficiency is not identical to natural disease. When tissue concentration of nutrient falls down to the critical level, it leads to abnormal metabolism and the abnormal metabolites present in tissues can be detected in urine and faeces. First changes of nutritional deficiency are recorded in rapidly metabolizing tissues e.g. skeletal muscle, myocardium and brain. Immature animals are more susceptible to nutritional disease. e.g. calves, chicks, piglets etc.

Types of deficiency

- Acute/chronic e.g. thiamine deficiency in pigs.
- Multiple deficiencies: e.g. poor quality food.
- Nutritional imbalance: e.g. imbalance in calcium: phosphorus (2:1) ratio.
- Protein malnutrition: e.g. malabsorption.
- Calorie deficiency: e.g. Loss of fat/ muscle wasting.

Factors responsible for nutritional deficiency

- Interference with intake e.g. anorexia, G.I. tract disorders.
- Interference with absorption e.g. intestinal hypermotility, Insoluble complexes in food (Fat/Calcium)
- Interference with storage e.g. hepatic disease leads to deficiency of vit. A.
- Increased excretion e.g. polyuria, sweating and lactation
- Increased requirement e.g. fever, hyperthyroidism and pregnancy
- Natural inhibitors e.g. presence of thiaminases in feed, leads to thiamine deficiency.

Calorie deficiency

Calorie deficiency in animals occurs due to food deprivation or starvation.

Food deprivation

Dietary deficiency of food in terms of quantity/quality leads to emaciation, loss of musculature, atrophy of fat, subcutaneous oedema, cardiac muscle degeneration and atrophy of viscera including liver and pancreas. The volume of hepatocytes reduced by 50% and mitochondrial total volume also reduced by 50%.

Starvation

Starvation is the long continued deprivation of food. It is characterized by fatty degeneration of liver, anemia and skin diseases. Young and very old animals are more susceptible to starvation while in pregnant animals it causes retarded growth of foetus. In animals, following changes can be seen due to starvation.

Intestinal involution

Absorptive surface is reduced with shrunken cells and pyknotic nuclei. Villi become shorter and show atrophy.

Atrophy of muscles

There is decrease in muscle mass.

Lipolysis

Increased cortisol leads to increased lipolysis resulting in formation of fatty acids in liver which in turn converts into ketones used by brain.

Gluconeogenesis

In early fasting blood glucose level drops down. The insulin level becomes low while glucagon goes high in starvation. The glucose comes from skeletal muscle, adipose tissue and lymphoid tissue during starvation. Twenty-four hours of food deprivation causes reduction in liver glycogen and blood glucose. Fatty acid from adipose tissue forms glucose and in mitochondria after oxidation it forms acetoacetate, hydroxybutyrate and acetone. These are also known as ketone bodies and are present in blood stream during starvation. This state is also known as ketosis e.g. ketosis/acetonemia in bovines. Lack of glucose in blood leads to oxidation of fatty acids which form ketone bodies as an alternate source of energy. They are normal/ physiological at certain level but may become pathological when their level is high.

Clinically it is characterized by anorexia, depression, coma, sweet smell in urine. Concentration of acetone increases in milk, blood and urine along with hyperlipimia and acidosis. A similar condition also occurs in sheep known as pregnancy toxaemia which is characterized by depression, coma and paralysis. This situation occurs when many foetus are present in uterus. There are fatty changes in liver, kidneys, and heart, with subepicardial petechiae or echymosis.

Protein deficiency

Generally, protein deficiency does not occur. However, the deficiency of essential amino acids has been reported in animals when certain ingredients are deficient in certain amino acids. e.g. maize is deficient in lysine and tryptophan that leads to slow growth; peanuts and soybean are deficient in methioine. Protein deficiency is characterized by hypoproteinemia, anemia, poor growth, delayed healing, decreased or cesation of cell proliferation, failure of collagen formation, atrophy of testicles and ovary, atrophy of thymus and lymphoid tissue.

Deficiency of Lipids

Generally, there is no deficiency of fat in animals. However, essential fatty acids, including linolenic acid, linoleic acid and arachdonic acid, deficiency may occur which causes dermatoses in animals. Fat has high calorie value and it is required in body because there are certain vitamins soluble in fat only.

Deficiency of Water

Deficiency of water may lead to dehydration and slight wrinkling in skin. Deficiency may occur due to fever, vomiting, diarrhoea, haemorrhage and polyuria, which can be corrected through adequate oral water supply or through intravenous fluid therapy.

Deficiency of Vitamins

Vitamin deficiency may occur due to starvation. There are two types of vitamins viz., fat soluble and water soluble. Fat soluble vitamins are vit. A, D, E and K and water soluble are vit B complex and C.

Vitamin A

It is also known as retinol. It is derived from its precursor carotene. It is found in abndance in plants having yellow pigment, animal fat, liver, cod liver oil, shark liver oil. β-carotene is cleaved in gut mucosa into two molecules of retinol (Vit. A aldehyde) which, after absorption, is stored in liver. Bile salts and pancreatic juice are responsible for absorption of vit. A from gut. Deficiency of vit. A occurs due to damage in liver.

Vit. A deficiency may lead to following disease conditions:

Squamous metaplasia of epithelial surfaces in esophagus, pancreas, bladder and parotid duct, which is considered pathognomonic in calves. Destruction of epithelium/ goblet cell in respiratory mucosa is generally replaced by keratin synthesizing squamous cells in vit. A deficient animals. There are abnormal teeth in animals due to hypoplasia of enamel and its poor mineralization. Vitamin A deficiency is also associated with still birth and miscarriages in pigs. It causes night blindness (Nyctalopia) in animals. Due to deficiency of Vit. A there are recurrent episodes of conjunctivitis/ keratitis. In poultry, there is distention of mucous glands, which opens in pharynx and esophagus because of metaplasia of duct epithelium leading to enlargement of esophageal glands due to accumulation of its secretions. The glands become spherical, 1-2 mm dia. over mucosa. It is considered pathognomonic for hypovitaminosis A. and is known as Nutritional roup (Fig. 2.22 a&b). Inflammation of upper respiratory tract lead to coryza. Urinary tract of cattle, sheep and goat suffers due to formation of calculi, which may cause obstruction in sigmoid flexure of urethra in males. Such calculi are made up of desquamated epithelial cells and salts and the condition is known as urolithiasis. Deficiency of vit. A may also lead to in abnormal growth of cranial bones and there may be failure of foramen ovale to grow leading to constriction of optic nerves which results in blindness in calves, increased CSF pressure, blindness at birth and foetal malformations. In sows, piglets are born without eyes (Anophthalmos) or with smaller eyes- (Microphthalmos).

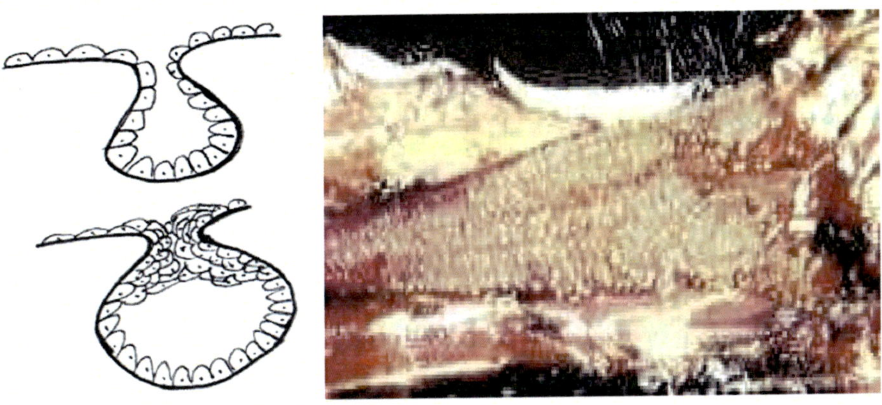

A **B**

Fig. 2.22: Nutritional roup- vitamin A deficiency

Vitamin D

Vitamin D occurs in three forms viz. vitamin D_2 or calciferol, Vit. D_3 or cholecaliciferol and Vit D_1 or impure mixture of sterols. About 80% Vit. D is synthesized in body skin through UV rays on 7-hydrocholesterol. In diet containing egg, butter, it is found in abundant quantity in milk, plants, grains etc. Active forms of vit. D are 25-hydroxy vit. D and 1, 25 dihydroxy vit D.

(Calcitriol) which is 5 to 10 times more potent than former. Vit D is stored in adipose tissue in body. The main functions of vit D are absorption of Ca and P from intestines and kidneys, mineralization of bones, maintenance of blood levels of Ca and P and immune regulation as it activates lymphocytes and macrophages.

- The deficiency of vitamin D is associated with rickets in young animals (Fig. 2.23), osteomalacia in adult animals and hypocalcemic tetany.

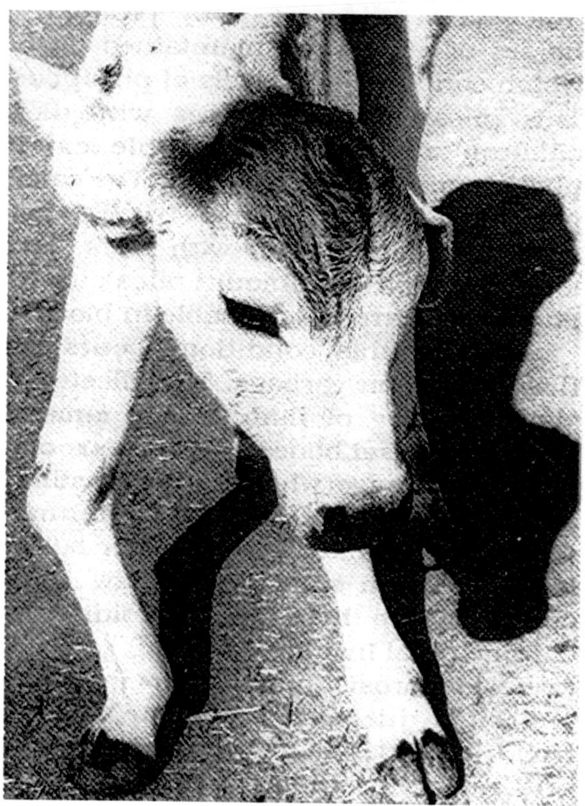

Fig. 2.23: Ricketts in a calf

- Excess of vitamin D leads to the formation of renal calculi, metastatic calcification and osteoporosis in animals.

Vitamin E (α- tocopherol)

Source of vitamin E is grains, oils, nuts, vegetables, and in body it is stored in adipose tissue, liver and muscles. It has antioxidant activity and prevents oxidative degradation of cell membrane.

- Deficiency of vit E causes degeneration of neurons in peripheral nerves. There is denervation of muscles leading to muscle dystrophy e.g. White muscle disease in cattle and Stiff lamb disease in sheep and

Myoglobinuria in horses. Deficiency of vit. E causes degeneration of pigments in retina and reduces life span of RBC, leading to anemia and sterility in animals. Crazy chick disease (Encephalomalacia) is also caused by vit E deficiency; the chicks become sleepy with twisting of head and neck. There is muscular dystrophy in chickens due to vit. E deficiency (Fig. 2.24).

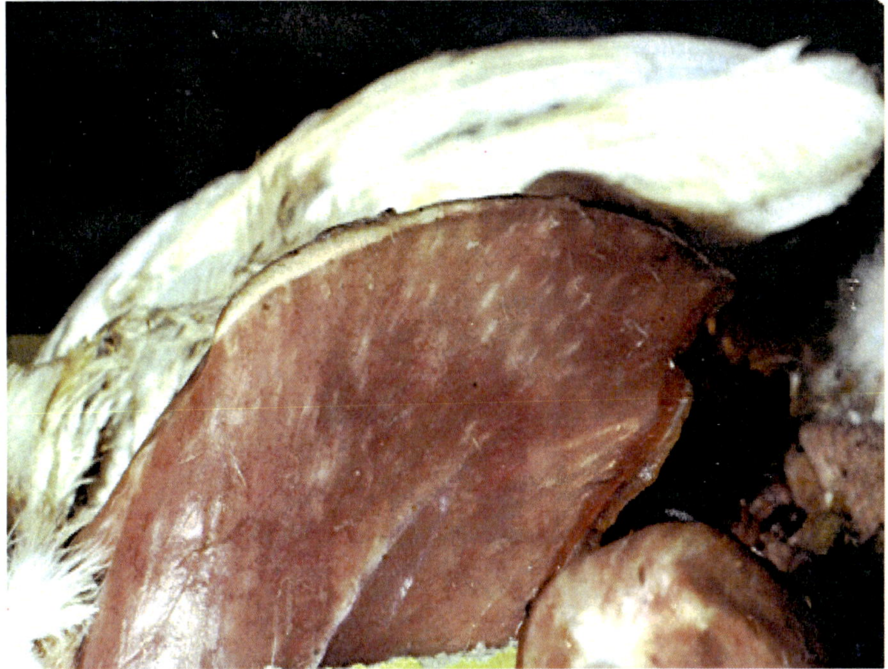

Fig. 2.24: Vitamin E deficiency- Muscular dystrophy

Vitamin K

Vit. K occurs in two forms namely vit. K_1 or phylloquinone found in green leaf and vegetables and Vit- K_2 or menadione which is produced by gut microflora. Its main function is coagulation of blood. Deficiency of vit K may leads to hypoprothrombinemia and haemorrhages.

Vitamin B

Vitamin B is a water soluble vitamin which has at least 9 sub types including B_1 or thiamine, B_2 or riboflavin, B_6 or pyridoxine, B_{12} or cyanocobalamin, niacin or nicotinic acid, folate or folic acid, choline, biotine and pantothenic acid.

Thiamine

In ruminants, synthesis of thiamine occurs in rumen. Sources of vit. B are pea, beans, pulses, green vegetables, roots, fruits, rice, wheat bran etc. Strong tea, coffee have antithiamine action. It is stored in muscles, liver, heart, kidneys and bones of animals. Thiamine plays active role in carbohydrate metabolism. Deficiency of thiamine may lead to Beriberi disease characterized by Ataxia and neural/lesions. Chastek paralysis in cats, fox and mink and stargazing attitude of chicks due to thiaminase (thiamine deficiency) in meal may be observed. Bracken fern poisoning in cattle and horses may cause deficiency of thiamine due to presence of thiaminase enzyme in bracken fern. Toxicity of thiamine splitting drugs like amprolium, a coccidiostate, may cause polioencephalomalcia in cattle and sheep. Cardiac dialation in pigs has also been observed due to vit. B_1 deficiency.

Riboflavin

Riboflavin is a component of several enzymes and is found in plants, meat, eggs and vegetables.

- Deficiency of riboflavin may cause Curled Toe Paralysis in chicks and swelling of sciatic and brachial nerves (Fig. 2.25).

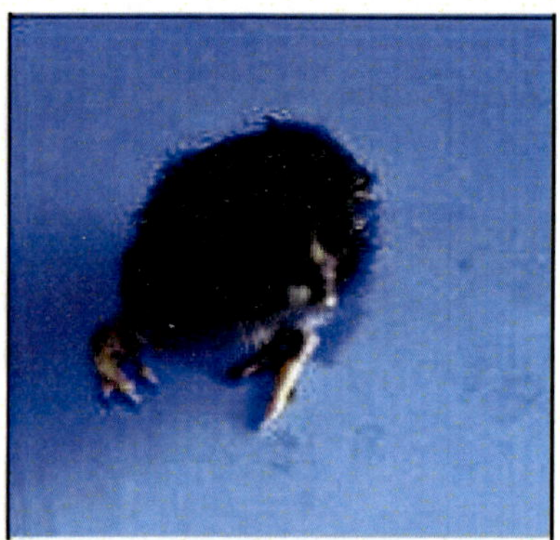

Fig. 2.25: Curled toe paralysis in a chick due to riboflavin deficiency

Niacin

Role of niacin (NAD/NADP, nicotinamide adenine dinucleotide) is in electron transport in mitochondria of cells. It is found in grains, cereals, meat, liver, kidneys, vegetables and plants.

- Deficiency of niacin is associated with skin disorders in man Pellegra; anorexia, diarrhoea, anemia in pigs and mucous hyperplasia, haemorrhage in gastrointestinal tract and black tongue in dogs which is also known as Canine pellegra.

Pyridoxine

It is found in egg, green vegetables, meat, liver etc.

- Deficiency of pyridoxine causes uremia, convulsions, dermatitis and glossitis

Pantothenic acid

- Pantothenic acid deficiency is associated with stunted growth of chicks.

Folate

- Folic acid is required in formation of erythrocytes and hence its deficiency leads to anemia.

Cyanocobalamin

Deficiency of cyanocobalamin may also lead to anemia, as it is also needed in RBC formation.

Biotin

Biotin deficiency causes paralysis of hind legs in calves and perosis in chicks (Fig.2.26).

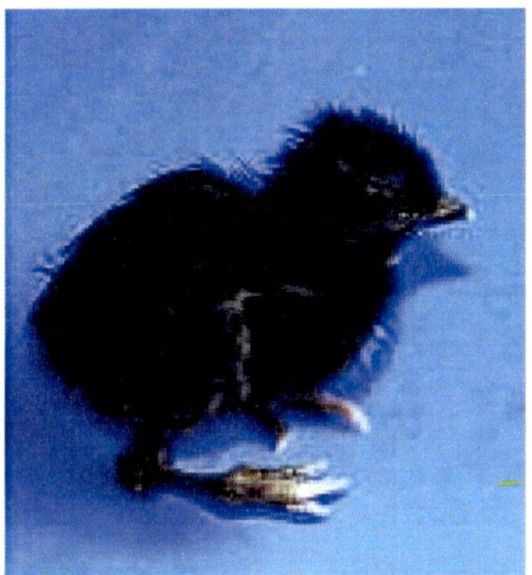

Fig. 2.26: Slipped tendon or perosis in a chick

Choline

Choline deficiency is associated with fatty changes in liver and perosis.

Vitamin C (Ascorbic acid)

It is found in green plants and citrus fruits. Deficiency of vit. C may cause retardation of fibroplasia, scurvy in G. pigs, haemorrhage, swelling, ulcers and delayed wound healing in animals.

Minerals

Various minerals are also necessary for survival of animals. Deficiency of any one of them or in combination may cause serious disease in animals. Some of the important minerals are

Sodium chloride

Sodium chloride is an essential salt which maintains osmotic pressure in blood, interstitial tissue and the cells because 65% of osmotic pressure is due to sodium chloride. Chloride ions of hydrochloric acid present in stomach also come from sodium chloride.

- The excess of sodium chloride causes gastroenteritis in cattle, gastroenteritis and eosinophilic meningoencephalitis in pigs and ascites in poultry.
- Deficiency of sodium chloride is characterized by anorexia, constipation, loss of weight in sows and pica, weight loss, decreased milk production and polyurea in cattle. Deficiency of salt occurs due to diarrhoea, dehydration and vomiting.

Calcium

Normal range of calcium is 10-11 mg/100 ml blood in body of animals. If it increases above 12 mg/100 ml blood, metastatic calcification occurs, while its level less than 8 mg/100 ml blood may show signs of deficiency characterized by tetany.

Absorption of calcium from gut is facilitated by vit. D. Paratharmone stimulates to raise blood Ca level from bones while calcitonin from thyroid stimulates its deposition in bones and thus reduces blood Ca levels.

- In pregnant cows, calcium deficiency occurs just after parturition. During gestation calcium goes to foetus from skeleton of cows, resulting in weak skeleton of dam. If calcium is not provided in diet, it may cause disease in dam characterized by locomotor disturbances, abnormal curvature of back, distortion of pelvis, tetany, incoordination, muscle spasms, unconsciousness and death. Such symptoms occur in animals when their blood calcium level falls below 6 mg/100 ml of blood and if it is less than 3 mg/100ml blood, death occurs instantly.

- Milk fever is a disease of cattle that occurs due to deficiency of calcium just after parturition. Cow suddenly becomes recumbent and sits on sternum with head bending towards flank and is unable of get up. No gross/ microscopic lesion is reported in this disorder. The calcium therapy recovers the animal immediately.
- The excess of calcium may cause metastatic calcification leading to its deposition in soft tissue of kidney, lungs and stomach.

Magnesium

It acts as activator of many enzymes e.g. alkaline phosphatase. It is required for activation of membrane transport synthesis of protein, fat and nucleic acid and for generation/ transmission of nerve impulses. The normal blood levels are 2 mg/100 ml of blood.

- Dietary deficiency leads to hypomagnesaemia and a level below 0.7 mg/100 ml causes symptoms in calves characterized by nervous hyperirritability, tonic and clonic convulsions, depression, coma and death.
- The post-mortem lesions of magnesium deficiency includes haemorrhage in heart, intestines, mesentery and congestion of viscera.
- Microscopic lesions include calcification of intimal layer of heart blood vessels (metastatic) muscles and kidneys. Grass tetany and Grass staggers occurs due to hypomagne-saemia and are characterized by hyper-irritability, abnormal gait, coma and death.

Phosphorus

Normal level of phosphorus is 4-8 mg/100 ml of blood. In bones, it is in the form of calcium phosphate. Deficiency of phosphorus may lead to hypophosphatemia and is characterized by pica, rheumatism and hemoglobinurea.

- Pica is licking/eating of objects other than food. It mainly occurs in cattle, buffaloes and camels, who eat bones, mud and other earthern materials. Such animals have heavy parasitic load in their gut.
- Rheumatism like syndrome is characterized by lameness in hind legs particularly in camels and buffaloes.

- Hemoglobinurea is characterized by the presence of coffee colour urine of animal due to extensive intravascular hemolysis Hemoglobin urea is thus known as postparturient hemoglobin urea.

Selenium

Deficiency of selenium causes hemolysis as it protects cell membrane of RBC and thus its deficiency leads to anemia. Blind Staggers occurs due to excess of selenium.

Iron

Deficiency of iron leads to anemia, which is hypochromic and microcytic but rarely occurs in animals.

Copper

Deficiency of copper results in anemia and steel wool disease in sheep, which is characterized by loss of crimp in wool. Enzootic ataxia with incoordination of posterior limb has been observed in goats.

Cobalt

Vit. B_{12} is synthesized by ruminal bacteria from cobalt in ruminants. Cobalt also stimulates erythropoiesis. Its deficiency may cause wasting disease, cachexia and emaciation in animals. The pathological lesions are comprised of anemia, hemosiderosis in liver, spleen and kidneys.

Manganese

Deficiency of manganese causes slipped tendon in chicken or perosis characterized by shortening of long bones in chickens. It occurs as the epiphyseal cartilage fails to ossify at 12 week of age and epiphysis becomes loose and thus gastrocnemious tendon slips medially. This condition is known as Slipped Tendon or Perosis (Fig. 2.26).

Zinc

Deficiency of zinc may cause parakeratosis in pigs at 10-20 weeks' age. Calcium in diet with phytate or phosphate forms a complex with zinc making it unavailable for absorption leading to its deficiency, which is characterized by rough skin of abdomen, medial surface of thigh, which becomes horny. It also causes fascial eczema in cattle, thymic hypoplasia in calves and immunodeficiency in animals.

Iodine

Deficiency of iodine causes goiter in newborn pigs characterized by absence of hair on their skin. Other signs of iodine deficiencies include abnormal spermatozoa, decreased spermatogenesis, loss of libido, reduced fertility, suboestrus, anoestrus, miscarriages, dystocia and hydrocephalus. Excess of iodine may lead to lacrimation and exfoliation of dandruff like epidermal scales from skin.

Fluorine

Excess of fluorine causes mottling in teeth and bones. The teeth become shorter, broader with opaque areas.

3

Disturbances in Circulation

Congestion/ Hyperemia

Hyperemia is increased amount of blood in circulatory system. It is of two types, active and passive. In active hyperemia blood accumulates in arteries while in passive hyperemia the amount of blood increases in veins (Figs. 3.1. to 3.4).

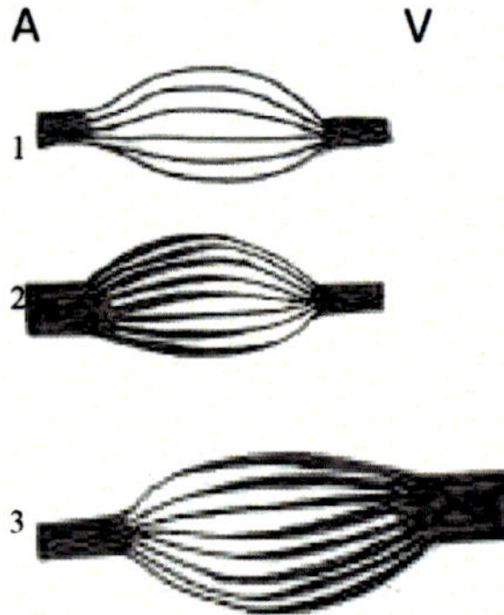

Fig. 3.1: Diagram showing congestion 1. Normal blood vessel A–arterial and V-Venous end, 2. Active congestion and 3. Passive congestion

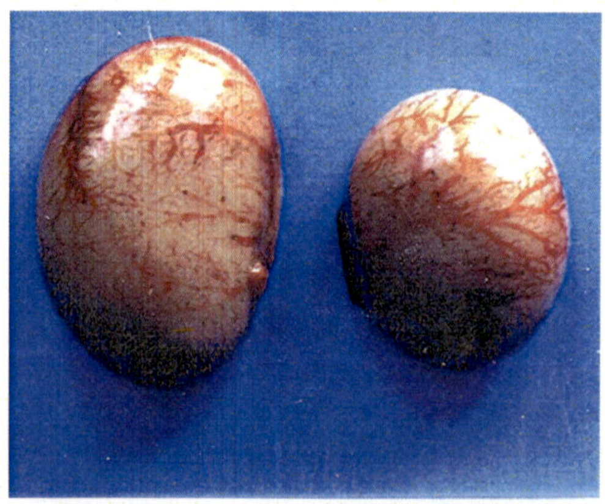

Fig. 3.2: Photograph of testes showing congestion

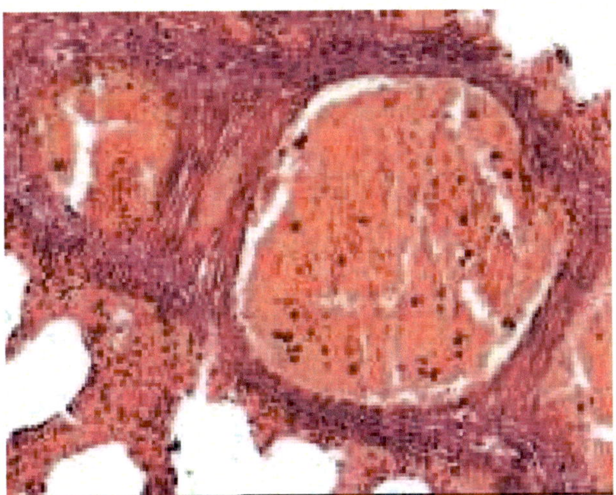

Fig. 3.3: Photomicrograph of lung showing congestion

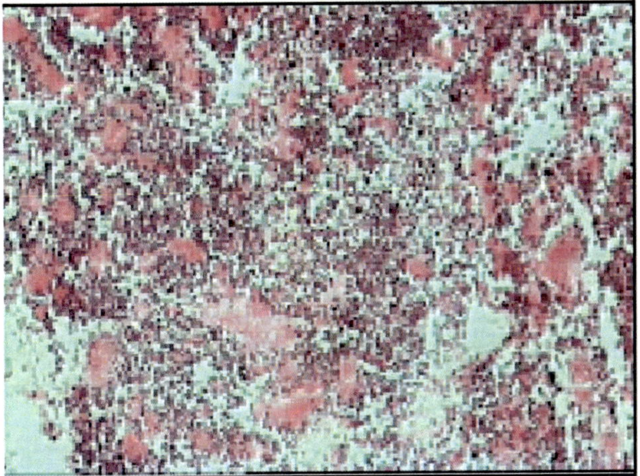

Fig. 3.4: Photomicrograph of lymph node showing congestion

Etiology

- As a result of inflammation.
- Obstruction of blood vessels.

Macroscopic features

- Organ becomes dark red/cyanotic.
- Size of organ increases.

- Weight of organ increases.
- Blood vessels become distended due to accumulation of blood.

Microscopic features

- Increased amount of blood in blood vessels.
- Veins/capillaries/arteries are distended due to accumulation of blood.
- Blood vessels become enlarged with blood and their number increases.

Haemorrhage

Escape of all the constituents of blood from blood vessels. It may occur through two processes i.e. rhexis- break in wall of blood vessel or through diapedesis in which blood leaves through intact wall of blood vessel. It occurs only in living animals (Fig. 3.5).

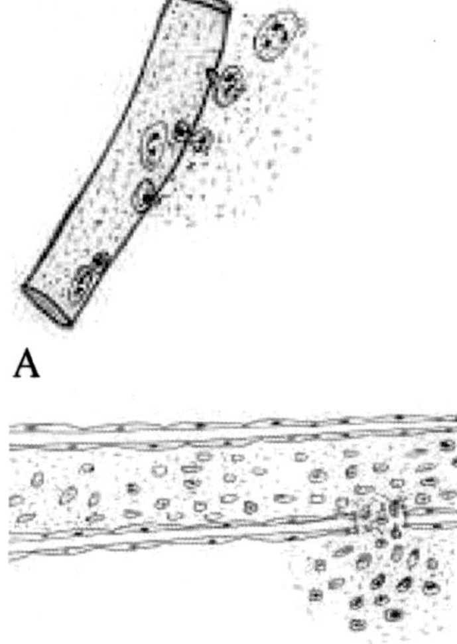

Fig. 3.5: Diagram showing haemorrhage through (A) diapedesis (B) rhexis

Etiology

- Mechanical trauma.
- Necrosis of the wall of blood vessels.
- Infections.
- Toxins.
- Neoplasm.

Macroscopic features

- Organ becomes pale due to escape of blood
- As per size, the hemorrhage is classified as under:

Pinpoint haemorrhage of about one mm diameter or pinhead size is known as *petechiae* (Fig. 3.6).

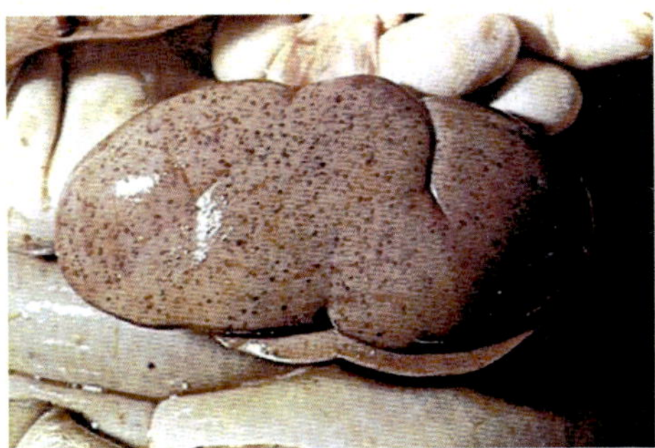

A

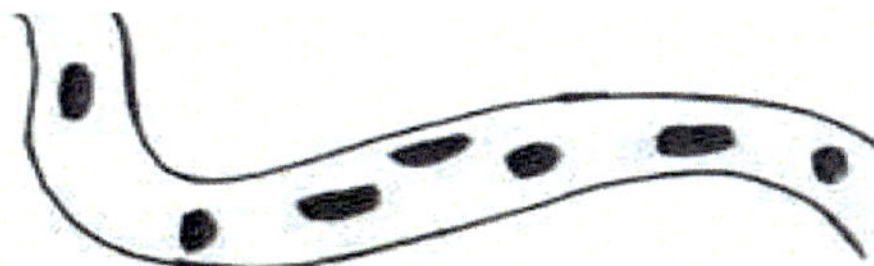

B

Fig. 3.6: Diagram showing (A) Petechial (B) Ecchymotic haemorrhage

More than one to 10 mm diameter haemorrhage are known as *ecchymoses* (Fig. 3.6).

Irregular, diffuse and flat areas of haemorrhage on mucosal or serosal surfaces are known as *suffusions*.

Haemorrhage appear in line in crests or folds on mucous membrane are known as *linear haemorrhage* (Figs. 3.7 & 3.8).

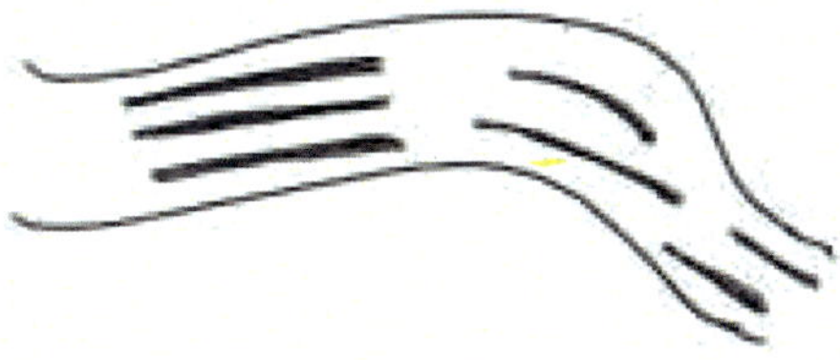

Fig. 3.7: Diagram showing linear hemorrhage

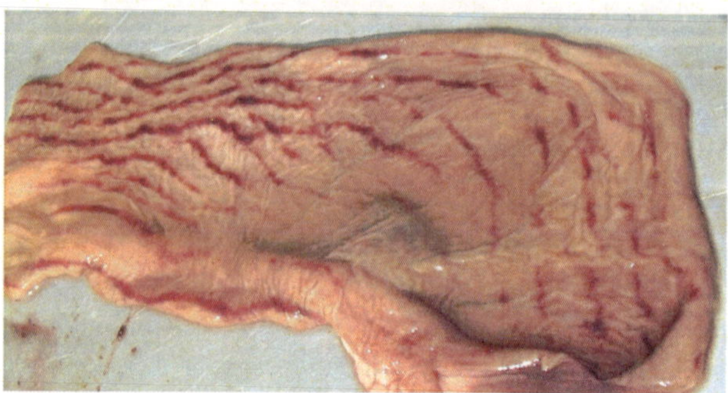

Fig. 3.8: Photograph of Large intestine showing linear haemorrhage

Hematoma is the accumulation of blood in spherical shaped mass (Fig.3.9).

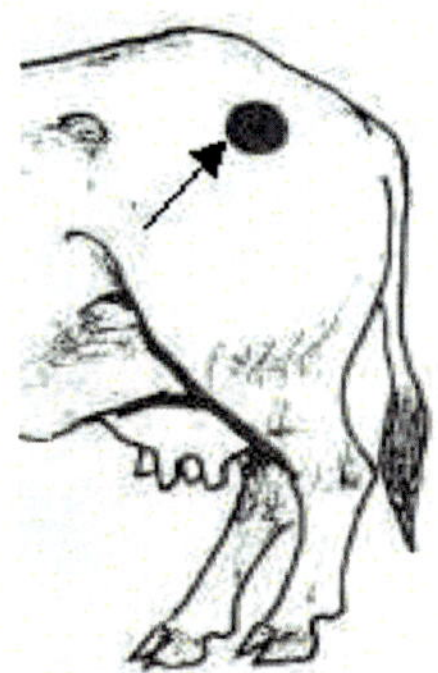

Fig. 3.9: Diagram showing hematoma

- According to location, the haemorrhage is classified as:

Hemothorax: Blood in thoracic cavity.

Hemopericardium: Blood in pericardial sac. When there is increased amount of blood in pericardial sac, it causes heart failure and is known as *cardiac temponade* (Fig. 3.10).

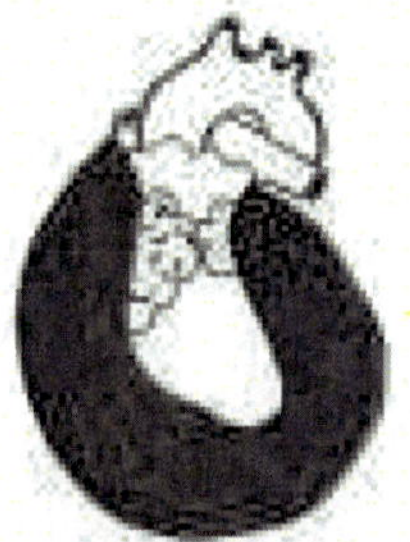

Fig. 3.10: Diagram showing cardiac temponade

Hemoperitonium: Blood in peritoneal cavity.

Hemoptysis: Blood in sputum.

Hematuria: Blood in urine.

Epistaxis: Blood from nose.

Metrorrhagia: Blood from uterus.

Melena: Bleeding in faeces.

Hematemesis: Blood in vomitus.

Microscopic features

- Blood constituents are seen outside the blood vessels.
- Break in blood vessels.
- Presence of red blood cells in tissues outside the blood vessels (Fig. 3.11).

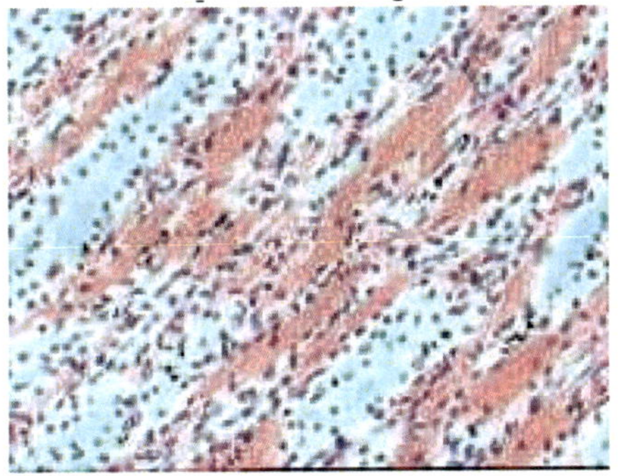

Fig. 3.11: Photomicrograph of kidney showing haemorrhage

Thrombosis

Formation of clot of blood in vascular system in the wall of blood vessel. It occurs due to endothelial injury leading to accumulation of thrombocytes, fibrinogen, erythrocytes and leucocytes (Figs. 3.12 & 3.13).

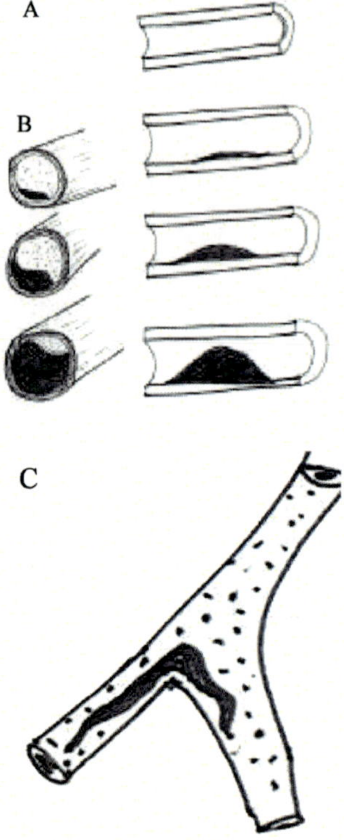

Fig. 3.12: Diagram of thrombi formation in wall of blood vessel **(A)** Normal **(B)** Thrombi formation **(C)** Saddle thrombi

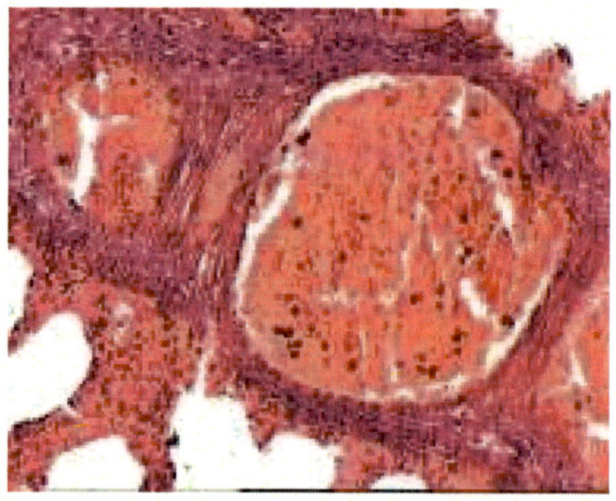

Fig. 3.13: Photomicrograph of thrombi in blood vessel of lung

Etiology

- Injury in endothelium of blood vessels.
- Alteration in blood flow.
- Alteration in composition of blood.

Macroscopic features

- Blood clot in wall of blood vessels.
- On removal of clot, rough surface exposed.
- Clot may be pale, red or laminated.
- Occlusive thrombus totally occlude blood vessels.
- Mural thrombus is on the wall of heart.
- Valvular thrombus is on valves of heart.
- Cardiac thrombus is in heart.
- Saddle thrombus is at the bifurcation of blood vessel just like saddle on back of horse.
- Septic thrombus contains bacteria.

Microscopic features

- Blood clot in blood vessel.
- Attached with wall of blood vessel.
- Alternate, irregular, red and gray areas in thrombi.

Embolism

Presence of foreign body in circulatory system which may cause obstruction in blood vessel (Fig. 3.14).

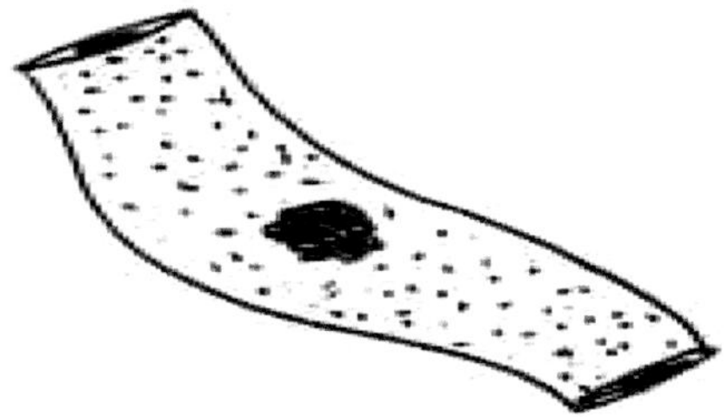

Fig. 3.14: Diagram of emboli in blood vessel

Etiology

- Thrombus, Fibrin.
- Bacteria.
- Neoplasm.
- Clumps of normal cells.
- Fat, Gas.
- Parasites.

Macroscopic features

- Emboli causing obstruction of blood vessels lead to formation of infarct in the area.
- Organ/ tissue becomes pale.
- Parasitic emboli e.g. *Dirofilaria immitis*

Microscopic features

- Presence of foreign material in blood.
- Dependent area necrotic due to absence of blood supply.

Ischemia

Ischemia is deficiency of arterial blood in any part of an organ. It is also known as local anemia.

Etiology

- External pressure on artery.
- Narrowing/obliteration of lumen of artery.
- Thrombi/emboli.

Macroscopic features

- Necrosis of dependent part.
- Occurrence of infarction.
- Dead tissue replaced by fibrous tissue.

Microscopic features

- Lesions of infarction

Infarction

Local **area** of necrosis resulting from ischemia. Ischemia is the deficiency of blood due to obstruction in artery (Figs. 3.15 & 3.16).

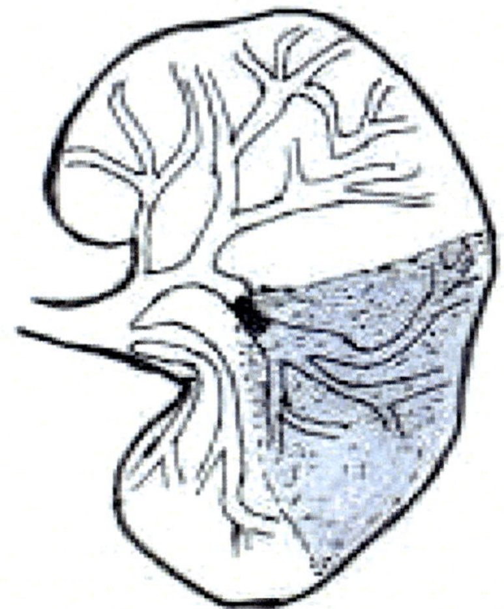

Fig. 3.15: Diagram of infarction in kidney

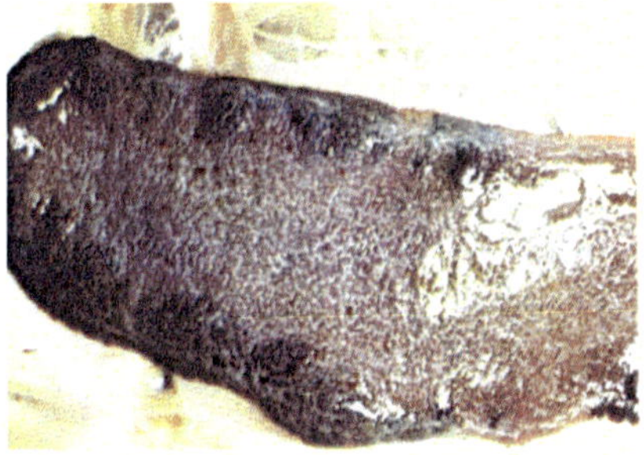

Fig. 3.16: Photograph of spleen showing infarction

Etiology

- Thrombi.
- Emboli.
- Poisons like Fusarium toxins.

Macroscopic features

- Necrosis in triangular area
- Red infarct is observed as red triangle bulky surface.
- Pale infarct is grey in colour and seen as triangle depressed surface.

Microscopic features

- Necrosis in cone shaped area.
- Obstruction of blood vessels.

Oedema

Accumulation of excessive fluid in intercellular spaces and / or in body cavity (Figs. 3.17 to 3.20).

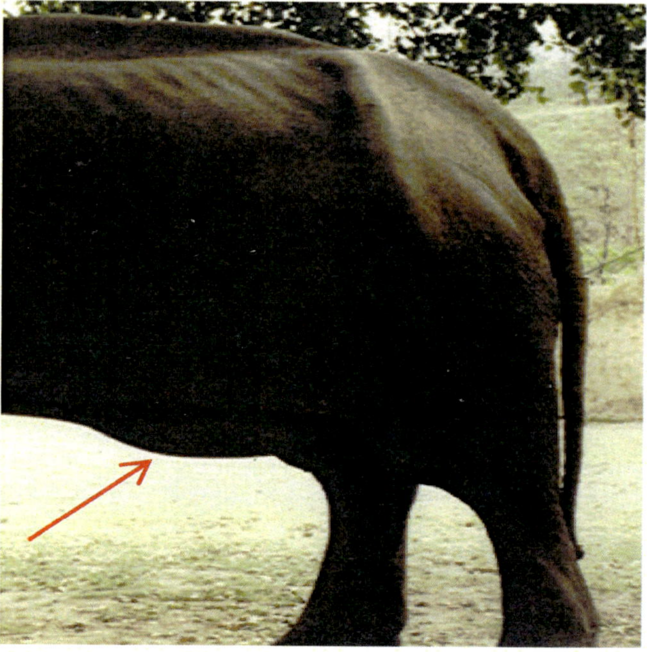

Fig. 3.17: Photograph of an elephant showing oedema in lower abdomen

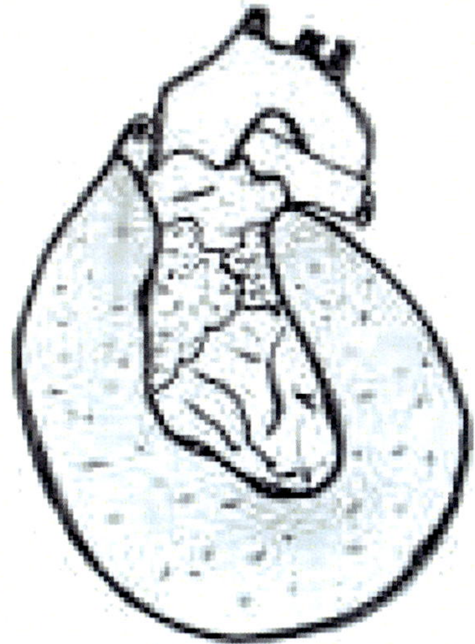

Fig. 3.18: Diagram of heart showing hydropericardium

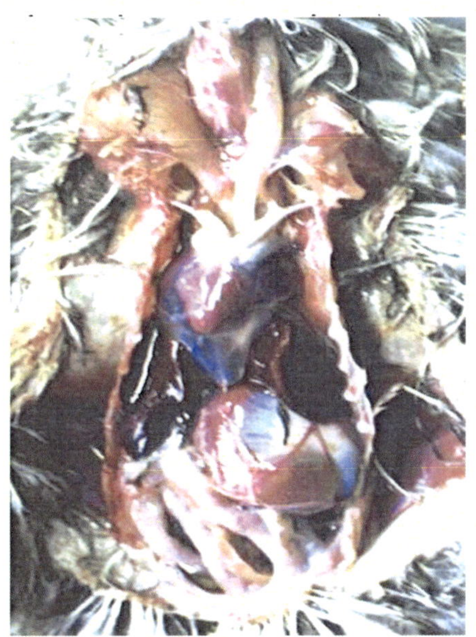

Fig. 3.19: Photograph of a dead bird showing hydropericardium

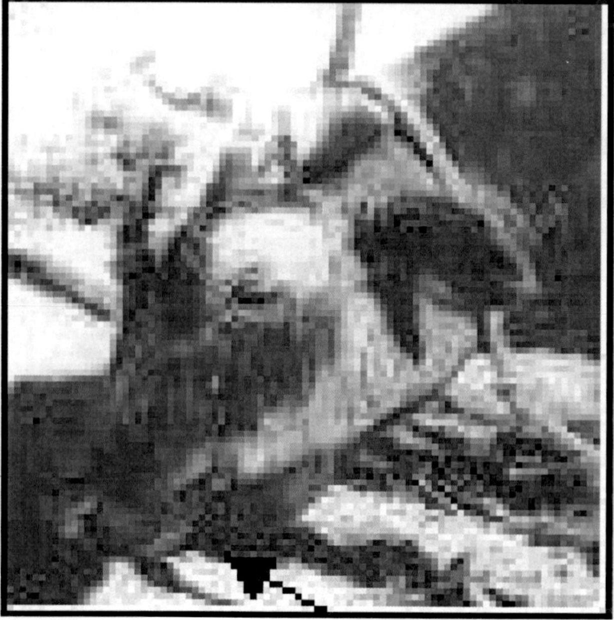

Fig. 3.20: Photograph of a bullock showing oedema of jaw

Etiology

- Deficiency of protein.
- Passive hyperemia.
- Increased permeability of capillaries.
- Obstruction of lymphatics.

Macroscopic features

- Swelling of tissue / organ / body.
- Weight and size of organ increased.
- Colour becomes light.
- Pitting impressions on pressure.
- Ascites is accumulation of fluid in peritoneum. It is also known as hydroperitonium.
- *Hydropericardium* is fluid accumulation in pericardial sac.
- *Hydrocele* is fluid accumulation in tunica vaginalis of the testicles.

- *Anasarca* is generalized oedema of body.
- *Hydrocephalus* is accumulation of fluid in brain.
- *Hydrothorax* is accumulation of fluid in thoracic cavity.

Microscopic features

- Intercellular spaces become enlarged.
- Serum/fluid deposits (pink in colour on H&E staining) in intercellular spaces.
- Cells separated farther.

Shock

Shock is a circulatory disturbance characterized by reduction in total blood volume, blood flow and by haemconcentration.

Etiology

- Primary shock

  Occurs immediately after injury.

  Injury / extensive tissue destruction. Emotional crisis.

  Surgical manipulation.

- Secondary shock

  Crushing injury involving chest and abdomen.

  Occurs after several hours of incubation.

  Release of histamine and other substances by injured tissue.

  Extensive haemorrhage. Burns.

  Predisposing factors like cold, exhaustion, depression.

Macroscopic features

- Acute general passive hyperemia.
- Dilatation of capillaries.
- Cyanosis.
- Numerous petechial haemorrhages.
- Oedema and loose connective tissue.

Microscopic features

- Capillaries and small blood vessels are distended due to accumulation of blood.
- Number of engorged blood vessels increased.
- Focal haemorrhage.
- Oedema, cells separated farther due to accumulation of transudate in intercellular spaces.

Sludged Blood

Sludged blood is agglutination of erythrocytes in the vascular system of an animal.

Etiology

- Fluctuation in blood flow.
- Slow rate of blood flow.

Macroscopic features

- Oedema.
- Emboli.
- Infarction.
- Necrosis.

Microscopic features

- Clumping of erythrocytes in pulmonary capillaries.
- Infarction, necrosis.
- Oedema.
- Erythrophagocytosis by reticuloendothelial cells.

4

Disturbances in Cell Metabolism

Cloudy Swelling

Swelling of cells occur with hazy appearance due to a mild injury. The cells take more water due to defect in sodium pump leading to swollen mitochondria which gives granular cytoplasmic appearance. It is the first reaction of cell to the mildest injury. Cloudy swelling is a reversible reaction (Figs. 4.1 & 4. 2).

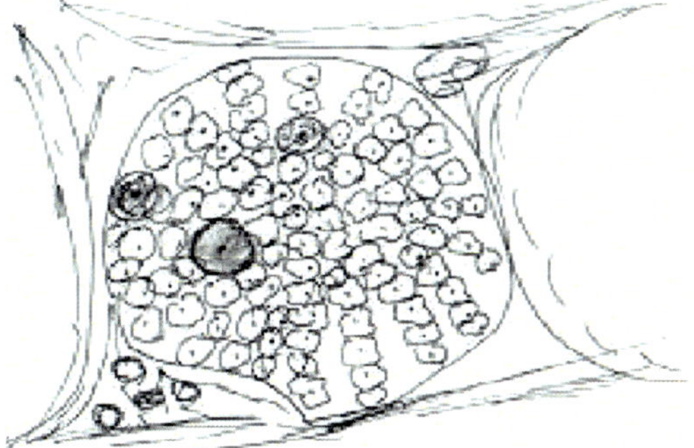

Fig. 4.1: Diagram showing cloudy swelling in liver

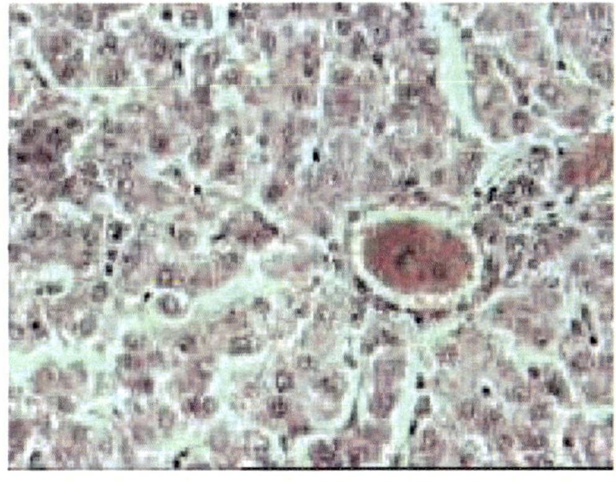

Fig. 4.2: Photograph showing cloudy swelling in liver

Etiology

- Can be caused by even mildest injury.
- Any factor causing interference with metabolism of the cell like bacterial toxins, fever, diabetes, circulatory disturbances etc.

Macroscopic features

- Organ becomes enlarged and rounded.
- Weight of organ increases.
- Bulging on cut surfaces.
- Amount of fluid increases in organ.

Microscopic features

- Swelling of cells, edges become rounded.
- Increased size of cells.
- Cytoplasm of the cells becomes hazy/cloudy due to increased granularity.
- Can be seen in liver, kidney and muscles.

Hydropic Degeneration

Cells swell due to intake of clear fluid. Such cells may burst due to increased amount of fluid and form vesicle. Hydropic degeneration can be seen in epithelium of skin and /or mucous membranes of body (Figs. 4.3 & 4.4)

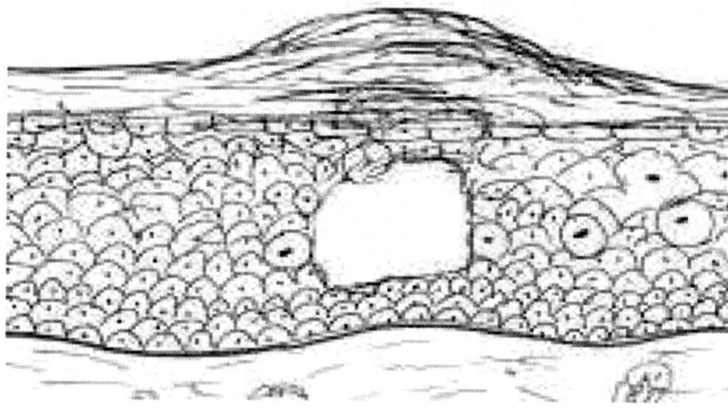

Fig. 4.3. Diagram showing hydropic degeneration and vesicle formation

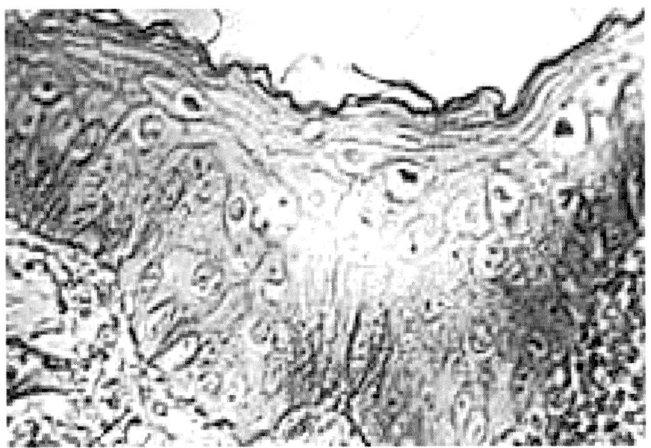

Fig. 4.4: Photomicrograph of skin showing hydropic degeneration

Etiology

- Mechanical injury.
- Burns.
- Chemical injury.
- Infections caused by virus like foot and mouth disease virus, pox virus etc.

Macroscopic features

- Vesicle formation.
- Accumulation of fluid under superficial layer of skin/mucus membrane.
- Heals rapidly within 2-4 days.
- No scar formation.
- Pyogenic organisms may convert it into pustule.

Microscopic features

- Cell size increases due to accumulation of clear fluid in cytoplasm.
- Droplets in cytoplasm as vacuoles.
- Cell bursts and epithelium protrudes leading to blister.
- Mostly affects prickle cell layer (Stratum spinosum) of skin.

Mucinous Degeneration

Excessive accumulation of mucin in degenerating epithelial cells. Mucin is a glassy, viscid, stringy and slimy is glycoprotein produced by columnar epithelial cells on mucus membranes. Such cells burst to release the mucin in lumen of organ and are called as goblet cells. When mucin is mixed with water, it is known as mucus (Figs. 4.5 & 4.6).

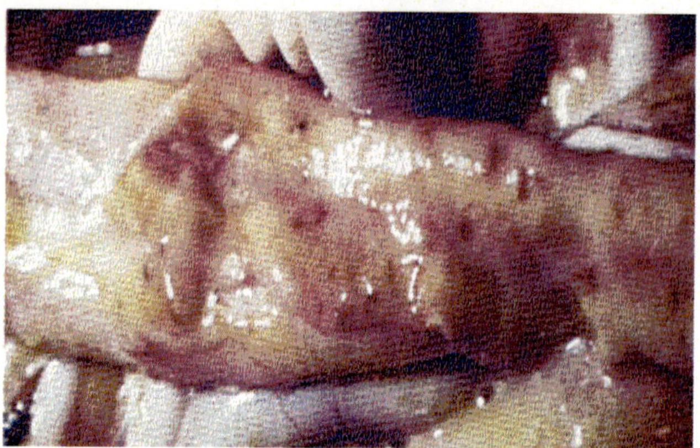

Fig. 4.5: Photograph of intestines showing mucinous degeneration

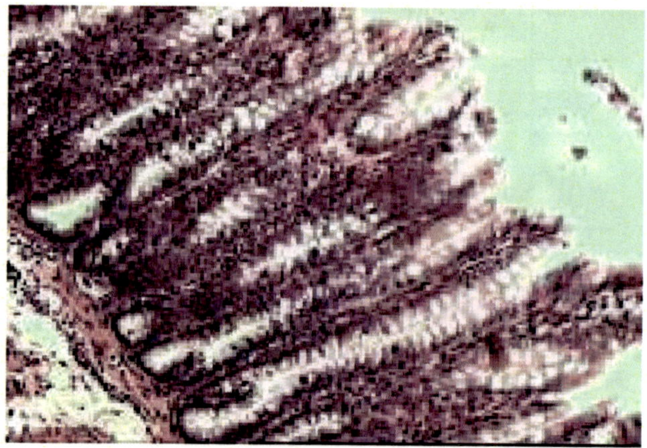

Fig. 4.6: Photomicrograph of intestines showing mucinous degeneration

Etiology

- Any irritant to mucus membrane like chemicals and infection.
- Bacteria e.g. E. coli.

- Virus e.g. Rotavirus.
- Parasite e.g. Ascaris.

Macroscopic features

- Over production of mucus in intestines which covers intestinal contents/ stool.
- Over production of mucus in genital tract during oestrus characterized by mucus discharge from vulva.
- Nasal discharge during respiratory mucosa involvement.
- Mucus is mucin mixed with water and slimy and stringy in nature.

Microscopic features

- Increased number of goblet cells.
- Goblet cells are elliptical columnar cells containing mucus.
- Mucin in lumen stains basophils through H & E staining.
- Seen on mucous surfaces only.

Mucoid Degeneration

Mucoid degeneration is mucin-like glycoprotein deposits in connective tissue.

Etiology

- In embryonic tissue e.g. umblical cord.
- In connective tissue tumors e.g. myxosarcoma.
- Myxedema due to thyroid deficiency.
- In cachexia due to starvation, parasitism or chronic wasting diseases.

Macroscopic features

- Shrunken tissue giving translucent jelly-like appearance.
- A watery, slimy and stringy material on cut surface.

Microscopic features

- Mucoid degeneration tissue stains blue
- Nuclei are hyperchromatic.

- Fibrous tissue is pale blue.
- Usually accompanied by fat necrosis.

Pseudomucin

Pseudomucin is secretion of ovaries and is observed in cystadenomas. However, it is not a disturbance of cell metabolism.

Etiology

- Cystadenoma, cystadenocarcinoma
- Paraovarian cysts.

Macroscopic features

- Transparent, slimy similar to mucin.
- It is not precipitated by acetic acid while mucin is precipitated.

Microscopic features

- Homogenous like plasma, stains pink with H&E stain.
- Extracellular.

Amyloid Infiltration

Deposition of amyloid between capillary endothelium and adjacent cells. Amyloid is a starch like substance which stains brown/blue/black with iodine and chemically it is protein polysaccharide (Fig. 4.7).

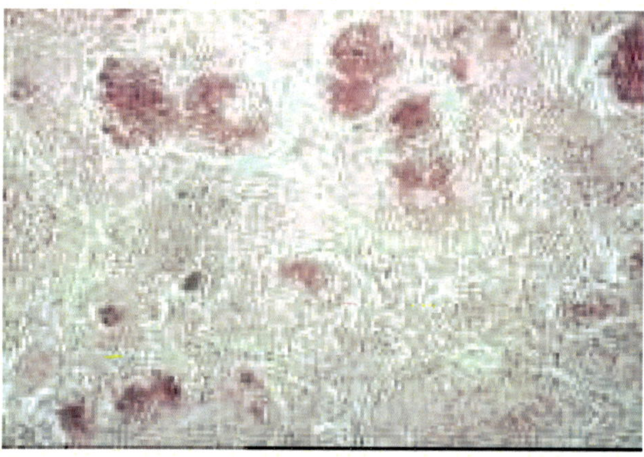

Fig. 4.7: Photomicrograph of spleen showing amyloid infiltration

Etiology

- Not exactly known.
- It is thought to be due to antigen-antibody reaction/deposition of immune complexes in between capillary endothelium and adjacent cells.

Macroscopic features

- Organ size increases with rounded edges, pits on pressure, cyanotic/ yellow in colour and fragile.
- Sago spleen due to deposition of grey, waxy sago-like material.

Microscopic features

- Amyloid stains pink on H& E stain.
- It is a permanent effect in body and remains the whole life without causing much adverse effects.

Hyaline Degeneration

Glossy substance (glass-like) solid, dense, smoothly homogenous deposits in tissues. Tissue becomes inelastic. It is a permanent change. Hyaline is very difficult to distinguish macroscopically (Fig. 4.8).

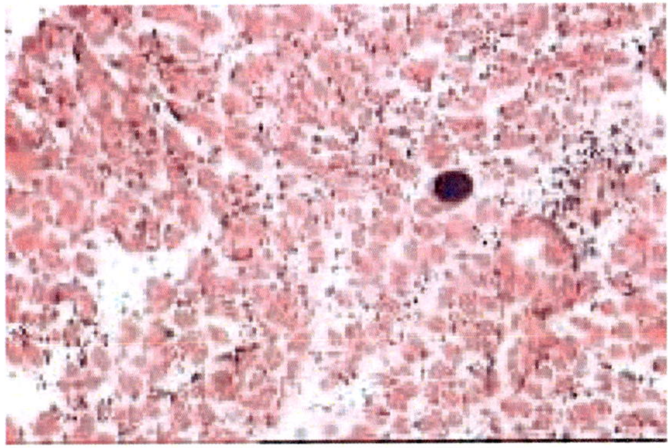

Fig. 4.8: Photomicrograph showing hyaline degeneration in muscles

Etiology

- Disturbance in protein metabolism.
- No specific cause.

Macroscopic and Microscopic Features

Connective Tissue hyaline

- In old scars, due to lack of nutrients; homogenous, strong acidophilic and pink in colour. There are no nuclei and no fibrils.

Epithelial Hyaline

- Starch-like bodies in prostate, lungs, kidneys.
- Microscopically characterized by round, homogeneous, pink, within an alveolus of lung.
- Homogenous, pink in kidney tubules/ glomeruli (Fig. 4.9).

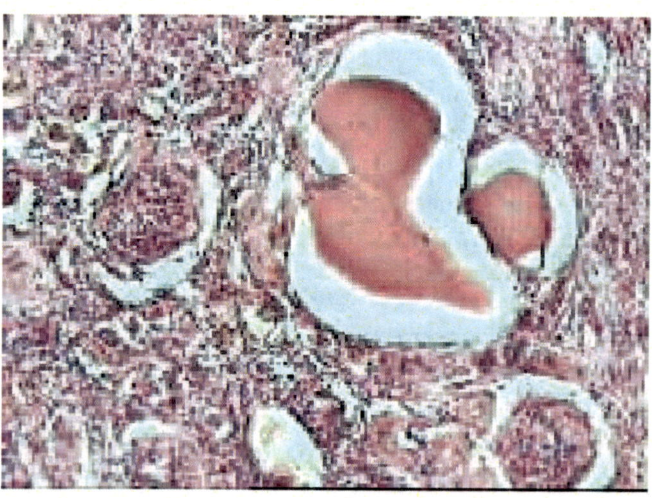

Fig. 4.9: Photomicrograph showing hyaline degeneration in kidney

Keratohyaline

- Occurs due to slow death of stratified squamous epithelial cells because of lack of nutrients. Keratinized epithelium is firm, hard and colourless. Microscopically, it is seen in epithelial pearls e.g. horn cancer, warts (Fig. 4.10).

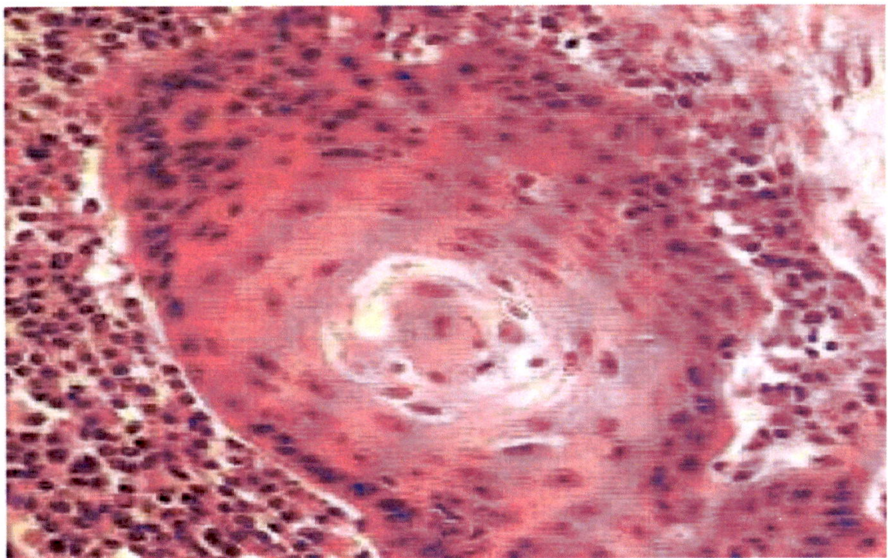

Fig. 4.10: Photomicrograph showing hyaline degeneration in skin (Epithelial pearl)

Fatty Changes

Intracellular accumulation of fat in liver, kidneys and heart. It is a reversible change.

Etiology

- Increased release of fatty acids.
- Decreased oxidation of fatty acids.
- Lipotrope deficiency.
- In ketosis, diabetes, pregnancy toxaemia.

Macroscopic features

- Enlargement of organ.
- Cut surfaces are bulging and greasy.
- Organ colour becomes light.

Microscopic features

- Intracellular deposition of fat droplets. (Fig. 4.11)
- In cytoplasm clear round/oval spaces with eccentrically placed nucleus.
- Stains yellow orange with sudan III

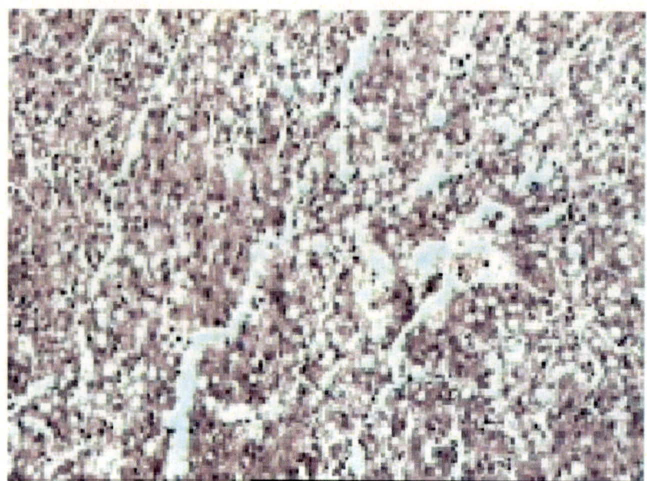

Fig. 4.11: Photomicrograph of liver showing fatty changes

Glycogen Infiltration (Glycogen Storage Disease)

Glycogen accumulates when increased amount of glycogen enters in the cells of kidneys, muscles and liver (Fig. 4.12).

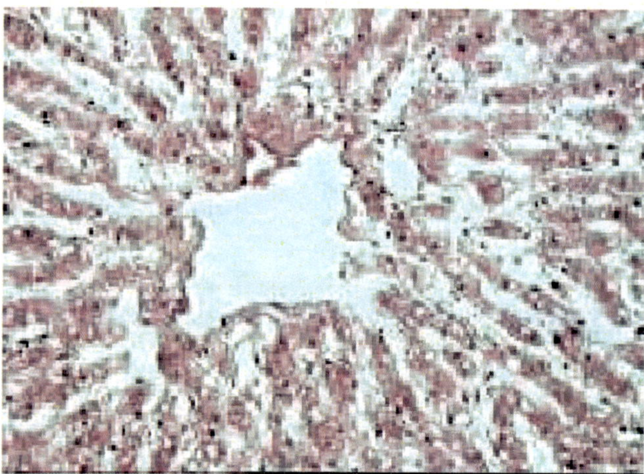

Fig. 4.12: Photomicrograph of liver showing glycogen infiltration

Etiology

- Diabetes mellitus.
- Impaired carbohydrate metabolism due to drugs e.g. corticosteroid therapy.

Macroscopic features

- Affected organ becomes enlarged.

Microscopic features

- Intracellular deposits of glycogen in cells of kidneys, liver and muscles.
- Small clear vacuoles seen in distal portion of proximal convoluted tubules, hepatocytes etc.
- It can be stained as bright red by Best's. Carmine and PAS and reddish brown by iodine.

5

Necrosis, Gangrene and Post-Mortem Changes

Necrosis

Local death of tissue /cells in living body is known as necrosis, It is characterized by the followings.

- *Pyknosis* is condensation of chromatin material, nuclei become dark, reduced in size and deeply stained.
- *Karyorrhexis* is fragmentation of nucleus.
- *Karyolysis* is dissolution of nucleus into small fragments, basophilic granules/fragments.
- *Chromatolysis* is lysis of chromatin material.
- *Necrobiosis* is physiological cell death after completion of its function e.g. RBC after 140 days.

Necrosis is further classified into coagulative, caseative, liquifactive and fat necrosis which are different from apoptosis (Figs. 5.1 to 5.3).

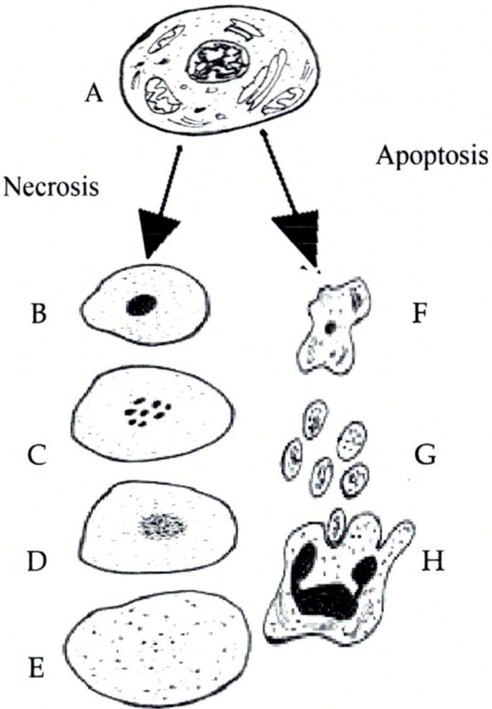

Fig. 5.1: Diagram showing pathogenesis of necrosis **(A)**Normal **(B)** Pyknosis **(C)** Karyorrhexis **(D)** Karyolysis **(E)** Chromatolysis, **(F)** Apoptosis **(G)** Blebs and **(H)** Phagocytosis

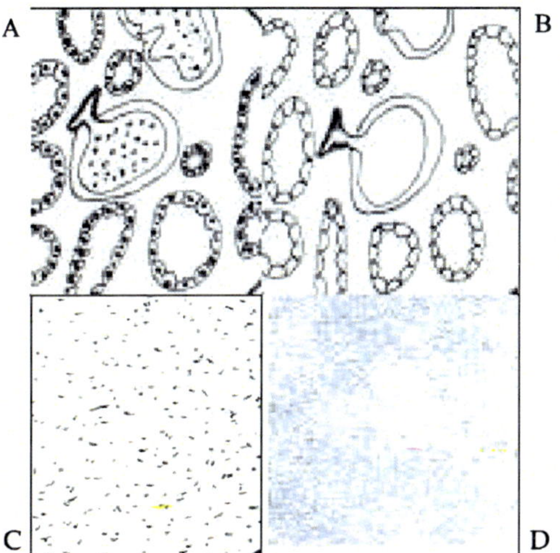

Fig. 5.2. Diagram showing necrosis **(A)** Normal **(B)** Coagulative **(C)** Caseative and **(D)** Liquefactive

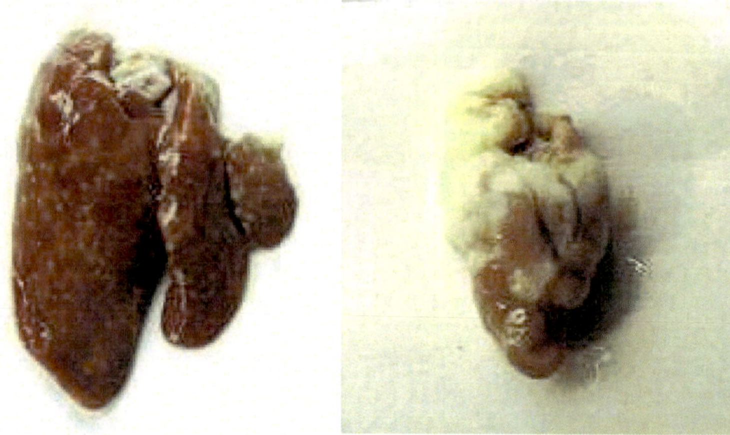

A B

Fig. 5.3: Photograph of **(A)** liver and **(B)** heart showing necrosis

Coagulative Necrosis

Local death of cells/tissue in living body characterized by loss of cellular details, while tissue architecture remains intact (Fig. 5.4).

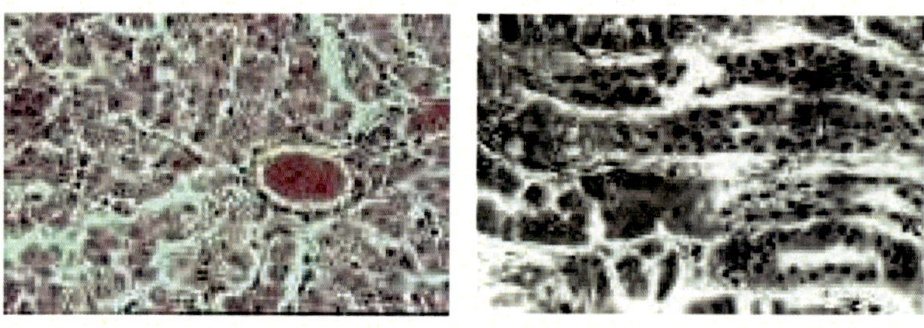

A B

Fig. 5.4: Photomicrograph of (A) liver and (B) Kidney showing coagulative necrosis

Etiology

- Infections.
- Ischemia.
- Mild irritant e.g. toxins/chemical poisons.
- Heat, trauma.

Macroscopic features

- Organ becomes grey/white in colour, firm, dense, depressed with surrounding tissue.

Microscopic features

- Cellular outline present, which maintains the architecture of tissue/ organ.
- Nucleus absent or pyknotic.
- Cytoplasm becomes acidophilic.

Liquifactive Necrosis

Local death of cells/tissues in living body characterized by rapid enzymatic dissolution of cells. The intracellular hydrolases and proteolytic enzymes of leucocytes play role in dissolution of cells (Fig. 5.5).

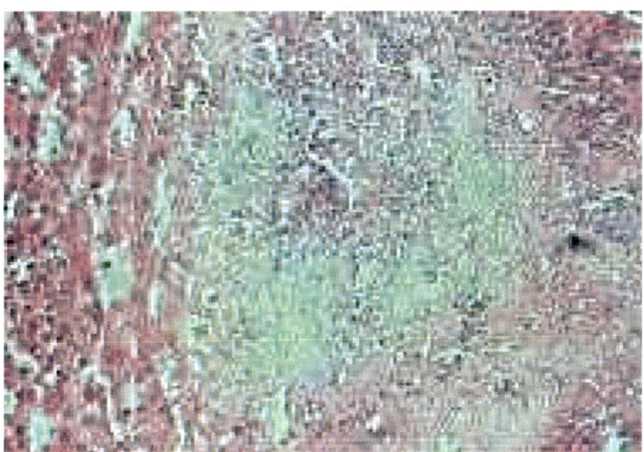

Fig. 5.5: Photomicrograph showing liquifactive necrosis

Etiology

- Pyogenic infections
- Infraction and traumatic injury
- Hypoxia; carbon monoxide and cyanide poisoning; thiamine deficiency in cat; vitamin E deficiency in chikens; and mouldy maize poisoning in horses

Macroscopic features

- Liquifactive necrosed tissue present in a cavity "Abscess".
- It contains small/large amount of cloudy fluid, which is creamy yellow (Pus).

Microscopic features

- Areas of liquifactive necrosis stains pink.
- Infiltration of neutrophils.
- Sometimes empty spaces but infiltration of neutrophils at periphery.

Caseative Necrosis

Local death of cells/tissue in living body; the dead cells/tissues are characterized by presence of firm, dry and cheesy consistency. It occurs due to coagulation of proteins and lipids (Fig. 5.6).

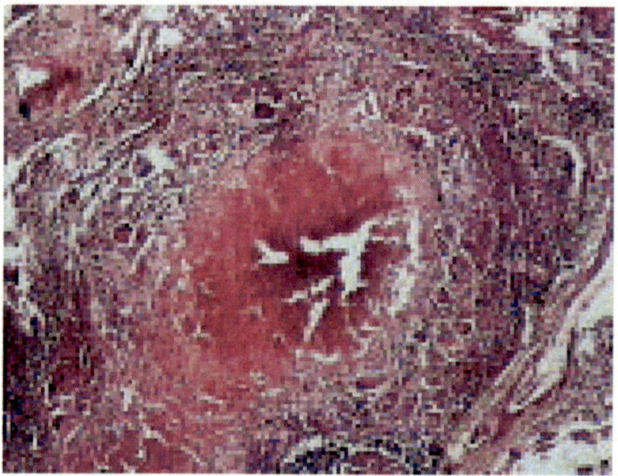

Fig. 5.6: Photomicrograph of tuberculous lung showing caseative necrosis

Etiology

- Chronic infections e.g. *Mycobacterium tuberculosis*.
- Systemic fungal infections.

Macroscopic features

- Dead tissue looks like milk curd or cottage cheese.
- Tissue dry, firm, agranular, white/grey/ yellowish in colour

Microscopic features

- Disappearance of cells; no cell details/ architecture.
- Purplish granules on H&E staining, blue granules from nucleus fragments, red granules from cytoplasm fragments.

Fat Necrosis

Local death of adipose cells in living body.

Etiology

- Trauma.
- Increased action of enzymes due to leakage of pancreatic juice.
- Starvation

Macroscopic features

- Chalky white mass deposits in organ.
- White opaque firm mass.

Microscopic features

- Adipose cell without nucleus (Fig. 5.7).
- Macrophage giant cells contain fat droplets.

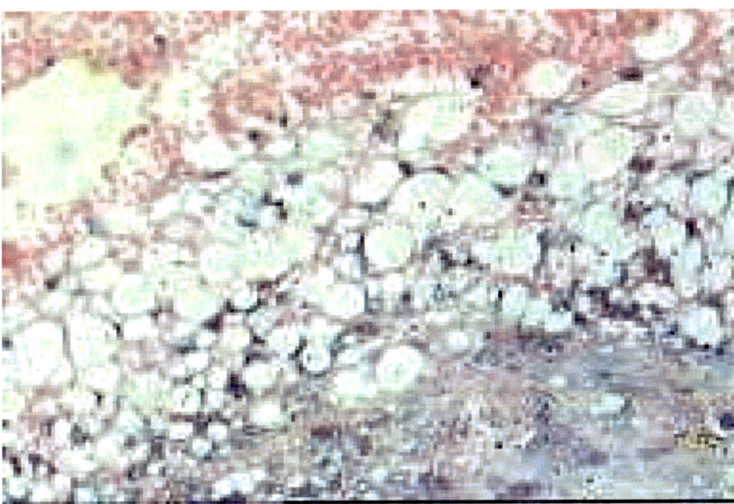

Fig. 5.7: Photomicrograph of fat showing necrosis

Table 5.1: Differential features of various types of Necrosis

	Coagulative	Liquifactive	Caseative	Fat
Macroscopic Features	1. Organ becomes gray/ white in colour, firm, dense, depressed with surrounding tissue	1. Liquifactive necrosed tissue present in a cavity "Abscess" 2. It contains small/large amount of cloudy fluid, which is creamy yellow (Pus)	1. Dead tissue looks like milk curd or cottage Cheese 2. Tissue dry, firm, agranular, white/gray/ yellowish in colour	1. Chalky white mass deposits in organ 2. White opaque firm mass
Microscopic Features	1. Cellular out line present, which maintains the architecture of tissue/ organ 2. Nucleus absent or pyknotic 3. Cytoplasm Becomes Acidophilic	1. Areas of Liquefactive necrosis stains pink. 2. Infiltration of Neutrophils 3. Sometimes empty spaces but infiltration of neutrophils at	1. Disappearance of cells; no cell details/ architecture 2. Purplish granules on H&E staining, blue granules from nucleus fragments, red granules from Cytoplasm fragments.	1. Adipose cell without nucleus 2. Macrophages giant cells contain fat droplets. 3. Presence of lime salts in tissues.

Apoptosis

Apoptosis is a finely tuned mechanism for the control of cell number in animals; the process is operative during foetal life, tumor regression and in the control of immune response. Apoptosis plays an shrinkage of cell, membrane blebbing, chromatin condensation and fragmentation of nucleic acid. Cells undergoing apoptosis often fragment into membrane bound apoptotic bodies that are readily phagocytosed by macrophages or neighbouring cells without generating an inflammatory response (Fig.5.8).

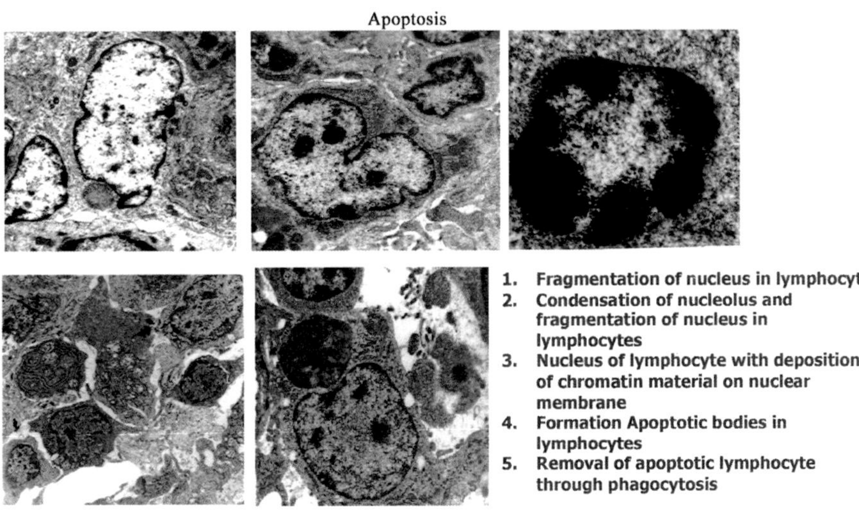

Fig. 5.8: Electron micro photographs of apoptosis

These changes distinguish apoptosis from cell death by necrosis. Necrosis refers to the morphology most often seen when cells die from severe and sudden injury such as ischemia, sustained hyperthermia or physical and chemical trauma. In necrosis, there are early changes in mitochondrial shape and function; cell losses its ability to regulate osmotic pressure, swells and ruptures. The contents of the cell are spilled into surrounding tissue, resulting in generation of a local inflammatory response.

Important role in the development and maintenance of homeostasis and in the maturation of nervous and immune systems. It is also a major defense mechanism of the body, removing unwanted and potentially dangerous cells such as self-reactive lymphocytes, virus infected cells and tumor cells. Most cells in animal have the ability of self-destruction by activation of an intrinsic cellular suicidal programme when they are no longer needed or are seriously damaged. The dying cell exhibits morphological alterations including

Necrosis is the consequence of a passive and degenerative process while the apoptosis is a consequence of an active process.

Execution of apoptosis requires the coordinated action of aspartate specific cysteine proteases (caspases) which are responsible for cleavage of key enzymes and structural proteins resulting in death of cell. Apoptosis is triggered by a variety of signals which activate the endogenous endonucleases to initiate the process of fragmentation of nuclear DNA into oligonucleosomal size fragments. Initially, the DNA fragments are large (50-300 Kb) but are later digested to oligonucleosomal size (multimers of 180-200 bp). The formation of this distinct DNA ladder is considered to be a biochemical hallmark of apoptosis.

There is rounding of nucleus with pyknosis and rhexis, chromatin coalesces to form a crescent along the nuclear membrane. Cell fragments to form blebs, which may have one or more organelles. Such changes occur in apoptotic cells within 20 min duration.

Apoptosis is generally synonymously used with "*programmed cell death*" but it differs from programmed cell death as apoptosis cannot be prevented by cycloheximide or actinomycin D, rather these chemicals accelerate the process of apoptosis while programmed cell death is prevented by these chemicals.

Gangrene

Necrosis of tissue is followed by invasion of saprophytes. Gangrene is mainly divided into three types: Dry, moist and gas gangrene.

Dry Gangrene

Dry gangrene occurs at extremities like tail, tip of ears, tip of scrotum, hoof etc. due to necrosis and invasion of saprophytes. The evaporation of moisture takes place resulting into dry lesions.

Etiology

- Mycotoxins from fungus Fusarium equiseti found on paddy straw in low lying areas with moisture (Degnala disease).

Macroscopic features

- Dry, fragmented crusts like lesions on tail, scrotum, ear (Figs. 5.9 & 5.10).

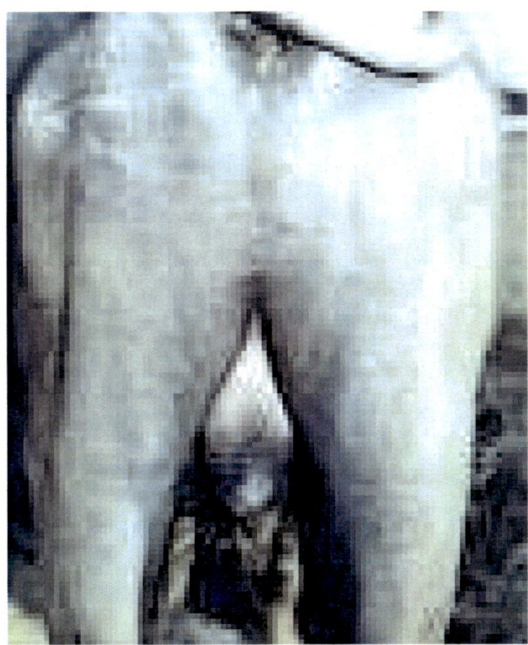

Fig. 5.9: Photograph of a buffalo bull showing dry gangrene at scrotum

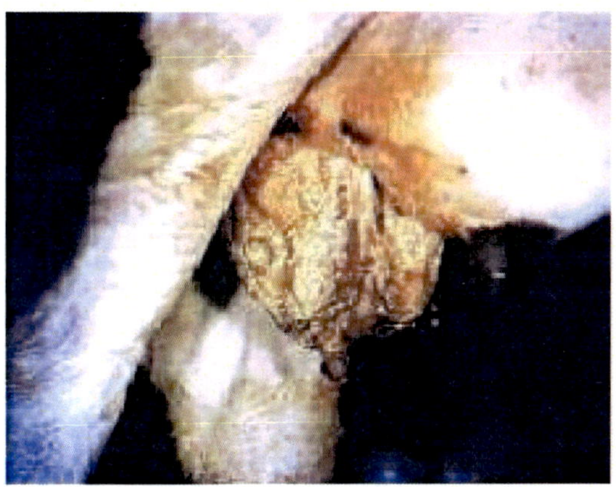

Fig. 5.10: Photograph of udder showing gangrene

- Hoof becomes detached due to necrosis and gangrene, sloughing, exposing the red raw surface (Figs. 5.11 & 5.12).
- Blackening of the affected area.

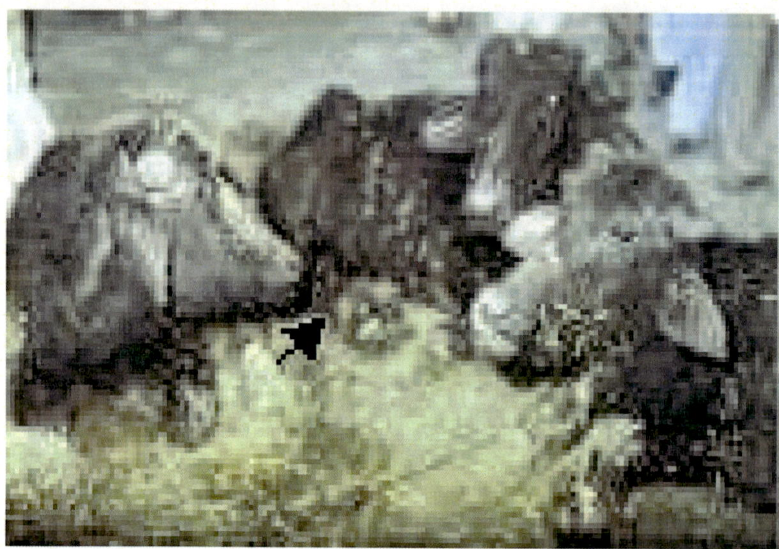

Fig. 5.11: Photograph of buffalo calves showing sloughing of hoofs due to Degnala disease

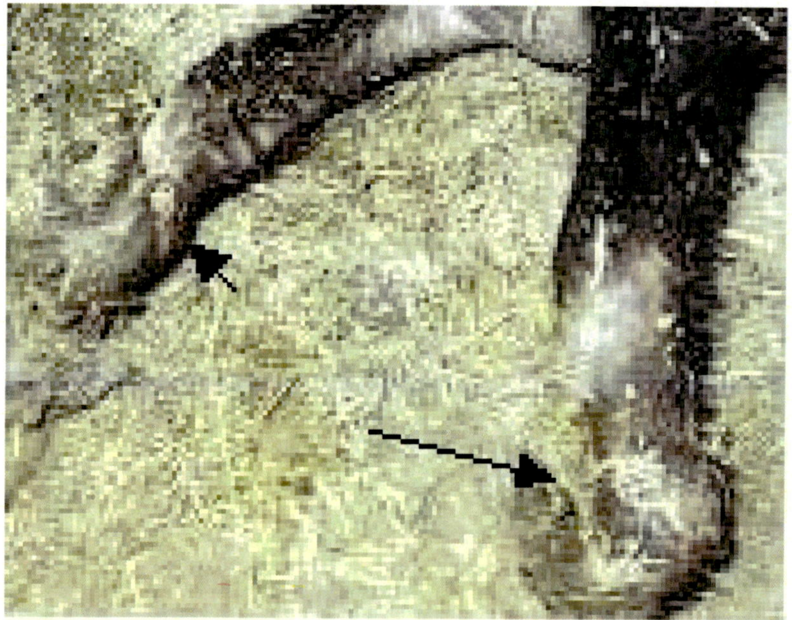

Fig. 5.12: Photograph of buffalo calves showing sloughing of hoofs due to Degnala disease

Microscopic features

- Necrosis and invasion of saprophytes in skin of tail, ear or scrotum.

Moist Gangrene

Moist gangrene mostly occurs in internal organs of body like lungs, intestine, stomach etc. It occurs due to necrosis and invasion of saprophytes leading to dissolution of the tissues (Figs 5.13 & 5.14).

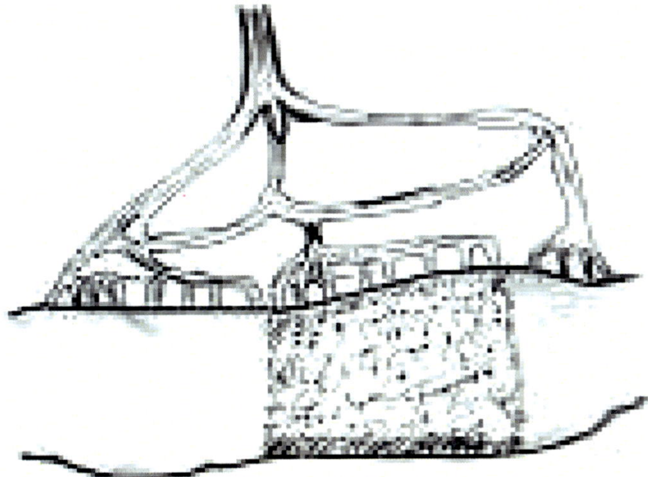

Fig. 5.13: Diagram showing moist gangrene in intestine

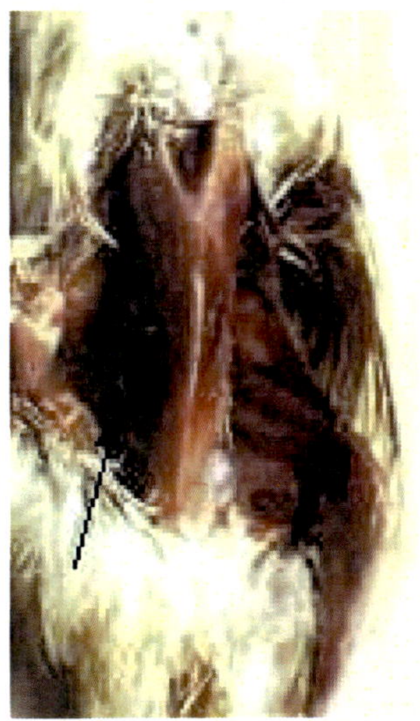

Fig. 5.14: Photograph showing moist gangrene in poultry

Etiology

- Drenching of milk, medicines etc. e.g. Aspiration pneumonia/ Drenching pneumonia.
- Volvolus/Intussusception or torsion in intestine.

Macroscopic features

- Greenish or bluish discolouration of the affected organ.
- Dissolution of affected part into fragments
- Presence of foreign material like milk, fibre, oil, etc.

Microscopic features

- Necrosis and invasion of saprophytes
- Presence of foreign material like milk, fibres, oil etc.

Gas Gangrene

Gas gangrene occurs in muscles particularly of thigh muscles of hind legs in heifers in case of black leg (Black Quarter; B.Q.) (Figs. 5.15 & 5.16).

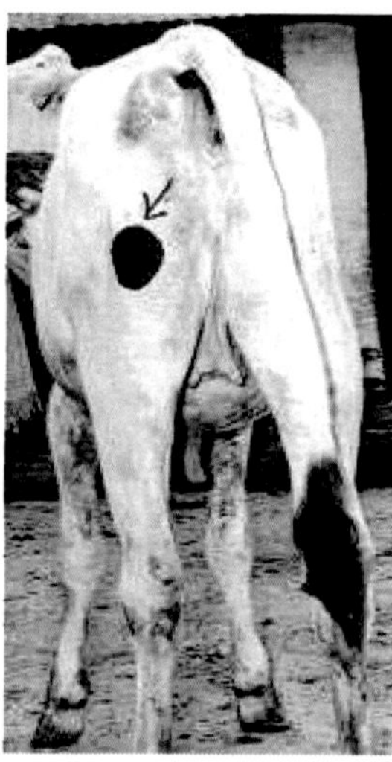

Fig. 5.15: Photograph showing gas gangrene in heifer

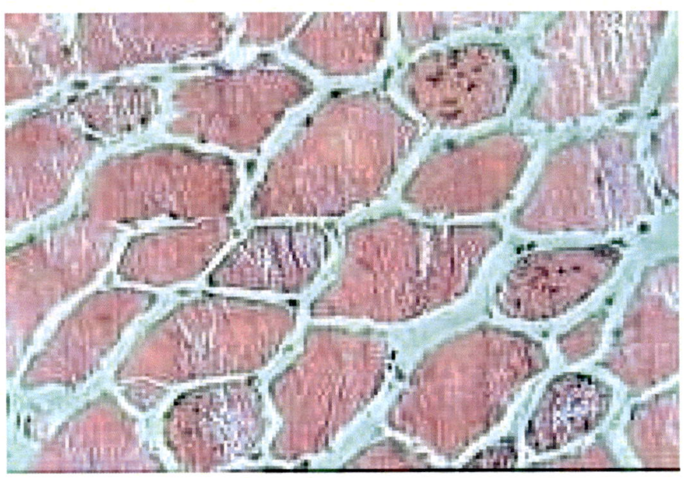

Fig. 5.16: Photomicrograph showing myositis/gas gangrene

Etiology

- Clostridium chauvei
- Gram positive, rod, anaerobe.
- Produces toxins under anaerobic conditions which cause disease.
- Stress, trauma, transportation predisposes animals.

Macroscopic features

- Oedema of Muscles in affected part particularly thigh region.
- Blackening of muscles due to production of H_2S by bacteria and its chemical reaction with iron of free hemoglobin producing iron sulphide.
- Presence of gas in the area giving crepitating sound on palpation.

Microscopic features

- Necrosis of muscles
- Presence of Gram positive rod shaped Clostridia
- Dissolution of muscle fibers due to saprophytes/ toxins of the organism.

Table 5.2: Differential features of various types of Gangrene

	Dry	**Moist**	**Gas**
Macroscopic features	1. Dry, fragmented crusts like lesions on tail, scrotum, ear	1. Greenish or bluish discoloration of the affected organ.	1. Oedema of Muscles in affected part particularly thigh region.
	2. Hoof becomes detached due to necrosis and gangrene, sloughing, exposing the red raw surface.	2. Dissolution of affected part into fragments	2. Blackening of muscles due to production of H_2S by bacteria and its chemical reaction with iron of free hemoglobin producing iron sulphide.
	3. Blackening of the affected area.	3. Presence of foreign material like milk, fiber, oil, etc.	3. Presence of gas in the area giving crepitating sound on palpation
Microscopic features	1. Necrosis and invasion of saprophytes in skin of tail, ear or scrotum	1. Necrosis and invasion of Saprophytes	1. Necrosis of muscles
		2. Presence of foreign material like milk, fibers, oil, etc.	2. Presence of Gram positive rod shaped Clostridia
			3. Dissolution of muscle fibers due to saprophytes/ toxins of the organism

Post-Mortem Changes

Alterations in cells/tissues occur after death of animal. The degree of such alterations and their speed depends upon the environmental temperature, size of animal, species of animal, external insulation and nutritional state of the animal. The postmortem changes occur rapidly in high environmental temperature, large, and fur/wool-bearing and fatty animals.

Autolysis

Autolysis is the digestion of tissue by its own enzymes and is characterized by uniform destruction of cells without any inflammatory reaction. After death, a state of hypoxia occurs leading to decreased ATP. The cell organelles degenerate and the membrane of lysosomes dissolve releasing the lysosomal enzymes in the cell responsible for digestion of cells/tissues. These enzymes cause disintegration of cell components into small granules in the cell. Microscopically, autolysis is characterized by uniform dead cells without any circulatory changes and inflammatory reaction.

Putrefaction

Putrefaction is decomposition of tissue after death by saprophytes leading to production of foul odour. After autolysis the saprophytes invade from external environment into the body, multiply and eventually digest the tissues with their enzymes. The tissue becomes fragile and produces foul odour.

Pseudomelanosis

Pseudomelanosis is greenish or bluish discolouration of tissues/organs after death. Saprophytes causing putrefaction also produce hydrogen sulfide which chemically reacts with iron portion of hemoglobin to produce iron sulfide. Iron sulfide is a black pigment and produces green, grey or black shades on combination with other tissue pigments.

Rigor Mortis

Rigor mortis is the contraction and shortening of muscles after death of animal leading to stiffening and immobilization of body. It occurs 2-4 hours after death and remains till putrefaction sets in. Rigor mortis begins in cardiac muscles first and then in skeletal muscles of head and neck with a progression towards extremities. It is enhanced by high temperature and increased metabolic activity before death; while it is delayed by starvation, cold and cachexia. Rigor appears quickly in case animal has died due to strychnine poisoning as a result of depletion of energy source ATP. Muscle fibres shorten due to contraction and remain in contraction in the absence of oxygen, ATP and creatine phosphate. Rigor mortis remains till 20-30 hours of death, the duration depends on autolysis and putrefaction. It disappears in same order as it appeared from head, neck to extremities. It can be used to determine the length of time after the death of animal.

Algor mortis

Algor mortis is cooling of body. As after death there is no circulation of blood, which maintains the body temperature, body becomes cool. However, it takes 2-4 hours, depending on the species, environmental temperature and type of animal.

Livor mortis

Livor mortis is the staining of tissues with hemoglobin after death of animals. It gives pinkish discolouration to the tissues.

Hypostatic congestion

Due to gravitational force, the blood is accumulated in dependent ventral parts of body. It is helpful in establishing of the state of the body at the time of death.

Post-mortem emphysema

It occurs due to decomposition by gas producing organisms including saprophytes. The gas is mainly accumulated in gastrointestinal tract causing rupture of the organ.

Post-mortem clot

It is clotting of blood after death of animal mainly due to excessive release of thrombokinase from dying leucocytes and endothelial cells. It is smooth in consistency having glistening surface that is red or yellow in colour. Post-mortem clot is uniform in structure and it does not attach to the wall of blood vessel as thrombus does. In anthrax, post-mortem clot does not appear. Post-mortem clot is of two types: Red or currant jelly clot forms when the components of blood are evenly distributed throughout the clot. It occurs due to rapid clotting of blood. The yellow or chicken fat clot occurs when the components of blood are not distributed evenly. The dorsal position is red and upper position in yellow due to WBC fibrin and serum. It occurs due to prolonged coagulation time of blood leading to sedimentation of red blood cells.

Displacement of organs

Displacement of internal organs due to rolling of dead animal. Mainly intestine/ stomach and uterus are affected with displacement which can be differentiated from ante-mortem displacement by absence of passive hyperemia.

Imbibition of bile

Cholebilirubin present in the gall bladder diffuses to the surrounding tissues/ organs and stains them with yellow/ greenish pigmentation.

6

Inflammation and Healing

Inflammation

Inflammation is a complex process of vascular and cellular alterations that occur in body in response to injury. The term inflammation has been derived from the Latin word inflammare, means to set on fire. Inflammation is considered as an important event in body that activates the existing defense mechanisms in circulating blood to dilute, naturalize or kill the irritant/ causative agent. Thus, it is said that immunity is the resistance of body, while inflammation is the activation of that immunity. It is beneficial to body except when chronic or immune origin. Inflammation starts with sublethal injury and ends with healing.

Etiology

- Any irritant/ injury.
- Bacteria, virus, parasite, fungus etc.
- Trauma.
- Physical or chemical injury.

Macroscopic features

- Inflammation is characterized by 5 cardinal signs;
- Redness;
- Swelling (Fig. 6.1);
- Heat;
- Pain;
- Loss of function

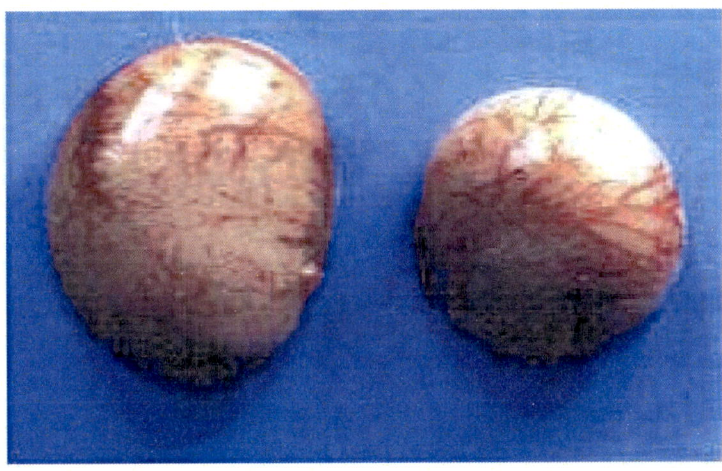

Fig. 6.1: Inflammation of testes showing redness and swelling

Microscopic features

- Acute inflammation is characterized by more intense vascular changes like congestion, oedema, haemorrhages, leakage of fibrinogen and leucocytes (Fig. 6.2).

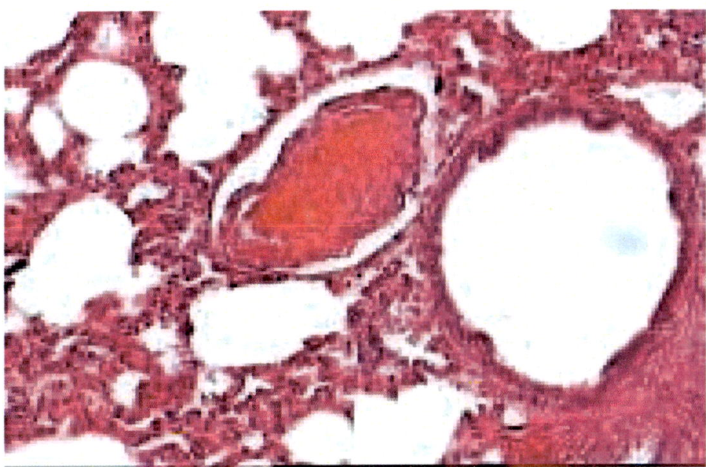

Fig. 6.2: Photomicrograph of acute inflammation showing intense vascular changes

- Chronic inflammation is characterized by more proliferative and/or regenerative changes such as proliferation of fibroblasts and regeneration of epithelium along with infiltration of leucocytes (Fig. 6.3).

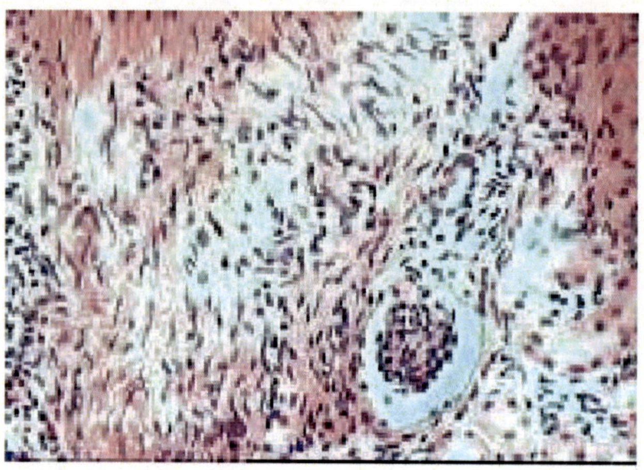

Fig. 6.3: Photomicrograph of chronic inflammation showing proliferative changes

Introduction and terminology

Inflammation may occur in any organ/tissue depending upon the type of injury and irritant. The inflammed state of an organ is called most often with a suffix "itis". Detailed nomenclature is as under for different organs/ tissues:

Abomasum	Abomasitis
Artery	Arteritis
Bileduct	Cholangitis
Bone & bone marrow	Osteomyelitis
Bone	Osteitis
Brain	Encephalitis
Bronchi	Bronchitis
Bursa	Bursitis
Caecum	Typhlitis
Cervix	Cervicitis
Colon	Colonitis
Conjunctiva	Conjunctivitis
Connective tissue	Cellulitis
Cornea	Keratitis
Crop	Ingluvitis
Durameter	Pachymeningitis
Ear	Otitis
Endocardium	Endocarditis

Eosophagus	Esophagitis
Epididymis	Epididymitis
Eustachian tube	Eustachitis
External ear	Otitis externa
Eyelid	Blepheritis
Eyes	Ophthalmitis
Fascia	Fascitis
Fat	Steatitis
Gall bladder	Cholecystitis
Glans penis	Balanitis
Gums	Gingivitis
Heart	Carditis
Inner part of uterus	Endometritis
Internal ear	Otitis interna
Intestine	Enteritis
Iris	Iritis
Joints	Arthritis
Kidney & pelvis	Pyelonephritis
Kidney	Nephritis
Lacrimal gland	Dacryadenitis
Larynx	Laryngitis
Ligament	Desmitis
Lip	Cheilitis
Liver	Hepatitis
Lungs	Pneumonitis/Pneumonia
Lymph nodes	Lymphadenitis
Lymph vessels	Lymphangitis
Meninges	Meningitis
Middle ear	Otitis media
Mouth cavity	Stomatitis
Muscle	Myositis
Myocardium	Myocarditis
Nails	Onychia
Nasal passage	Rhinitis
Nerve	Neuritis
Omasum	Omasitis
Ovary	Oophoritis
Oviduct	Salpingitis
Palates	Lampas / palatitis
Pancreas	Pancreatitis

Pericardium	Pericarditis
Peritoneum	Peritonitis
Pharynx	Pharyngitis
Piameter	Leptomeningitis
Pleura	Pleuritis
Prepuce	Posthitis
Rectum	Proctitis
Reticulm	Reticulitis
Retina	Retinitis
Rumen	Rumenitis
Salivary glands	Sialadenitis
Sinuses	Sinusitis
Skin	Dermatitis
Spermatic cord	Funiculitis
Spinal cord	Myelitis
Spleen	Spleenitis
Stomach	Gastritis
Synovial membrane of joints	Sinovitis
Tendon	Tendinitis
Testes	Orchitis
Tongue	Glossitis
Trachea	Tracheitis
Ureter	Ureteritis
Urethra	Urethritis
Urinary bladder	Cystitis
Uterus	Metritis
Vagina	Vaginitis
Vein	Phlebitis
Vertebra	Spondylitis
Vessel	Vasculitis
Vulva	Vulvitis

Pathogenesis of Inflammation

Inflammation starts with sublethal injury and ends with healing; in between there are many events that take place which are described as under:

Transient vasoconstriction

The blood vessels of the affected part become constricted for movement of blood as a result of action of irritant (Fig. 6.4a).

Vasodialation and Increase in permeability

The blood vessels become dilated. Endothelium becomes more permeable and Releases procoagulant factors and prostaglandins. Fluid and proteins come out due to leakage in endothelium.

Fluid contains water, immunoglobulins, complement component, biochemical factors of coagulation and mediators of inflammation (Fig. 6.4B).

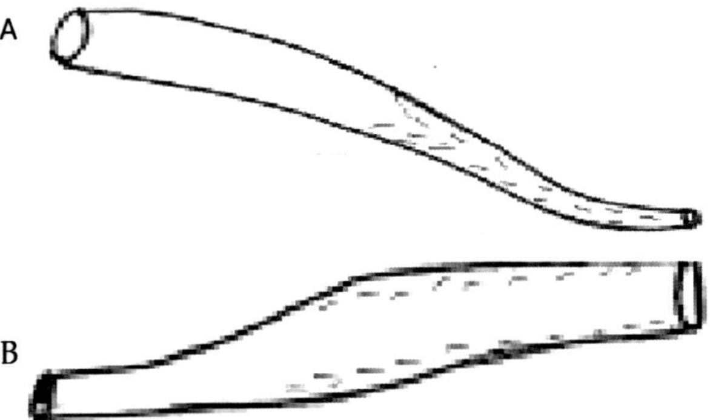

Fig. 6.4: Diagram of a blood vessel showing **(a)** Vasoconstriction and **(b)** Vasodilation.

Blood flow decrease

Due to stasis of blood in blood vessel, there is increase in leakage of fluids / cells outside the blood vessels. It gives rise to congestion/ hyperemia.

There is margination of leucocytes also known as pavementation (Fig. 6.5).

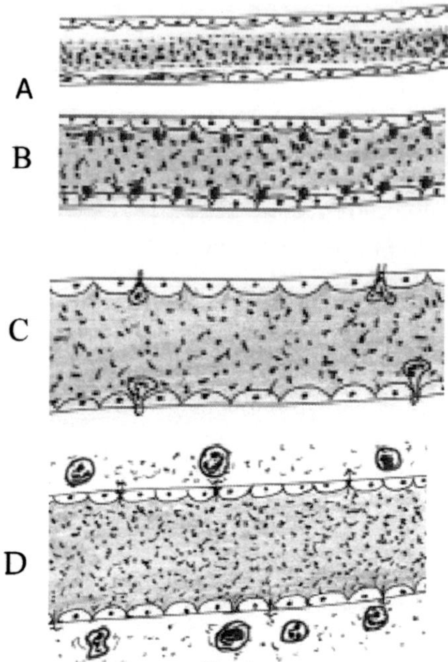

Fig. 6.5: Diagram of blood vessel showing altered blood flow (a) Normal (b) Decreased blood flow (c) Pavementation and (d) increased permeability

Cells in perivascular spaces

Due to pseudopodia movement, leucocytes come out from the dilated blood vessels through intact and swollen endothelium and this process is known as "diapedesis". Cells also come out through break in blood vessel and this process is called as "rhexis" (Fig. 6.6).

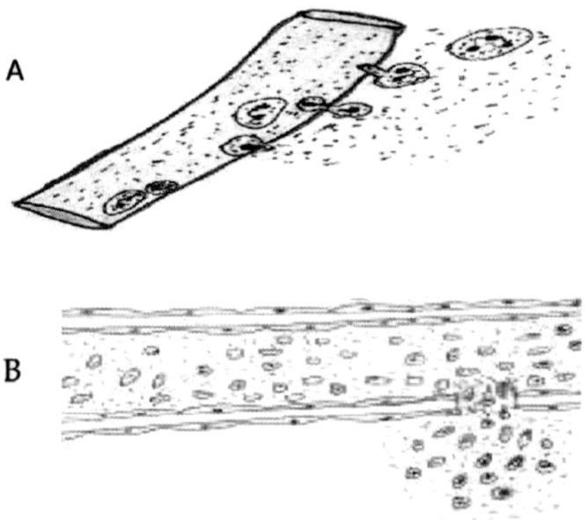

Fig. 6.6: Diagram of blood vessels showing (a) diapedesis and (b) rhexis

Leucocytes degranulate in perivascular tissue spaces

When Leucocytes reach tissue spaces, they release chemical mediators of inflammation, antimicrobial factors in tissues such as cationic proteins, hydrogen peroxide, hydrolytic enzymes, lysozymes, proteases, kinins, histamine, serotonin, heparin, cytokines, and complement (Fig. 6.7).

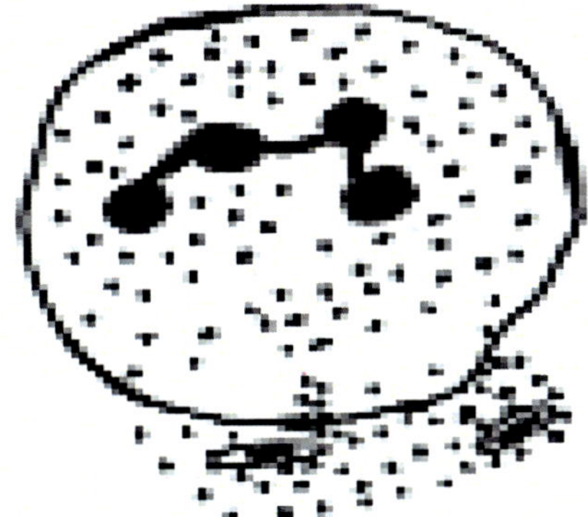

Fig. 6.7: Diagram of polymorphonuclear cell showing degranulation

Irritant is removed and damaged tissue healed By the process of inflammation irritant is neutralized/removed or killed. Fluids are absorbed through lymphatics and debris is removed by phagocytosis. Blood vessel becomes normal. If the irritant is strong and not normally removed by the inflammatory process, it remains at the site and gets covered by inflammatory cells and after some time by fibrous cells in order to localize the irritant. e.g. granuloma.

Vascular Changes

In inflammation, there is transient vasoconstriction followed by vasodilation increased capillary permeability and decrease in blood flow. Circulatory changes are more pronounced in acute inflammation (Figs. 6.8 to 6.11).

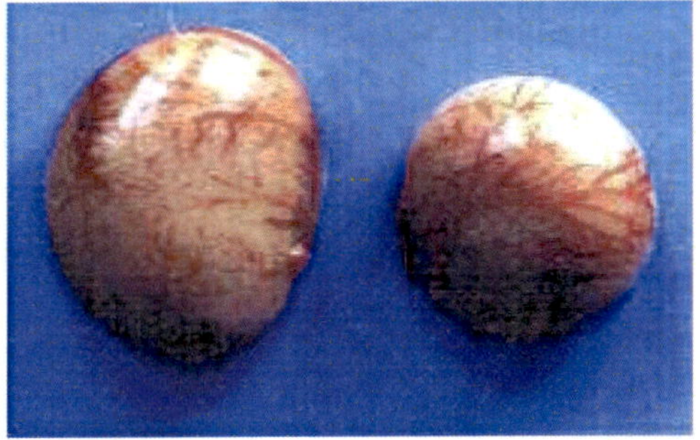

Fig. 6.8: Photograph of testicles showing congestion

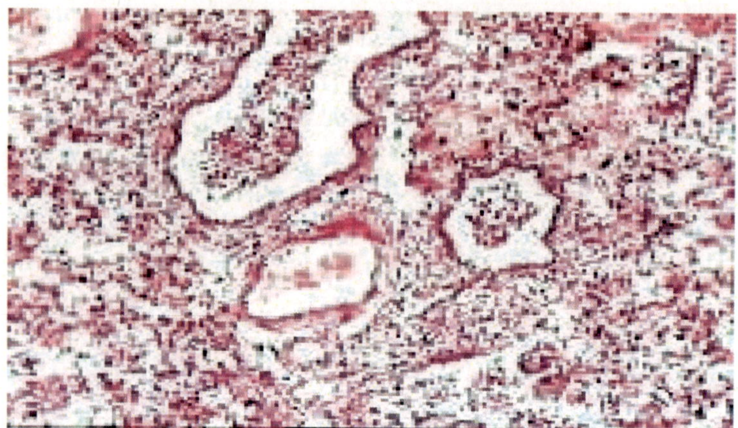

Fig. 6.9: Photomicrograph of lung showing acute inflammation

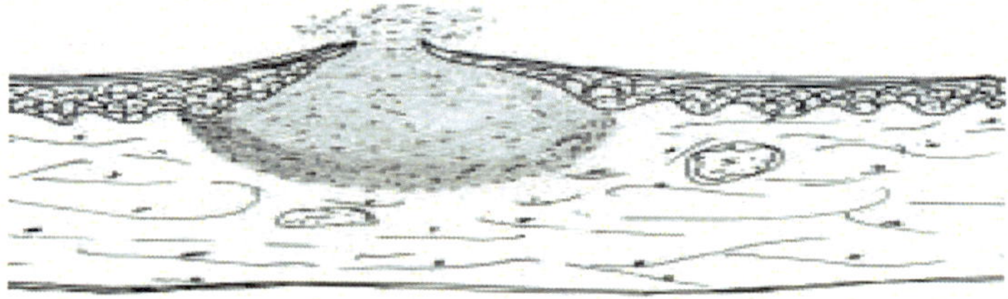

Fig. 6.10: Diagram of an abscess

Etiology

- Any irritant/ injury causing inflammation.

Macroscopic features

- Congestion of the affected organ/tissue.
- Oedema.
- Haemorrhage.

Microscopic features

- Congestion of blood vessels.
- Oedema, presence of fibrin net work.
- Infiltration of leucocytes such as neutrophils, lymphocytes, macrophages, eosinophils etc.

Cellular Changes

In inflammation, there is infiltration of leucocytes in the inflammed area in order to provide defense to the body and to kill or neutralize the etiological factors.

Etiology/ Occurrence

- Any irritant/ injury causing inflammation.

Macroscopic features

- Formation of pus/ abscess if there is increased number of neutrophils in the inflammed area.
- Area becomes hard, painful, with swelling/ nodule.

Microscopic features

- Presence of leucocytes in the inflammation area.
- Presence of the type of cell may also determine the type of inflammation.

Cells of inflammation are polymorphonuclear cells, lymphocytes, macrophages, eosinophils, mast cells, plasma cells, giant cells, etc.

Polymorphonuclear cells

They are also known as neutrophils (mammals) and heterophils (birds). Size of these cells vary from 10μ to 20μ. They are attracted by certain chemotactic factors like bacterial proteins, C_3a, C_5a, fibrinolysin and kinins. These cells are produced in bone marrow and are short life of only 2-3 days. Mature cells have multilobed nucleus and two types of granules. Primary granules are the azurophilic granules present in lysosomes containing acid hydrolases, myeloperoxidases and neuraminidases. Secondary or specific granules have lactoferin and lysozymes. These cells degranulate through Fc receptor, binding with non-specific immune complexes or opsonins (Fig. 6.12).

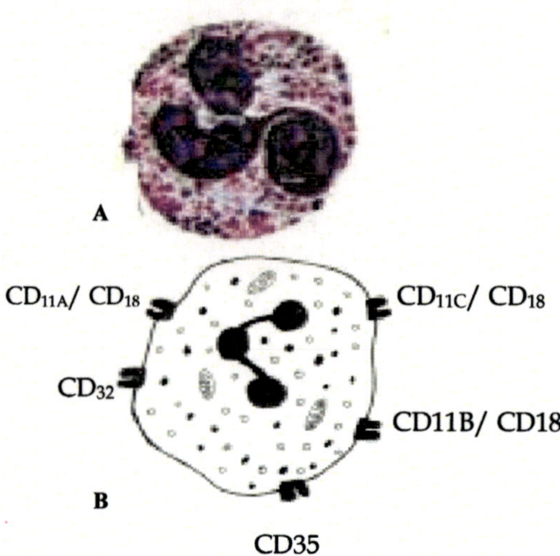

Fig. 6.12: A. Photomicrograph of polymorpho-nuclear cell **B.** diagram of polymorphonuclear cell showing different receptors

Lymphocytes

Lymphocytes are produced in primary lymphoid organs like thymus, bursa of Fabricious and bone marrow and their maturation takes place in secondary lymphoid organs like spleen, lymphnodes, tonsils, and mucosa associated lymphoid tissue etc. These cells may survive for years and in some cases for whole life of an animal. There are two types of lymphocytes seen on light microscopy i.e. small and large. Small lymphocytes are mainly T-helper or T-cytotoxic cells having nuclear cytoplasm ratio (N:C). The larger lymphocytes have low N:C ratio and are mainly B cells and NK cells. There are large numbers of molecules present on cell surface of lymphocytes which are used to distinguish the type of cells. These are known as markers and are identified by a set of monoclonal antibodies and are termed as Cluster of Differentiation (CD system of classification) e.g. CD_4 T-helper cells, CD_8 T-cytotoxic cell, CD_2 and CD_5 Pan-cell marker and CD_7 NK cells.

B-lymphocytes are characterized on the basis of presence of mature immunoglobulins (IgG, IgA, IgM, IgE, IgD) on their surface. They comprise only 5-15% of total peripheral blood lymphocytes. The B-cells having IgM, IgG, IgD are present in blood while IgA-bearing B-lymphocytes are present in large numbers on mucosal surfaces. The B-lymphocytes can be further divided into B_1 and B_2; B_1 are present predominantly in peritoneal cavity and are predisposed for autoantibody production while B_2-cells are conventional antibody-producing cells (Fig. 6.13).

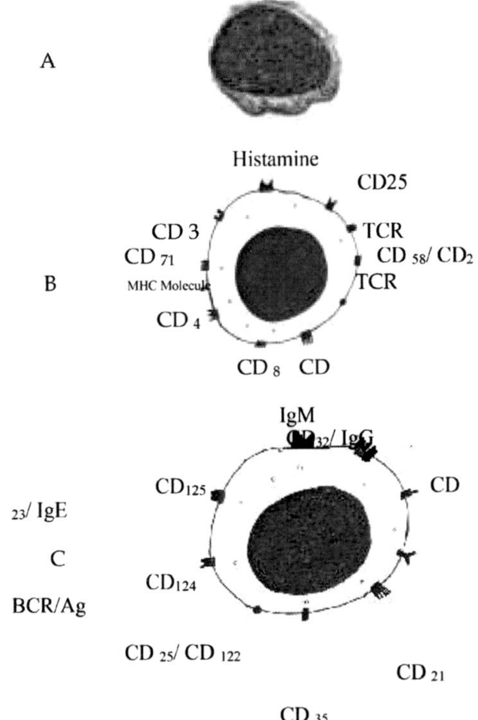

Fig. 6.13: A. Photomicrograph of lymphocyte, **B.** Diagram of T-lymphocyte and **C.** B-lymphocyte showing different receptors.

Natural Killer (N.K.) cells are also present in 10-15% of total peripheral blood lymphocytes. These are defined as the lymphocytes which do not have any conventional surface antigen receptor i.e. TCR or immunoglobulin. In other words, they are neither T nor B cells. The NK cells do not have CD_3 molecule but CD_{16} and CD_{56} are present on their surface. These cells may kill tumor cells, virus containing cells and targets coated by IgG non specifically. They excrete gamma interferon interleukin 1 and GM- CSF.

Macrophages

The mononuclear macrophages are the main phagocytic and antigen presenting cells which develop from bone marrow stem cells and may survive in body till life. The professional phagocytic cells destroy the particulate material while antigen presenting cells (APC) present the processed antigen to the lymphocytes. They have horseshoe shaped nucleus and azurophilic granules. They have a well developed Golgi apparatus and many intracytoplasmic lysosomes which contain peroxidases and hydrolases for intracellular killing of microorganism.

Macrophages have a tendency to adhere to glass or plastic surface and are able to phagocyte the bacteria and tumor cells through specialized receptors. These cells also have CD_{14} receptors for lipopolysaccharide (LPS) binding protein normally present in serum and may coat on Gram negative bacteria. There are CD_{64} receptor for binding of Fc portion of IgG responsible for opsonization, extracellular killing and phagocytosis. Antigen presenting cells (APC) are associated with immunostimulation, induction of T-helper cell activity and communication with other leucocytes. Some endothelial and epithelial cells may, under certain circumstances, also acquire the properties of APC when stimulated by cytokines. They are found in skin, lymphnodes, spleen and thymus (Fig. 6.14).

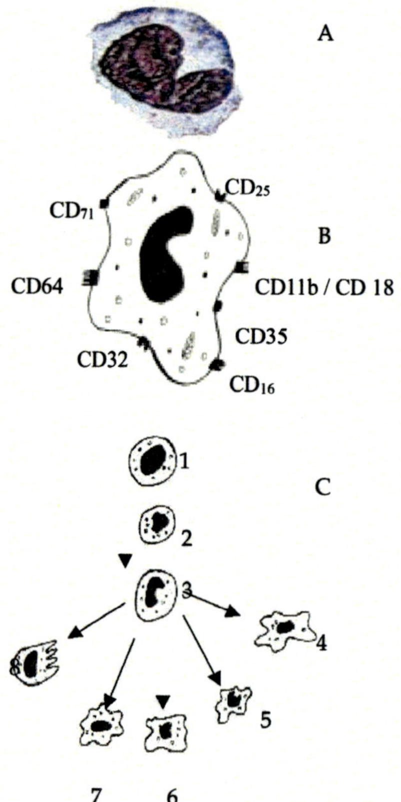

Fig. 6.14. A. Photomicrograph of macrophage/ monocyte **B.** Diagram of macrophage showing different receptors and **C.** Diagram showing different stages and types of phagocytic cells: **1.** Stem cell **2.** Promonocyte **3.** Monocyte **4.** Microglia in brain **5.** Histiocyte in connective tissue **6.** Kupffer cell in liver **7.** Alveolar macrophages and **8.** Oosteoclasts in bone

Eosinophils

Eosinophils comprise 2-5% of total leucocyte count in peripheral blood. They are responsible for killing of large objects which cannot be phagocytosed such as parasites. However, they may also act as phagocytic cells for killing bacteria but it is not their primary function. These cells have bilobed nucleus and eosinophilic granules. The granules are membrane-bound with crystalloid core. These granules are rich in major basic protein which also releases histaminase and aryl sulfatase and leucocyte migration inhibition factor (Fig. 6.15).

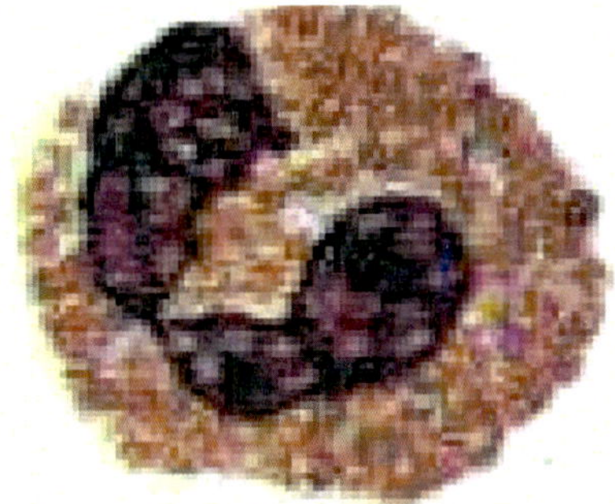

Fig. 6.15: Photomicrograph of eosinophil

Mast cells/ Basophils

There are 0.2% basophils in peripheral blood which have deep violet blue coloured granules. The tissue basophils are known as mast cells. They are of two types, mucosal mast cells and connective tissue mast cells. Basophilic granules present in these cells are rich in heparin, SRS-A and ECF-A. When any antigen or allergen comes into contact with cells, it crosses links with IgE bound on the surface of mast cells and stimulates the cells to degranulate and release histamine which plays an active role in allergy (Fig. 6.16).

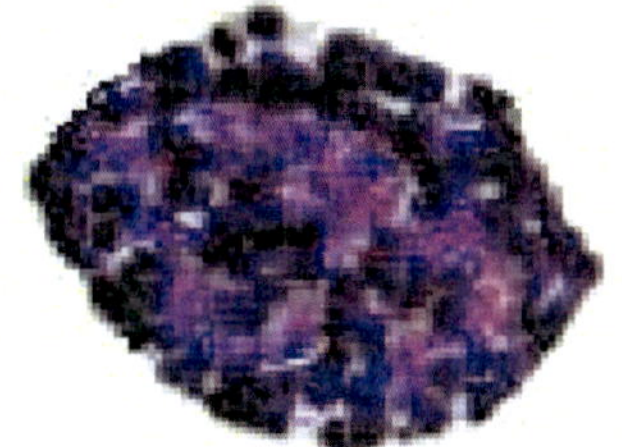

Fig. 6.16: Photomicrograph of Basophil

Platelets

Platelets are derived from bone marrow and contain granules. These cells help in clotting of blood and are involved in inflammation. When endothelial surface gets damaged, platelets adhere and aggregate on damaged endothelium and release substances to increase permeability, attract leucocytes and activate complement.

Plasma cells

The plasma cells are modified B-lymphocytes meant for production of immunoglobulins. Plasma cells have smooth spherical or elliptical shape with increased cytoplasm and eccentrically placed cart wheel-shaped nucleus. The cytoplasm stains slightly basophilic and gives a magenta shade of purplish red. In the cytoplasm, there is a distinct hyaline homogenous mass called Russell body which lies on the cisternae of the endoplasmic reticulum. This is the accumulation of immunoglobulin produced by these cells. Such cells are present in almost all types of inflammation (Figs. 6.17 & 6.18).

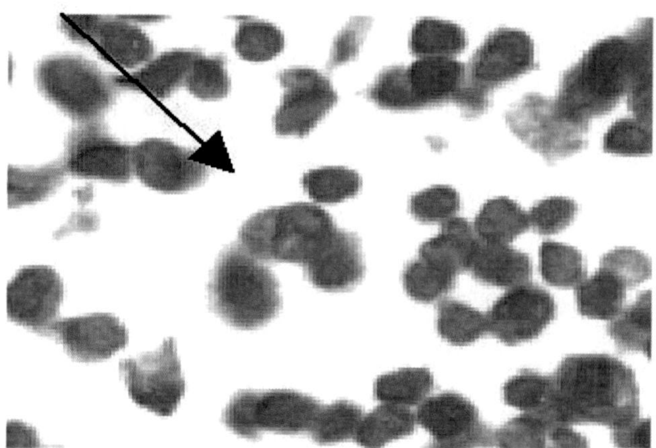

Fig. 6.17: Photomicrograph of Plasma cells

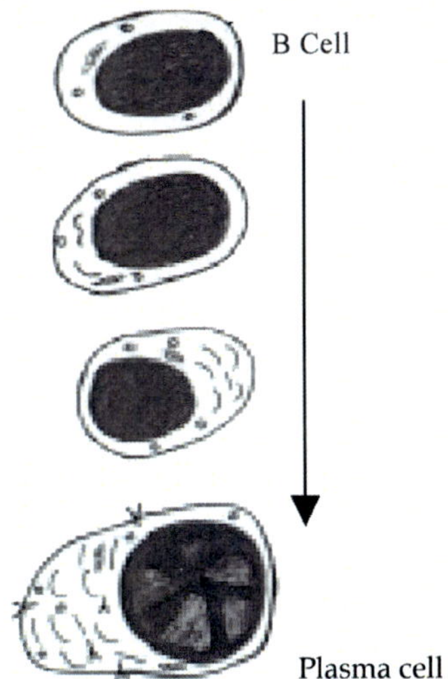

Fig. 6.18: Diagram of Plasma cells

Epithelioid cells

They are the activated macrophages mostly present in granuloma when macrophages become large and foamy due to accumulation of phagocytosed material (bacteria) and degenerated tissue debris. These cells are considered as hallmark of granulomatous inflammation. They are elongated with marginal nucleus that looks like columnar epithelial cell and hence the name "Epithelioid" cells (Fig. 6.19).

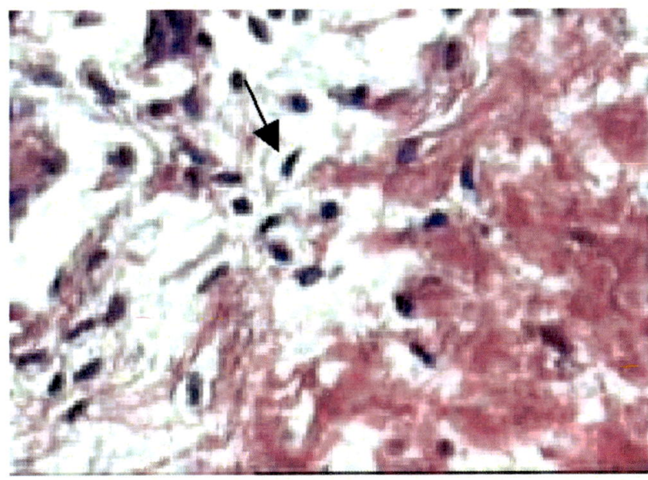

Fig. 6.19: Photomicrograph of epithelioid cells

Giant cells

The giant cells are multinucleated macrophages fused together to kill the microorganisms. They are formed by the fusion of many macrophages to phagocytose larger particles such as yeast, fungi and mycobacteria. They have usually more than one nucleus and abundant cytoplasm. Such cells are formed when macrophages fail to phagocytose the particulate material. They are of several types as listed blow (Figs. 6.20 & 6.21).

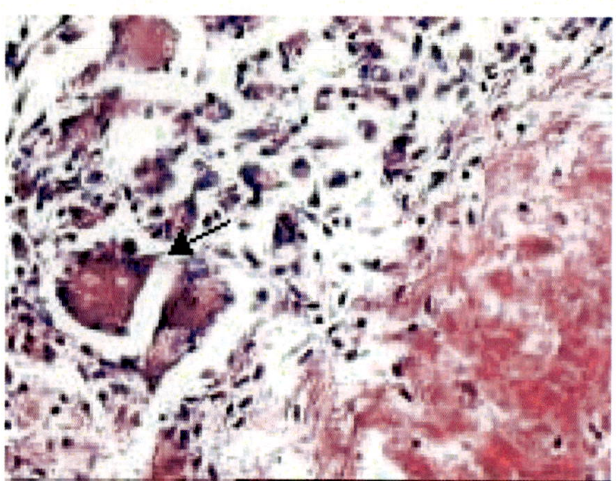

Fig. 6.20. Photomicrograph of giant cell

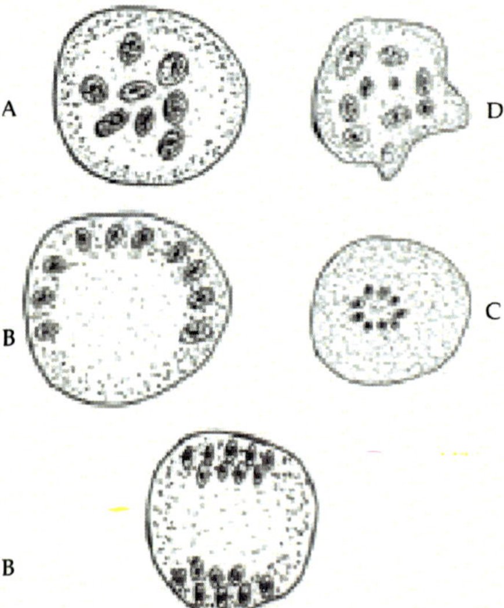

Fig. 6.21 Diagram of giant cells: **A.** foreign body **B.** Langhan's **C.** Touton, and **D.** Tumor giant cell

Foreign body giant cells: They have many nuclei, upto 100, which are uniform in size and shape and resemble the macrophage nucleus. The nuclei are scattered in the cytoplasm. Such cells are seen in chronic infectious granulomas of tuberculosis.

Langhan's giant cells: They are horseshoe shaped giant cells having many nuclei and are characteristically present in tubercle. The nuclei resemble that of macrophages and epithelioid cells. The nuclei are mostly arranged at periphery giving horseshoe shape.

Touton giant cells: They are multinucleated cells having vacuolation in the cytoplasm due to increased lipid content. They mostly occur in xanthoma.

Tumor giant cells: These are larger, pleomorphic and hyperchromatic cells having numerous nuclei with different size and shape. Nuclei of such cells do not resemble that of macrophages or epithelioid cells. They are not true giant cells and not formed from macrophages but are found in cancers as a result of fast division of nuclei in comparison to cytoplasm.

Fibroblasts

Fibroblast proliferates to replace its own tissue and others which are not able to regenerate. The new fibroblasts originate from fibrocyte as well as from the fibroblasts through mitotic division. Collagen fibres begin to appear on 6th day as an amorphous ground substance or matrix. They are characteristic of chronic inflammation and repair. Fibroblasts are elongated cells having long nuclei, sometimes looking like the smooth muscle fibres. The proliferation of fibroblasts is extremely active in neonates and slow and delayed in old animals. The fibroplasia can be enhanced by removal of necrosed tissue debris and by fever (Fig. 6.22 & 6.23).

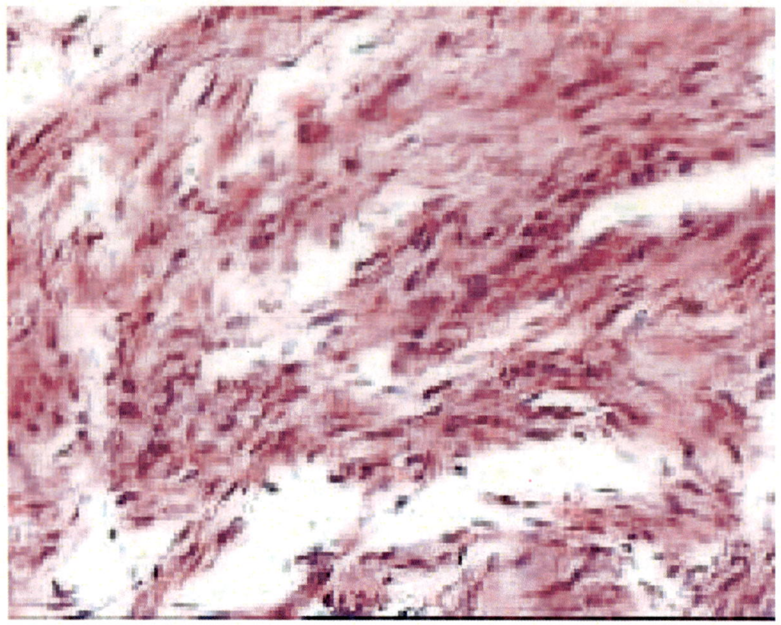

Fig. 6.22. Photomicrograph showing proliferation of fibroblasts

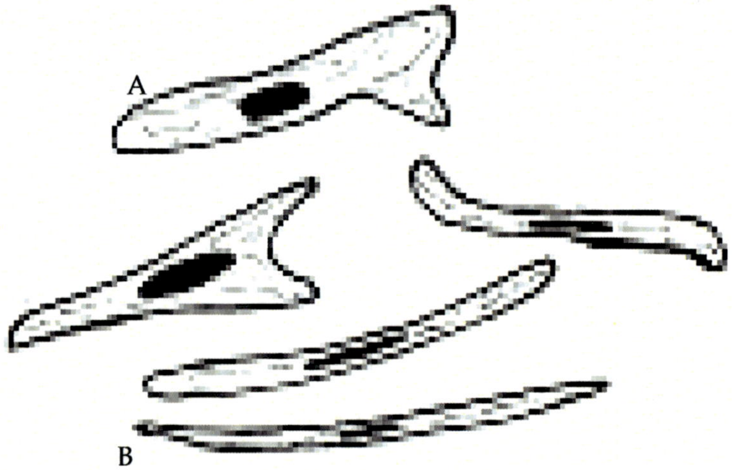

Fig. 6.23. Diagram of **A.** fibroblasts and **B.** fibrocytes

Chemical Changes

There is a long list of chemical mediators responsible for acute inflammation. These are endogenous biochemical compounds, which can increase the vascular permeability, vasodilation, chemotaxis, fever, pain and cause tissue damage. Such chemical mediators are released by cells, plasma or damaged tissue and are broadly classified as: cell and plasma derived chemical mediators of inflammation.

Cell Derived Mediators

Vasoactive amines

Histamine

Histamine is found in basophilic granules of mast cells or basophils and in platelets. It is released through stimuli due to heat, cold, irradiation, trauma, irritant, chemical and immunological reactions and anaphylotoxins C3a, C5a and C4a. Histamine is also released due to action of histamine releasing factors from neutrophils, monocytes and platelets. It acts on blood vessels and causes vasodilation, increased vascular permeability, itching and pain.

Serotonin (5-Hydroxy-tryptamine)

It is present in tissues of gastrointestinal tract, spleen, nervous tissue, mast cells and platelets. It also acts on blood vessels to cause vasodilation and increased permeability but its action is mild in comparison to histamine.

Arachidonic acid metabolites

Arachidonic acid is a fatty acid, which either comes directly from the diet or through conversion of linoleic acid to arachidonic acid. Arachidonic acid is activated by C5a to form its metabolites through either cyclo-oxygenase or lipo-oxygenase pathways. Cyclo-oxygenase is a fatty acid enzyme which acts on arachidonic acid to form prostaglandin endoperoxidase (PGG) which is further transformed into prostaglandins like PGD_2, PGE_2 PGF_2; thromboxane A_2 (Tx A_2) and prostacyclin (PGI_2). Prostaglandins act on blood vessels to cause vasodilation, increased permeability bronchodilation except $PGF_2\alpha$, which is responsible for vasodilation and bronchoconstriction. Thromboxane A_2 is a vasoconstrictor, bronchoconstrictor, and causes aggregation of platelets leading of increased function of inflammatory cells. Prostacylin is found to be responsible for vasodilation, bronchodilation and inhibitory action on platelet aggregation.

Lipo-oxygnese acts on arachidonic acid to form hydroperoxy eico-satetraenoic acid (5HPETE) which is further converted into 5HETE, a chemotactic agent for neutrophils and leucotrienes (LT) or slow reacting substance of anaphylaxis (SRS-A). The leucotrienes include an unstable form leucotriene

A (LTA), which is soon converted into leucotriene B (LTB), a chemotactic and adherence factor for phagocytic cells, and leucotriene C, D and E (LTC, LTD, LTE) causing contraction of smooth muscles leading to vasoconstriction, bronchoconstriction and increased vascular permeability.

Lysosomal components

Lysosomal granules are released by neutrophils and macrophages to cause degradation of bacterial and extracellular components, chemotaxis and increased vascular permeability. These lysosomal granules are rich in acid proteases, collagenases, elastases and plasminogen activator.

Platelet activating factor (PAF)

Platelet activating factor (PAF) is released from IgE sensitized mast cells, endothelial cells and platelets. It acts on platelets for their aggregation and release, chemotaxis, bronchoconstriction, adherance of leucocytes and increased vascular permeability. In low amount PAF causes vasodilation while in high concentration it leads to vasoconstriction.

Cytokines

Cytokines are hormone-like substances produced by activated lymphocytes (Lymphokines) and monocytes (Monokines). These are glycoprotein in nature with low molecular weight (8-75KD) and are composed of single chain. They differ from hormones which are specifically produced by endocrine glands to maintain homeostasis through endocrine action as cytokines are produced by many different cell types and act on different cells of body with very high functional activity. They cause autocrine, paracrine and endocrine action leading to tissue repair and resistance to infection. Cytokines are broadly classified as interleukins, interferon, cytotoxins and growth factors.

Multicellular organisms have developed defense mechanisms to maintain an internal environment conducive to cell proliferation & proper functioning. However, this environment also encourages growth of foreign cells & also uncontrolled proliferation of abnormal cells. Therefore, it is crucial to have systems in place to eliminate these invaders, abnormal cells, or toxins once they have invaded the protective barriers of the body. In vertebrates, the immune system, including T- & B-lymphocytes, mononuclear & polymorphonuclear phagocytes, & phagocytic cells, plays a crucial role in eliminating infections. The phagocytic cells kill the invaders extracellularly, while B-lymphocyte secrete antibodies which aid in phagocytosis. Antibodies trigger cell lysis by activating proteins, creating pores in infected cell membranes, & lysing cells with Cytotoxic Lymphocytes & Natural Killer (NK).

1. The immune system must meet specific conditions to function effectively.
2. The immune system must be able to differentiate between foreign & self-component. The antigen receptors of B- & T-lymphocytes are highly specific & are enormously diverse. They allow distinguishment of more than 10^8 different antigenic structures. B-lymphocytes secrete antibodies that tag antigen-expressing particles or cells for phagocytes, killer cells, or complement system activation. T-cell receptor molecules specifically restrict interaction with target cells, preventing the development of lymphocytes with antigen receptors that react against body components. This prevents the development of self reacting lymphocytes.

In the event of an infection or abnormality the immune system needs to recruit, activate, & cause proliferation of cells in order to defend the body. Also the response needs to stop after the infection is eradicated so that the repair mechanisms take control.

The defense processes are highly dependent on intercellular mediators, with cytokines being a major constituent. They facilitate the access of immune cells to the infection site & the elimination of debris. The term "Cytokine" is derived from the Greek words "Cyto" meaning "Cell" & "Kinin" meaning "hormones". Included under the term "Cytokines" are the Colony-Stimulating Factors, Interleukins, Monokines, & Lymphokines (CSFs), Tumor Necrosis Factor (TNF), Interferons (IFNs), & Chemokines.

1. Cytokines are glycopeptide or polypeptide signaling molecules with molecular weight ranging from from 5 to 70,000 Daltons. Initially the term "Lymphokines", coined by Dumonde in 1969 was used as at the beginning they were thought to be produced by lymphocytes only; however, it soon became evident that apart from lymphocytes other leukocytes as well as cells of non-hematopoietic origin, virtually all nucleated cells are capable of secreting them. They facilitate communication between cells & the external environment, act as mediators of immune as well as inflammatory reactions. Cytokines are key factors in determining health because they dynamically regulate immune cell development, proliferation, & response. Different cell types can emit a single cytokine, which can then operate on various cell types to produce a variety of biological functions. Variations in the concentrations of cytokines in different bodily fluids, including blood, serum, feces, saliva, & perspiration, can be very useful in determining the diagnosis, stage, & prognosis of different illnesses. Like traditional hormones, cytokines act through target cell receptor thereby altering the

cell functions. But cytokines differ from traditional hormones & lastly, a fundamental aspect of cytokine biology is that every cytokine has a variety of effects on a variety of tissues & acts reciprocally to either enhance or reduce the production of other cytokines that have opposite or comparable effects.

2. A traditional hormone is released from a single cell type but the same cytokine can be released from several cell types.
3. Most cytokines function locally in the region of their synthesis, either by binding to & affecting a nearby cell (paracrine action) or by affecting the same cell that produced them (autocrine action), in contrast to most traditional hormones, which act on distant tissues (endocrine action). Although certain cytokines may function peripherally, following a traditional endocrine pattern.
4. Although cytokine levels may rise sharply in response to an infection or trauma, the circulating concentrations are normally relatively low (in the picomolar range). The majority of traditional hormones, on the other hand, have a resting concentration that is 1,000 times greater (nanomolar range).

Cytokines also play an important role in Cancer Immunotherapy. In preclinical mouse cancer models, cytokines that regulate the immune response have been demonstrated to be effective. Treatments authorized for hairy cell leukemia include interferon (IFN)-α & interleukin (IL)-2, which are used to treat metastatic renal cancer & advanced melanoma, respectively. Clinical studies have also been conducted to assess IL-12, IL-15, IL-21, & granulocyte macrophage colony-stimulating factor (GM-CSF). Clinical trials are being conducted on cytokines in conjunction with checkpoint inhibitors, anticancer monoclonal antibodies to boost the antigen-dependent cellular cytotoxicity (ADCC) of these antibodies, anti-CD40 to promote tumor-specific immune responses. Although cytokines act in conjunction with the immune system to protect the body but in certain cases like in some infections, autoimmune diseases & in various malignancies, hereditary conditions, as well as due to certain medical treatments the body may develop potentially fatal systemic inflammatory syndrome caused by massive release of cytokines. Cytokines Release Syndrome (CRS) is a condition characterized by the excessive release of cytokines due to immune cell activation, leading to a dysregulated inflammatory response that can be life-threatening to the host. It is associated with various diseases & therapies including Anaphylaxis, Acute Respiratory Distress Syndrome (ARDS), Systemic Inflammatory Response Syndrome

(SIRS), Chimeric Antigen Receptor-T (CAR-T) Cell Therapy & Sepsis, which accounts for up to 19.7% of all deaths worldwide. Organ failure & death may result from abnormal or elevated cytokine production, such as during a cytokine storm. For example, the poor prognosis of critical Corona Virus Disease 2019 (COVID-19) patients was caused by "Cytokine Storm Syndrome." Circulating Cytokine levels act as a crucial marker in clinical medicine.

Properties of Cytokines

1. Pleiotropic. It is the ability of a single cytokine to affect many cell types. For instance, IL-2, which was first identified as a T-cell growth factor, also influences the proliferation & differentiation of B-cells & natural killer (NK) cells.
2. Redundancy. Distinct cytokines can trigger the same activity. For example, TNF-α & IL-1 both function as mediators of inflammation.
3. Multifunctionality which refers to the possibility that a single cytokine can control many immunological processes.
4. Cytokines may act either by Autocrine, Endocrine or Paracrine mode of action.

Classification of Cytokines

Cytokines are proteins that can be classified into various categories, including TNFs, ILs, lymphokines, monokines, IFNs, CSFs, & TGFs. Cytokines may also be classified as pro-inflammatory or anti-inflammatory. Pro-inflammatory cytokines stimulate inflammatory reactions & stimulate immunocompetent cells, while Anti-Inflammatory cytokines inhibit inflammation & suppress immune cells. Pro-inflammatory cytokines include interferons, IL-1β, IL-6, IL-8, IL-12, & TNF-α while Anti-Inflammatory cytokines Conversely include TGF-β, IL-4, IL-6, IL-10, IL-11, IL-13, & IL-1 receptor antagonist (IL-1RA). Both Pro- & Anti-Inflammatory characteristics may be seen in some cytokines, such IL-6.

Mechanism of Action

Cytokines attach to the external cell receptors of the target cells. Tyrosine kinase, an intracellular protein kinase, is activated by the cytokine receptor complex. This, in turn, causes the phosphorylation (& activation) of several other intracellular kinases. The majority of cytokines cause DNA transcription to begin in the target cell by activating these related kinases, which sets off a series of processes that eventually lead to a transcription protein entering the nucleus & binding to a particular DNA regulatory site. Protein synthesis of the particular proteins that mediate the response of that cytokine occurs. These cytokines are large molecules hence they are unable to cross the blood-brain barrier. It has been suggested that enter the central nervous system at sites where the blood-brain barrier is missing. Another hypothesis suggests that peripheral cytokines produce neurotransmitters or small active molecules in blood vessels supplying the brain, which then diffuse into the brain & exert significant effects. Peripherally produced cytokines, particularly IL-1, stimulate regional peripheral nerves, such as the vagus, which carry the message of infection & inflammation to the central nervous system. This signal is then hypothesized to stimulate the release of central interleukins, initiating systemic responses such as fever, fatigue, & anorexia.

Cytokines in Inflammation

Inflammation is a complex biological response well regulated by cytokines, & imbalances between tissue homeostasis & inflammatory cytokines, along with unregulated Pro- & Anti-Inflammatory cytokine levels can lead to significant negative health impacts. Inflammation is caused by Parenchymal & Stromal cells within a tissue or organ in addition to immune cells like Neutrophils, Macrophages, B & T-Lymphocytes etc. The main mediators of inflammation are cytokines, which are secreted by one cell & recognized by other cells that exhibit the relevant receptors. In response cytokines trigger distinctive & intricate signaling cascades that result in an appropriate cellular response, such as cell division, proliferation, or the release of enzymes & other mediators that regulate the cellular environment & offer ways to prolong the effects of cytokines. Certain cytokines, known as the Pro-Inflammatory cytokines, are known to openly stimulate inflammation, whereas other cytokines, known as Anti-Inflammatory cytokines, work to inhibit the effects of proinflammatory cytokines. For instance, B lymphocytes may be effectively activated by IL-4, IL-10, & IL-13. But IL-4, IL-10, & IL-13 are also very effective anti-inflammatory drugs. Because they can inhibit the genes that produce pro-inflammatory cytokines including TNF, IL-1, & chemokines, they are anti-inflammatory cytokines.

Pro-Inflammatory Cytokines

The inflammatory response is primarily controlled by cytokines, which initiate an acute phase response to protect the host from irritation, injury, & infection. These pro-inflammatory cytokines, such as IL-1β, IL-6, IL-8, IL-12, IFN-γ, & TNF-α, communicate to surrounding tissues about infection or injury, & can enter the systemic circulation, leading to immune cell activation

& significant host physiology changes like fever & acute-phase reaction. Pro-inflammatory cytokines include the chemokines which facilitate the passage of leukocytes from circulation into tissues. The principal chemokine is the Neutrophil Chemoattractant IL-8, which activates neutrophils to degranulate & cause tissue damage. IL-1 & TNF induce endothelial adhesion molecules, essential for leukocyte adhesion to the endothelial surface. Proinflammatory cytokine-mediated inflammation is a cascade of gene products usually not produced in healthy individuals. Cytokines IL-1 & TNF stimulate the expression of these genes, acting synergistically. These cytokines initiate the cascade of inflammatory mediators by targeting the endothelium, whether induced by infection, trauma, ischemia, immune-activated T cells, or toxins. Pro-inflammatory cytokines, released from macrophages, have immune properties that can protect the host against bacteria & other microorganisms in the environment or the skin & intestinal tract. Macrophages are the first line of defense against bacterial infections, triggering adaptive immune responses. They release pro-inflammatory cytokines like IL-1, IL-6, IL-8, IL-12, IL-18, IFN-α/γ, & TNF-α, which induce inflammatory activity in macrophages. IL-1 has direct cytostatic & cytocidal effects, IL-6 is a major mediator for immune & inflammatory responses, IL-12 enhances T-cell responsiveness, & IFNs mediate host protection against viral infection. These cytokines are coordinatedly released from activated macrophages and modulate the immune response to protect the host.

Excessive pro-inflammatory responses can cause chronic inflammation, disrupting biological homeostasis, leading to health issues like cancer, diabetes, cardiovascular, gastrointestinal, Parkinson's, & aging-related diseases. Pro-inflammatory interferons are crucial in the pathogenesis of autoimmune diseases. Pro-inflammatory cytokines like IL-1, IFN-γ, & TNF-α also stimulate tumor growth & metastasis. These cytokines also induce adhesion molecules & metalloproteinases, enabling tumor invasion. Regulating these excessive pro-inflammatory responses is crucial to prevent pathological states due to abnormal immune mediator expression.

Anti-Inflammatory Cytokines

Anti-Inflammatory cytokines include IL-1, IL-4, IL-6, IL-10, IL-11, IL-13, & TGF-β, are immunoregulatory molecules that suppress the excessive inflammatory response of pro-inflammatory cytokines. IL-10, a potent anti-inflammatory cytokine, inhibits pro-inflammatory cytokine production & has anti-inflammatory effects on eosinophils, basophils, & mast cells thereby playing a crucial role in allergy & asthma control. Other Anti-inflammatory cytokines such as IL-4, IL-10, IL-13, & TGF-B suppress the production of pro-inflammatory cytokines like IL-1, TNF, chemokines like IL-8, & vascular adhesion molecules. Except for interleukin (IL)-1 Receptor Antagonist (IL-1ra), which may be an exception, all anti-inflammatory cytokines also have some proinflammatory characteristics as well. Anti-inflammatory cytokines can inhibit the synthesis of proinflammatory cytokines like IL-1 & TNF. CD41 T helper lymphocytes can differentiate into two types: Th1- & Th2-type cells, based on the cytokines produced. CD81 cytotoxic T cells also have a similar functional system. Th1-type cells secrete high levels of cytokines like IL-2, TNF-a, & IFN-g, activating macrophages & promoting cell-mediated immune responses against invasive pathogens. Th2-type cells produce anti-inflammatory cytokines like IL-4, IL-5, IL-6, IL-10, & IL-13, promoting humoral immune responses against extracellular pathogens. Mutual cross-inhibition between Th1- & Th2-type cytokines polarizes functional Th cell responses into cell-mediated or humoral immune responses. Regulation of T-cell activation by anti-inflammatory cytokines is a crucial early control element in this process.

Cytokines Elevated in Various Types of Inflammation

1. Inflammation Induced by Lack of Blood

Tumor necrosis factor-α (TNF-α), interleukin-1β (IL-1β), & IL-6 will all rise in response to inflammation brought on by a blood clot, such as an ischemic stroke. The cytokines Interferon-γ, TNF-α, & IL-1β will all rise as a result of atherosclerotic inflammation. The cytokines IL-1β, TNF-α, & IL-6 rise in response to myocardial infarction, or a heart attack.

2. Inflammation Due to an Immunological Disorder

Generalised immune mediated inflammation results in an increase in TNF-α, IL-6, IL-8, & IL-12 cytokines. Type 2 Diabetes & other insulin resistance-related inflammation cause increased levels of interferon-γ, IL-1β, TNF-α, IL-6, IL-8, & IL-12. Systemic Lupus Erythematosus-related inflammation cause increased levels of TNF-α, IL-6, Interferon-α & -γ, as well as a number of other cytokines. Osteoarthritis-related inflammation will increase levels of TNF-α, IL-6, IL-8, & numerous other cytokines. Rheumatoid arthritis-related inflammation will increase levels of IL-1β, TNF-α, IL-6, IL-12, & a number of other cytokines.

3. Inflammation Caused By Cancer

Colon cancer, especially colitis-associated malignancy induces inflammation & increases the levels of cytokines such as interferon-α, IL-1β, TNF-α, IL-6, & IL-8. Lung cancer-induced inflammation raises levels of TNF-α, IL-6, IL-8, interferon-γ, & a number of other cytokines. Inflammation due to stomach cancer increases the levels of IL-1β, TNF-α, IL-6, IL-8, & numerous more. Breast cancer-induced inflammation raises levels of TNF-α, IL-1β, IL-6, IL-8, & a number of other cytokines. The cytokines IL-1β, TNF-α, IL-6, IL-8, IL-12, & others rise in response to an oesophageal cancer, whereas interferon-γ will decrease.

4. Inflammation Caused by an Infectious Agent

The inflammatory cytokines IL-1β, TNF-α, IL-6, & IL-8 will all rise in response to a bacterial infection. Fungal infections induce inflammation that is characterized by increased levels of TNF-α, IL-6, IL-8, & interferon-γ. The following cytokines will be elevated during a viral infection: Interferon-α, Interferon-γ, IL-1β, TNF-α, IL-6, IL-8, IL-12. The presence of a protozoan parasite infection shows marked increase in levels of the cytokines TNF-α & IL-1β.

5. Inflammation Due to A Chemical Agent

The cytokines IL-1β, TNF-α, IL-8, & Interferon-γ rise in an inflammatory response brought on by exposure to polycyclic aromatic hydrocarbons. Exposure to dioxin results in inflammation which increase the levels of TNF-α & IL-1β. Smoke-related inflammation will result in increased levels of TNF-α, IL-6, & IL-8 cytokines while the levels of IL-1β & interferon-γ remain almost normal.

6. Inflammation Due to A Physical Injury

Trauma-induced inflammation will result in elevated levels of IL-6 & IL-8 & decreased levels of IL-12 nevertheless the levels of IL-1β, TNF-α, Interferon-α, & Interferon-γ remain almost normal. The cytokines IL-1β, TNF-α, & Interferon-γ rise in an inflammatory response to a hemorrhagic stroke, & the levels of IL-6 & IL-8 will also rise significantly.

List of Cytokines

Name	Cells of Origin	Functions
IL-1	Monocytes, Macrophages & Dendritic cells	Maturation & Proliferation of B-Cells, Co-Stimulation of T_H Cells, Activation of NK Cells, Induce acute phase reaction in trace amount
IL-2	T_H1 Cells	Growth & Differentiation of T-Cells
IL-3	NK Cells, Activated T_H Cells, Mast Cells, Eosinophils, Endothelial Cells	Differentiation, Proliferation of Myeloid Cells
IL-4	T_H2 Cells, Activated & Memory CD4+ Cells, Macrophages, Mast Cells	Proliferation, Differentiation of B-Cells, Synthesis of IgG1 & IgE, Proliferation of T-Cells
IL-5	T_H2 Cells, Eosinophils & Mast Cells	Differentiation of B-Cells, Production of IgA
IL-6	B-Cells, T_H2 Cells, Macrophages, Endothelial Cells, Astrocytes	Differentiation of B-Cells into Plasma Cells, Antibody Secretion by Plasma Cells, Differentiation of Hematopoietic Stem Cells & T-Cells
IL-7	Stromal Cells of Bone Marrow & Thymus	Differentiation & Proliferation
IL-8	Lymphocytes, Macrophages, Endothelial Cells & Epithelial Cells	Chemotactic for Neutrophils
IL-9	T_H2 Cells, CD4+ Helper T-Cells	Potentiation of IgM, IgE, IgG, Stimulation of Mast Cells
IL-10	T_H2 Cells, CD8+ T-Cells, B-Cell subset, Macrophages, Mast Cells	Cytokine production by Macrophages, Activation of B-Cells, Inhibition of Production of INF-γ, TNF-β, IL-2 by T_H1 Cells, Stimulation of T_H2 Cells
IL-11	Stromal Cells of Bone Marrow	Production of Acute Phase Proteins, Formation of Osteoclasts
IL-12	B-Cells, T-Cells, Macrophages & Dendritic Cells	Along with IL-2 stimulates differentiation of Cytotoxic T-Cells, Increased production of IL-10, INF-γ, TNF-α
IL-13	N-K Cells, Activated T_H2 Cells, Mast Cells	Inhibition of T_H1 Cells, Growth & Differentiation of B-Cells into Effector Cells for IgE Production, Production of Inflammatory Cytokines by Macrophages
IL-14	Some Malignant B-Cells, T-Cells	Controls Growth, Proliferation of B-Cells, Inhibition of Immunoglobulin Production
IL-15	Macrophages, Other Mononuclear Phagocytic Cells, Certain Virus Infected Cells	Proliferation of N-K Cells
IL-16	CD8+ T-Cells, Epithelial Cells, Eosinophils	Chemoattractant for CD4+ T-Cells [14][88]

Name	Cells of Origin	Functions
IL-17	T_H17 Cells	Angiogenesis, Differentiation of Progenitor cells into Osteoclasts, Production of Inflammatory Cytokines
IL-18	Macrophages	Potentiation of N-K Cells, Production of INF-γ
IL-19	Monocytes	Enhances the production of Cytokines by T_H2 Cells. Production of IL-10 by Monocytes. Role in Atopy & Allergy
IL-20	Keratinocytes, Monocytes	Regulation of Proliferation & Differentiation of Keratinocytes
1L-21	N-K Cells, Activated T_H Cells	Co-stimulation, Activation & Proliferation of CD8+ T Cells, Augments Cytotoxic activity of N-K, Augments CD-40 induced B-Cell Proliferation, Differentiation & Isotype Switching, Differentiation of T_H17 Cells
IL-22	T_H17 Cells	Production of Acute Phase Proteins, Activates STAT1 & STAT3
IL-23	Dendritic Cells, Macrophages	Indices Angiogenesis, Reduces CD8T- Cell Infiltration
IL-24	Keratinocytes	Tumor Suppression, Wound Healing, Promotes Cell Survival
IL-25	T_H2 Cells, Mast Cells	Induces production of IL-4, IL-5, IL-13 which stimulates proliferation of Eosinophils
IL-26	Monocytes	Induces Secretion of IL-10, IL-8, Expression of CD-54 on the surface of the cells.
IL27	Antigen Presenting Cells	Regulates activity of B& T-Cells
IL-28		Immune Response against Viruses
IL-29		Host defense against microbes
IL-30		Forms chain of IL-27
IL-31	Activated T-Cells	Role in Inflammatory Response by the Skin
IL-32		Induces secretion of TNF-α, IL-8,CXCL2 by Monocytes & Macrophages
IL-33		Induces Type-2 Cytokine production by T_H2 Cells
IL-34		Growth of Monocytes
IL-35	Regulatory T-Cells	Suppression of activation of T_H Cells
IL-36	Phagocytes	Regulation of INF-γ Synthesis by N-K & T-Cells
IL-37	Phagocytes	Regulate Innate Immunity leading to Immunosuppression
IL-38	Cells of Placenta, Skin, Spleen, Thymus	Inhibition of Synthesis of IL-17 & IL-22
IL-39	B-Lymphocytes	Differentiation & Expansion of Neutrophils
IL-40	Bone Marrow, Fetal Liver, Activated B-Cells	Humoral Immunity

Name	Cells of Origin	Functions
IL-41	Activated Monocytes, Stromal Cells, Mucosa of Respiratory & Digestive Tract, Adipocytes	Level increased in Gout, Regulates the release of IL-4 & IL-13

Interferons

Interferons are glycoproteins having antiviral action and inhibit the virus replication in cells.

These are of five types like alpha (α), beta (β), gamma (γ), omega (ω), and tau (ι).

Table 6.2: Interferons

Sl. No.	Interferon	Source	Action
1.	Interferon alpha (IFN- α)	Lymphocytes, Monocytes, Macrophages	Inhibit viral growth, activates macrophages
2.	Interferon beta (IFN-β)	Fibroblasts	Inhibit viral growth, activates macrophages
3.	Interferon gamma (IFN-γ)	Th-1 cells, Cytotoxic T-cells, NK cells, Macrophages	Stimulates B-cells, production, enhances NK Cells activity activates macrophages and phagocytosis. Promotes antibody-dependent and cell-mediated cytotoxicity.
4.	Interferon Omega	Lymphocytes, Monocytes	Virus infected cells to check viral growth
	(IFN-ω)	Trophoblasts	Activate Macrophages
5.	Interferon tau (IFN- ι)	Trophoblasts	Virus growth, Immunity to faetus through placenta.

Tumor Necrosis Factor or Cytotoxins

Tumor necrosis factor or cytotoxins are produced by macrophages and T-cells and are associated with apoptosis in tumors. Tumor necrosis factor beta (TNF-β) is produced by T-helper 1 cells and activates CD8+ T-cells, neutrophils, macrophages, endothelial cells and B-lymphocytes. Tumor necrosis factor alpha (TFN-α) is produced by macrophages, T- cells, B-cells and fibroblasts and it activates macrophages and enhances immunity and inflammatory reaction.

Chemokines

Chemokines are small proteins divided into two α and β subfamilies. Alpha-chemokines include IL-8, which is produced by fibroblasts, macrophages, endothelial cells, lymphocytes, granulocytes, hepatocytes and keratinocytes. It acts as chemotactic agent for basophils, neutrophils and T-cells. The neutrophils get activated and release their granules and leucotrienes. There is increased respiratory burst. Besides, it also acts on basophils and lymphocytes. Macrophage inflammatory protein MIP-1 of β-chemokines are produced by macrophages, T and B-lymphocytes, mast cells and neutrophils. It acts on monocytes, eosinophils, B and T-lymphocytes. Beta-chemokines include macrophage inflammatory protein (MIP-1), Monocyte chemoattractant protein (MCP) and RANTES protein. The MCP is produced by macrophages, T-cells, fibroblasts, keratinocytes and endothelial cells and activates the monocytes, basophils and some T-cells.

Growth factors

Many cytokines are also known as growth factors which act on cells and stimulate them to proliferate. Thus they play a very important role in inflammation and healing. In nature these are glycoprotein which controls the proliferation and maturation of several blood cells. The growth factors also include interleukin 3, 7, 11, and 15. The granulocyte colony stimulating factor (G-CSF) is produced by fibroblasts, endothelial cells and macrophages. It acts on granulocyte progenitors and regulate their maturation and production of superoxide. Macrophage colony stimulating factors (M-CSF) are the glycoproteins released by lymphocytes, macrophages, fibroblasts, epithelial cells and endothelial cells. They act on monocyte progenitors for their proliferation and differentiation and promote their killing activity.

Granulocyte macrophage colony stimulating factor (GM-CSF) is released from macrophages, T-lymphocytes, endothelial cells and fibroblasts and facilitates phagocytosis, antibody dependent cell cytotoxicity (ADCC) and superoxide production. It activates eosinophils to enhance superoxide production and macrophages for increased phagocytosis and tumoricidal activity. Transforming growth factor (TGF) are five related proteins (TGF-B_1, B_2, B_3 in mammals; B_4 and B_5 in poultry) released from neutrophils, macrophages, T-and B-lymphocytes and they inhibit the proliferation of macrophages, T - and B-lymphocytes and stimulates the proliferation of fibroblasts.

Plasma Derived Mediators

Plasma derived mediators of inflammation are kinins, clotting, fibrinolytic and complement systems; each of them has initiators and accelerators in plasma depending upon their need through feedback mechanism. During inflammation Hagman factor (Factor XII) is activated through leakage in endothelial gaps in increased permeability of blood vessels. The activated factor XII acts on kinin, clotting and fibrinolytic systems and end product of these systems activate complement to generate C3a and C5a, which are potent mediators of inflammation.

Kinin system

Through activation of factor XII, kinin system generates the bradykinin which causes contraction of smooth muscles. The activated factor XII (XIIa) acts on prekallikrein activator which in turn converts the plasma prekallikrein into kallikrein.

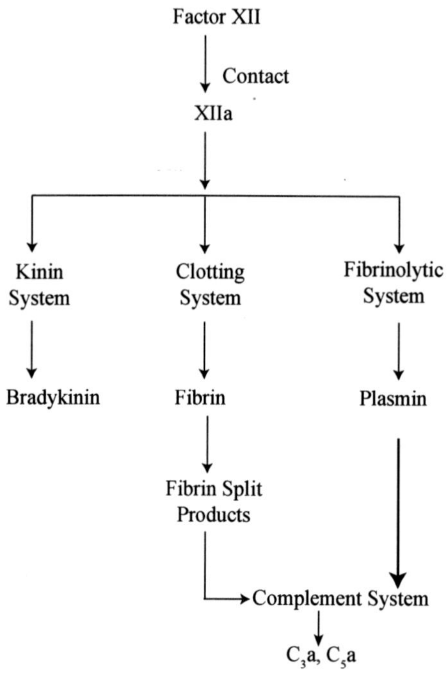

The bradykinin is formed from kininogen through the action of kallikrein. The bradykinin acts on smooth muscles leading to their contraction. Bradykinin is also found to be responsible for vasodilation, increased vascular permeability and pain.

Clotting Mechanism

The activated Hagman factor (XIIa) initiates the cascade of clotting system and factor XI

Clotting system

Clotting System

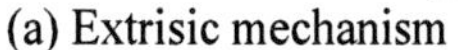

(a) Extrisic mechanism

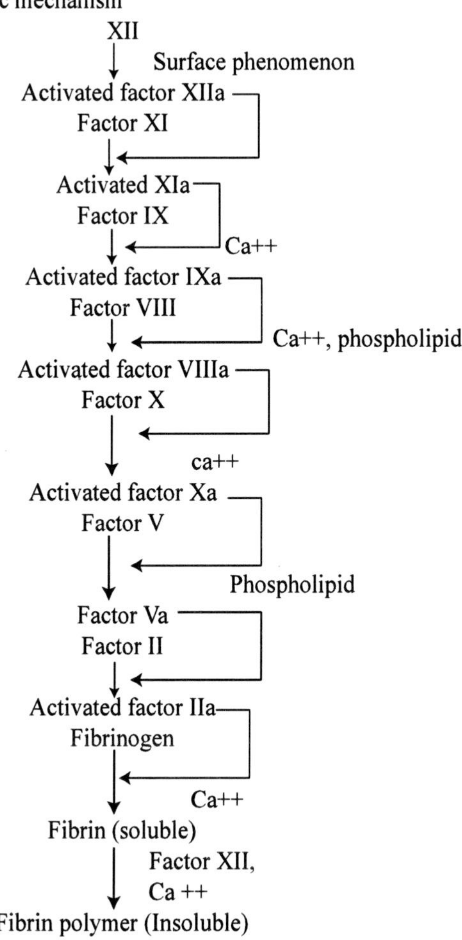

(b) Intrisic mechanism

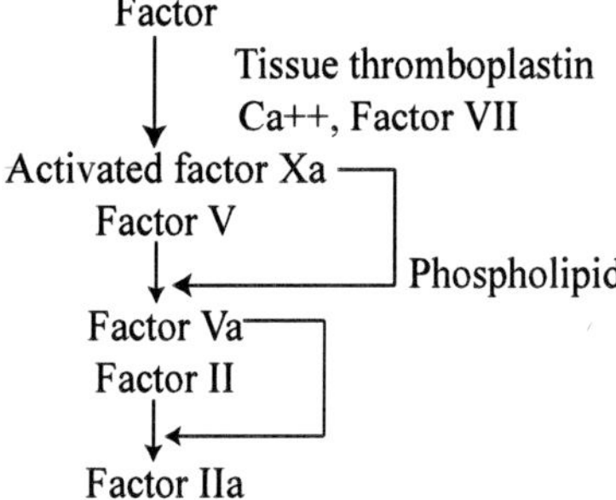

Into XIa which along with factor VIIa changes factor X into Xa. Factor Xa along with factor Va converts prothrombin into thrombin which acts on fibrinogen to form fibrin responsible for clotting of blood.

Fibrinolytic System

Plasminogen activator is released from endothelial cells and leucocytes and acts on plasminogen present as a component of plasma proteins to form plasmin. The plasmin is responsible for breakdown of fibrin into fibrinopeptides or fibrin split products, conversion of C_3 to C_{3a} and stimulates the kinin system to generate bradykinin.

Complement System

Complement is activated through classical and alternate pathways; the classical pathway includes activation of complement through antigen-antibody complexes while the alternate pathway gets activated via non-immunologic agents such as bacterial toxins. Complement system on activation generates 3 anaphylotoxin through either of pathway including C3a, C5a and C4a, which are responsible for release of histamine from the mast cells, increased vascular permeability and chemotaxis for leucocytes. The complement components are activated by antigen antibody complex and form AAC1423 which causes opsonization and enhances phagocytosis. C567 acts as chemotactic factor for phagocytic cells. AAC $_{1\text{-}7}$ renders the cell susceptible for lymphocytotoxicity by T-cell. The complement AAC $_{1\text{-}9}$ causes lysis of erythrocytes and Gram negative bacteria. However, Gram positive bacteria are resistant to complement lysis.

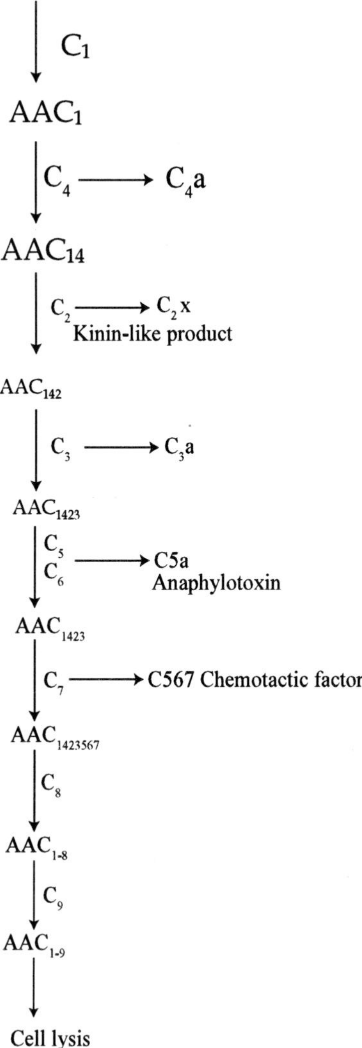

Phagocytosis

Phagocytosis is the process of engulfment and digestion of particulate matter by certain cells of body (phagocytes; phagocytic cells). Mainly there are two types of the cells which perform the phagocytosis including polymorphonuclear neutrophils (PMN) or microphages and monocytes or tissue mononuclear cells also known as macrophages. The process of phagocytosis is almost similar by these micro and macrophages and involves 4 stages (Fig. 6.24):

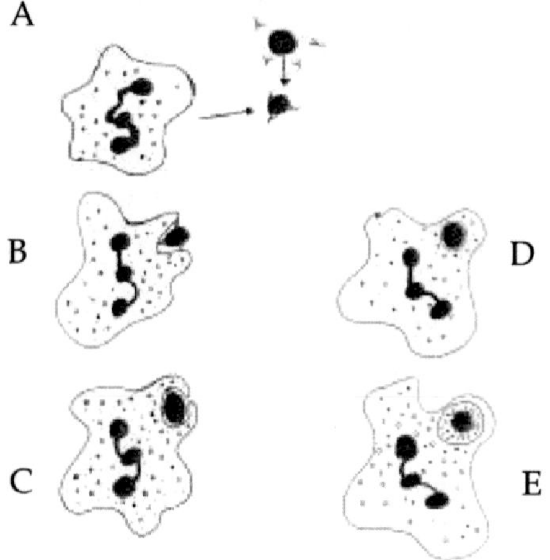

Fig. 6.24: Diagram showing phagocytosis. **A.** Opsonization and Chemotaxis **B - C.** Engulfment and **D-E.** Digestion.

I. Chemotaxis

The phagocytic cells, neutrophils and monocytes are present in circulating blood while there are several tissue macrophages found in inflammation. Vasodilation and decreased blood flow leads to disturbances in blood stream resulting in margination of leucocytes. At that time endothelial cells of blood vessels express certain proteins known as selectins and integrins that bind with neutrophils. Since they are attracted by certain chemical mediators, these cells are directed to migrate towards the chemical mediators. This directed migration of phagocytic cells is known as chemotaxis. Various chemotactic agents for different phagocytic cells are as under:

Chemotactic agents	**Phagocytic cells**
C_{3a}, C_{5a}, C_{567} Leucotriene B_4	Neutrophils
Bacterial proteins, LPS.	
C_{3a}, C_{5a}, C_{567} Bacterial Products	Macrophages/monocytes
Neutrophilic cationic protein	
Cytokines, Kinins	
ECF-A, Parasitic proteins, Complement C_{3a}, C_{5a}	Eosinophils

The chemotactic agents diffuse at the site of tissue damage to attract the phagocytic cells. However, large dose of chemotactic molecules may make the phagocytic cells insensitive to chemoattraction and such non-responsive cells may migrate from the damaged area after completion of phagocytosis.

II. Adherence and opsonization

The phagocytic cells and foreign particle like bacteria are suspended in body fluid with negative charge that repel each other. The negative charge on foreign particle is neutralized by coating of positively charged protein and such proteins are immunoglobulins (IgG) and $C_{3b,}$ the complement component. Thus, the particle coated with IgG or C_{3b} reduces its surface charge and it is attracted towards phagocytic cells. The molecules (IgG or C_{3b}) coatings on particulate matter to facilitate phagocytosis are known as opsonins and this process is termed as opsonization. The word opsonin is derived from Greek language and means sauce, implying that it makes the particles more tastier to phagocytic cells. The phagocytic cells have receptors for Fc portion of IgG and C_3b protein that facilitates the adherence of the particles on the surface of the cells. Another mechanism is trapping of particulate material through pseudopodia movement of the phagocytic cells.

III. Ingestion

The phagocytic cell forms pseudopodia around the particles to cover it from outside. The particle is bound to the surface of cells through opsonization and is drawn inside the cytoplasm through engulfment. The phagocytic cell forms vacuole by enveloping the particle which is known as phagocytic vacuole. The plasma membrane covering phagocytic vacuole breaks and the ingested particle lies free in cytoplasm of phagocytic cell. The lysosome present in cell cytoplasm binds with phagocytic vacuoles to form phagolysosome or phagosome.

There is degranulation on the particle and liberation of hydrolytic enzymes and antibacterial substances to kill the ingested particle.

IV. Digestion

The ingested particles are destroyed by the phagocytic cells through two separate mechanisms, the respiratory burst and by action of lysosomal enzymes

Respiratory Burst

Soon after the ingestion of particulate material phagocytic cell increases its oxygen consumption nearly 100 fold and also activates the cell surface enzyme NADPH-oxidase. This activated enzyme converts NADPH to $NADP^+$ with release of electrons.

$$NADPH + O_2 \xrightarrow{NADPH-Oxidase} NADP^+ + 2\ O^- + H^+$$

One molecule of oxygen accepts a single donated electron, leading to the generation of one molecule of superoxide anion. $NADP^+$ increases the hexose monophosphate shunt and converts sucrose to a pentose, carbon dioxide and energy for utilization of the cellular functions. Two molecules of superoxide anions interact to generate one molecule of hydrogen peroxide under the influence of enzyme superoxide dismutase.

$$2\left(2O^-\right) + 2\ H^+ \xrightarrow{Superoxide\ dismutase} H_2O_2 + O_2$$

Superoxide anions do not accumulate in the cell because under the influence of dismutase enzyme they rapidly convert into hydrogen peroxide. However, there is accumulation of hydrogen peroxide in the cells which is also converted into bactericidal compounds the hypohalids through the action of myeloperoxidase.

$$H_2O_2 + Cl^- \xrightarrow{Myeloperoxidase} \begin{matrix} H_2O_2 + OCl^- \\ (Hypochloride) \end{matrix}$$

Hypochloride kills bacteria by oxidizing their proteins and enhancing the bactericidal activities of the lysosomal enzymes.

Lysosomal enzymes

Once the phagolysosomes are formed, the lysosomal enzymes are released in the particulate matter that can kill the bacteria. Many Gram positive and Gram negative bacteria are destroyed by the lysosomal enzymes. However, there are certain bacteria like Brucella, Listeria which are so resistant that they even grow inside the cell and may become fatal to the cell. Dying neutrophils release elastases and collagenase which act as chemotactic factors for macrophages. The macrophages destroy the particulate material/ bacteria by both oxidative and non-oxidative mechanisms. In cattle, macrophages, after activation, synthesize the nitric oxide synthatase. This enzyme acts on L-arginine by using oxygen and NADPH to produce nitric oxide and citrulline. Nitric oxide is not highly toxic but it reacts with superoxide anions released during respiratory burst to produce very toxic derivatives such as $NO_{2,}$ N_2O_3 ONOO and NO_3 which can kill the ingested bacteria and cause severe tissue damage. Macrophages are also used by the body as scavenger cells to remove the dead or dying cells.

When the foreign particulate material persists for longer period, macrophages accumulate in large number around it to kill and remove from the system. The phagocytosed particles are so potent that they kill the macrophages also. Then after destruction of macrophages it is rephagocytosed. This continuing destruction of macrophages leads to excessive release of lysosomal enzymes and reactive oxygen and nitric oxide metabolites resulting in chronic tissue damage and chronic inflammation. In such situation, macrophages become elongated looking like epithelial cells and such cells are termed as epithelioid cells. If these cells are also unable to destroy the ingested material then they combine/ fuse together to form multinucleated giant cells.

Types of Inflammation

Inflammation is classified according to the duration as of acute, subacute and chronic form. The acute inflammation is characterized by the presence of more vascular alterations while chronic inflammation is identified on the basis of presence of more proliferative changes, fibrosis and less vascular alterations (Fig. 6.25-A&B & 6.26).

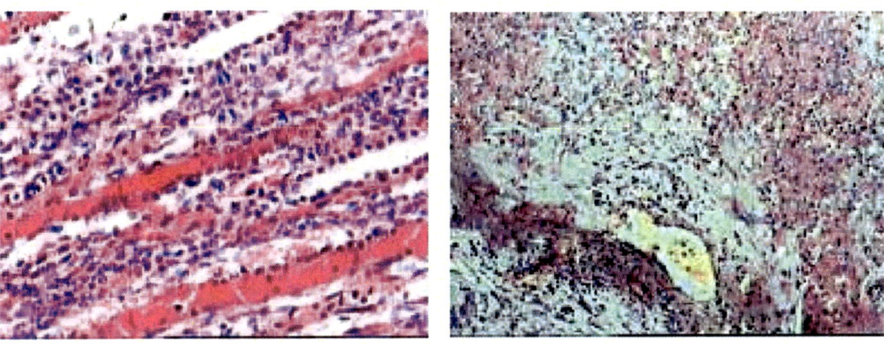

A B

Fig. 6.25: Photomicrograph showing **A.** acute and **B.** Chronic inflammation

Sl. No.	Changes	Acute	Subacute	Chronic
1.	Vascular changes	+++	++	+
2.	Proliferative changes	+	++	+++

On the basis of the presence of exudate, the inflammation is divided into catarrhal, serus, fibrinous, suppurative, eosinophilic, lymphocytic, haemorrhagic, granulomatous etc., described as under (Fig. 6.26):

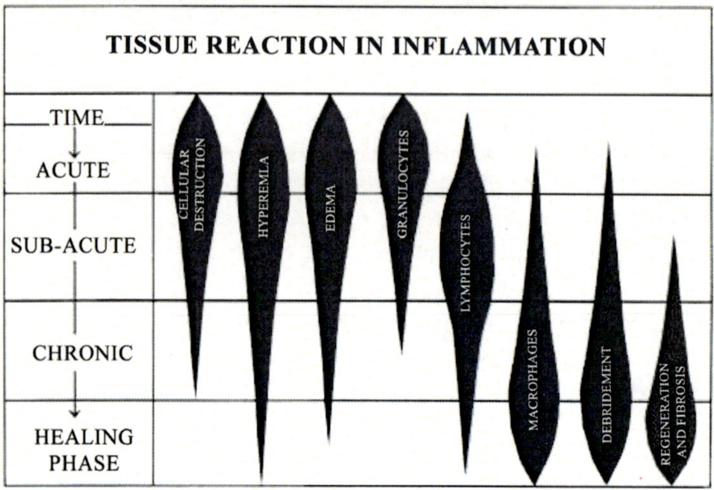

Fig. 6.26. Diagram showing tissue reaction in inflammation

Catarrhal Inflammation

Catarrhal inflammation occurs on mucus surfaces and is characterized by the presence of increased amount of mucin as principal constituent of exudates e.g. catarrhal enteritis, catarrhal rhinitis (Fig. 6.27 & 6.28).

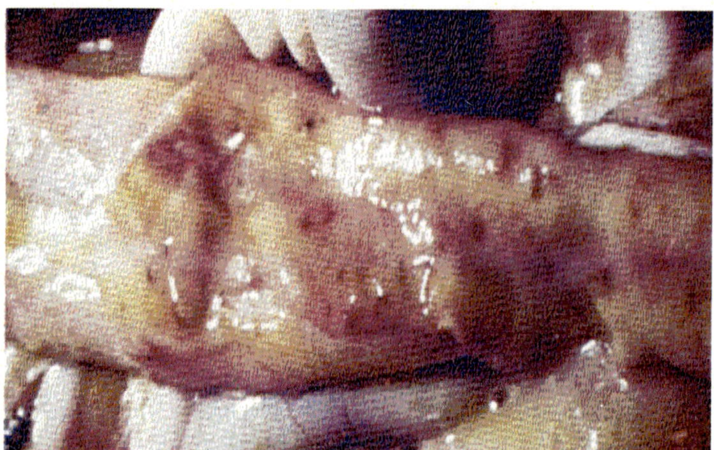

Fig. 6.27: Photograph of intestine showing catarrhal inflammation

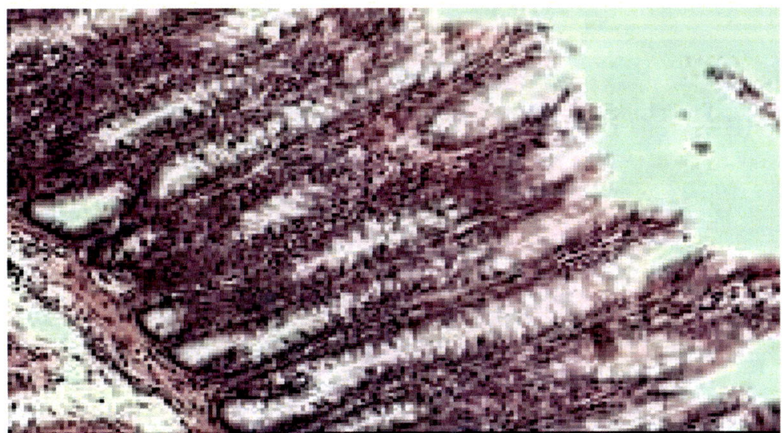

Fig. 6.28: Photomicrograph of intestine showing catarrhal inflammation

Etiology

- Mild irritant on mucous membrane e.g. Rotavirus infection in calves.
- Cold exposure causes excessive mucous discharges from nasal mucosa.

Macroscopic features

- Congestion.
- Presence of increased amount of slimy, stringy mucin along with stool.
- Mucus nasal discharge, if respiratory mucosa is involved.
- Mucous vaginal discharges in uterine disorders or as physiological phenomenon.

Microscopic features

- Increased number of goblet cells on mucous surface.
- Increased amount of mucin, which takes basic stain.
- Hyperplasia of epithelial cells on mucous surface.
- Infiltration of neutrophils, lymphocytes and macrophages.

Serus Inflammation

Serus inflammation occurs due to any mild irritant and is characterized by the presence of serum/ plasma as main constituent of the exudates (Figs. 6.29 & 6.30).

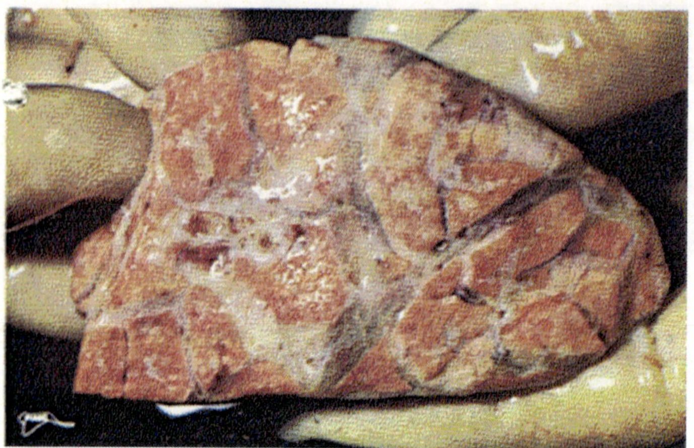

Fig. 6.29: Photograph of lung showing serous inflammation

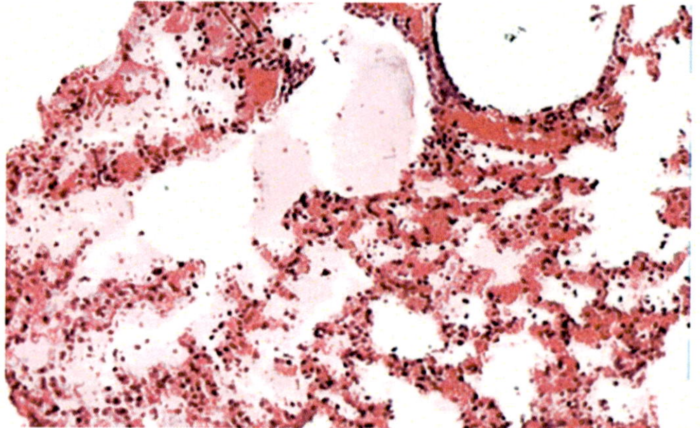

Fig. 6.30: Photomicrograph of lung showing serous inflammation

Etiology

- Mild irritants e.g. chemicals.
- Physical trauma.
- Infection:

  Virus e.g. Pox, FMD

  Bacteria e.g. Pasteurlla multocida

Macroscopic features

- Congestion.
- Watery exudate in cavity/vesicle/in intercellular spaces.
- On rupture of vesicle clear fluid comes out.

Microscopic features

- Congestion.
- Presence of serus exudate-acidophilic in tissue.
- Infiltration of neutrophils/lymphocytes/ mononuclear cells.

Fibrinous Inflammation

Fibrinous inflammation is characterized by the presence of fibrin as main constituent of the exudates (Figs. 6.31 & 6.32).

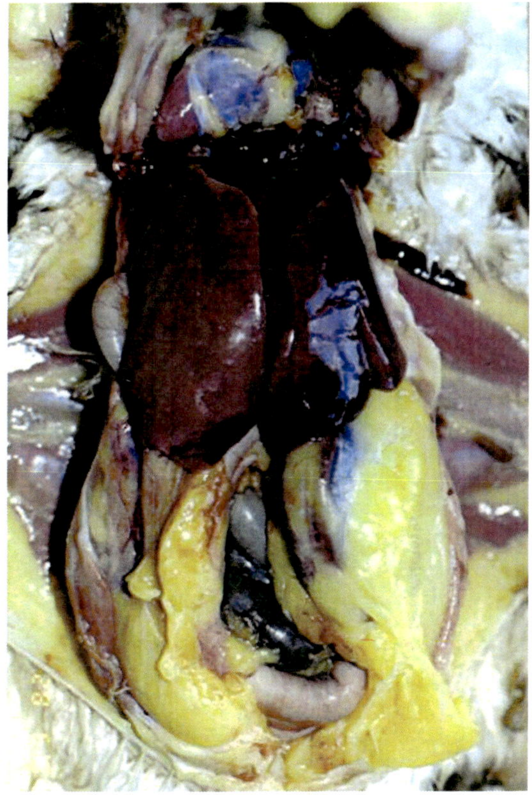

Fig. 6.31: Photograph of liver showing fibrinous inflammation

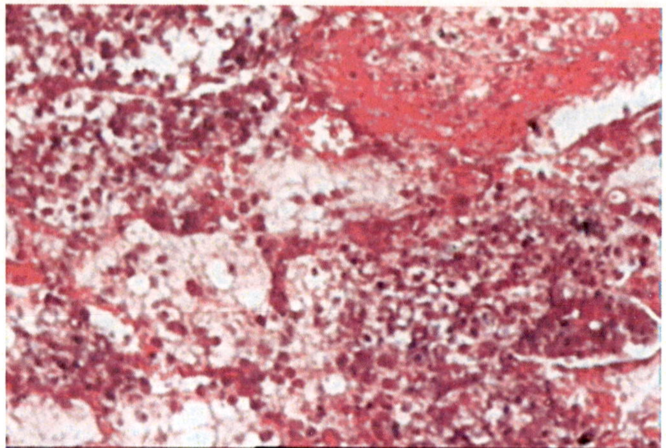

Fig. 6.32: Photomicrograph of lung showing fibrinous inflammation

Etiology

- Chemicals.
- Thermal injury.
- Bacteria e.g. Corynebacterium diphtheriae.
- Viruses e.g. Herpes virus, influenza virus.

Macroscopic features

- Organ becomes firm and tense.
- Surface of organ loses its shine.
- Produces adhesions in between two layers or two organs.

False membrane/crupous membrane present, which can be removed easily e.g. fibrinous membrane over heart and liver due to colisepticemia in birds.

Microscopic features

- Congestion.
- Presence of fibrin network (thread-like) on the surface or in the organ.
- Infiltration of inflammatory cells like neutrophils, lymphocytes and macrophages.

Suppurative Inflammation

Suppurative inflammation is characterized by the presence of neutrophils (polymorphonuclear cells) as principal constituent of the exudates (Figs. 6.33 & 6.34).

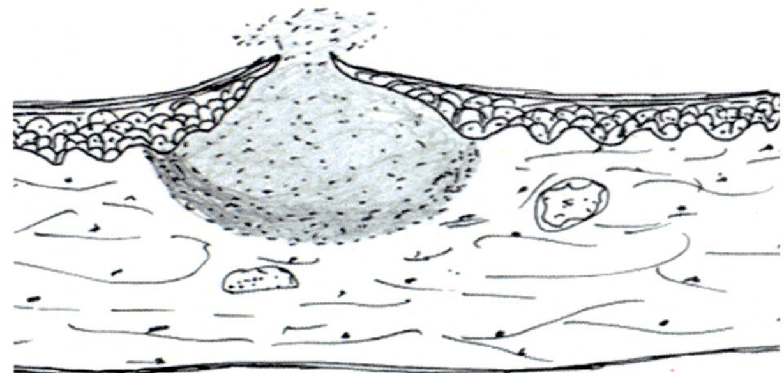

Fig. 6.33: Diagram of skin showing suppurative inflammation

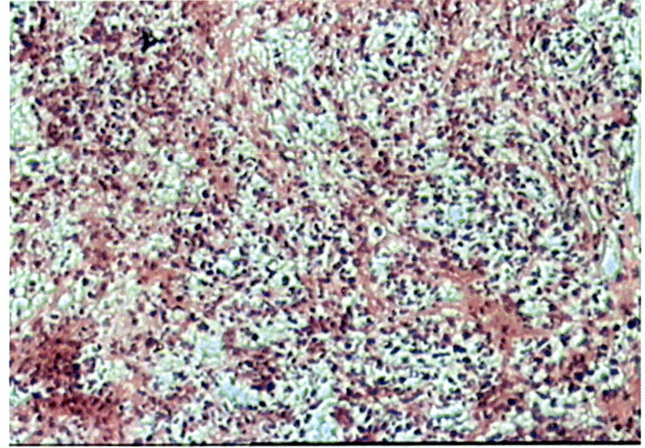

Fig. 6.34: Photomicrograph of skin showing suppurative inflammation

Etiology

- Bacterial infection e.g. Staphylococci.
- Chemicals e.g. turpentine.

Macroscopic features

- Presence of pus in lesion
- Pus is white yellow/greenish, thin, watery or viscid/material.

- When pus present in a cavity it is known as abscess while the presence of pus diffusely scattered throughout the subcutaneous tissue is known as Phlegmon or cellulitis.

Microscopic features

- Congestion.
- Presence of neutrophils as main constituent of the exudate.
- Liquifactive necrosis of the cells / tissue.

Haemorrhagic Inflammation

Haemorrhagic inflammation is characterized by the presence of erythrocyte as principal constituent of the exudate (Figs. 6.35 & 6.36).

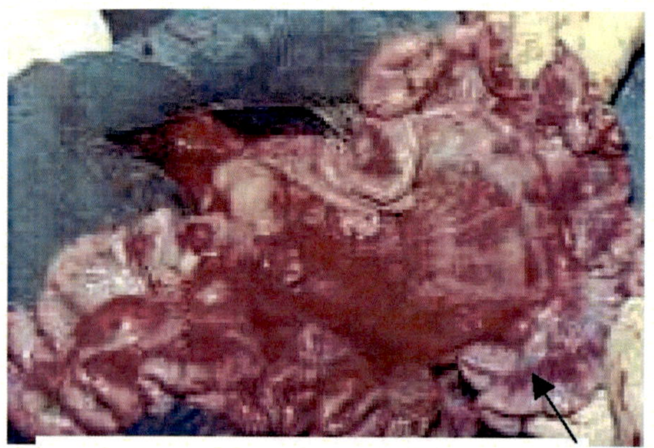

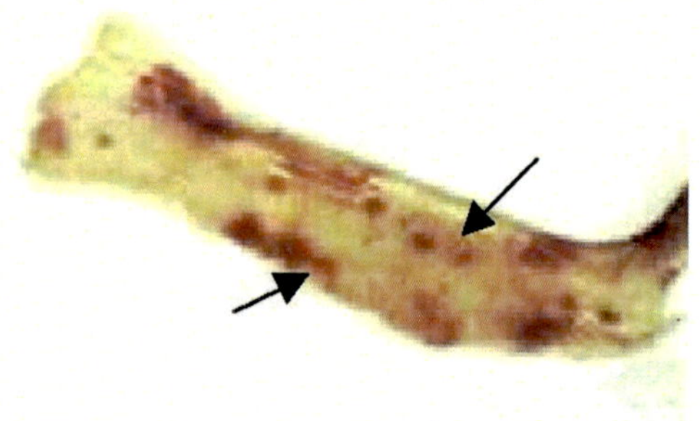

Fig. 6.35: Photograph of intestines showing haemorrhagic inflammation

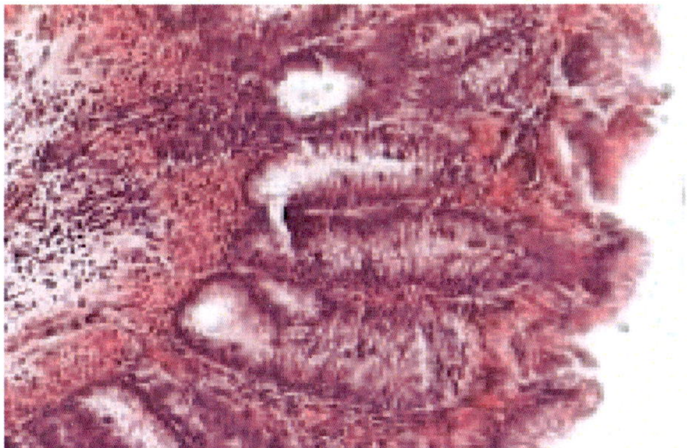

Fig. 6.36: Photomicrograph of intestines showing haemorrhagic inflammation

Etiology

- Extremely injurious chemicals e.g. phenol.
- Bacterial infection e.g. Anthrax, H.S.
- Viral infection e.g. R.P., Blue tongue.

Macroscopic features

- Colour of organ/tissue becomes red/cyanotic.
- Exudate contains clots of blood.
- Petechial, echymotic haemorrhages on the surfaces of organs.
- Mucous membranes become pale / anemic.

Microscopic features

- Presence of erythrocytes outside the blood vessels in extracellular spaces along with neutrophils/ lymphocytes/ macrophages.
- Serus/serofibrinous exudates.

Lymphocytic Inflammation

Lymphocytic inflammation is characterized by the presence of lymphocytes as principal constituent of the exudate (Fig. 6.37).

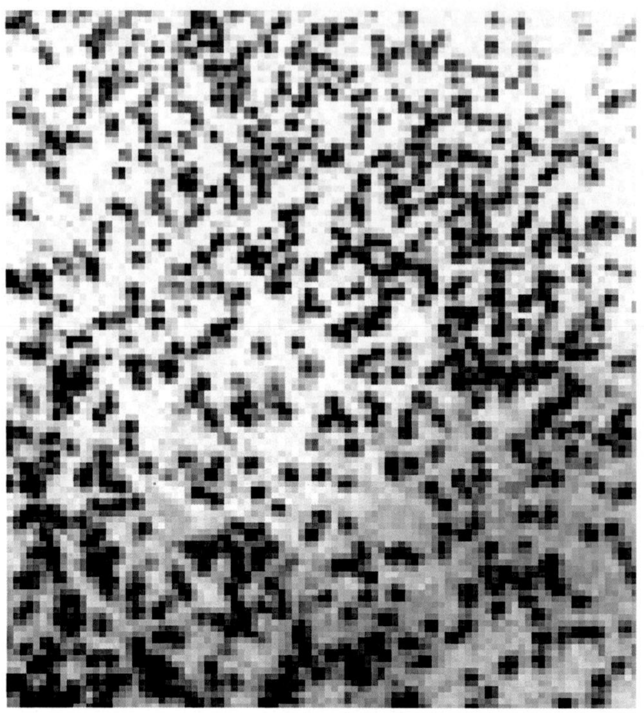

Fig. 6.37: Photomicrograph showing lymphocytic inflammation

Etiology

- Viral / Bacterial infections.
- Toxic conditions.

Macroscopic features

- No characteristic gross lesion; sometimes there is formation of small modules on serosa of the affected organ.
- Enlargement of lymphnodes.
- Congestion.
- Presence of white/grey lymphoid nodules in organ.

Microscopic features

- Presence of lymphocytes in abundant number as principal constituent of the exudate.
- Congestion.

- Accumulation of lymphocytes around the blood vessels, "Peri vascular cuffing"
- Aggregation of lymphocytes leading to lymphofollicular reaction.

Granulomatous Inflammation

Granulomatous inflammation is a chronic condition, characterized by the presence of granuloma in the organs. The granuloma consists of central caseative necrosis surrounded by lymphocytes, macrophages, epithelioid cells, giant cells and fibrous connective tissue (Figs. 6.38 & 6.39).

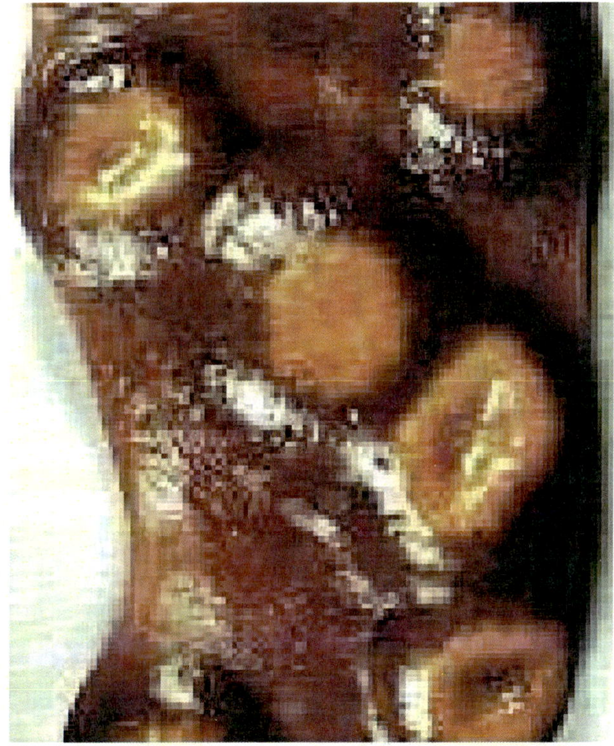

Fig. 6.38: Photograph of spleen showing granulomatous inflammation

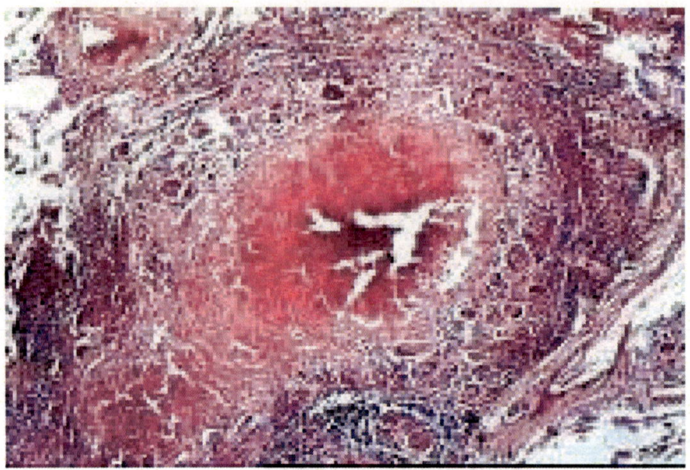

Fig. 6.39: Photomicrograph of lung showing granulomatous inflammation

Etiology

- Chronic bacterial infection e.g. tuberculosis.
- Fungal infections e.g. blastomycosis.

Macroscopic features

- Presence of hard, tiny, nodules in the organ.
- Lungs become hard, patchy.
- Lymph nodes become hard and fibrus.
- Later the affected organ is calcified and gives cracking sound on cut.

Microscopic features

- Presence of granuloma in the tissue/ organ.
- Central caseative necrosis, surrounded by epithelioid cells, macrophages, lymphocytes, giant cells and covered by fibrous connective tissue capsule.
- Caseative area contains causative organisms also, which can be demonstrated by special staining e.g. Tuberculous organisms by Acid-fast staining.
- Calcification of necrosed area at later stage looking black/ violet colour on H & E stain.

Tble 6.2: Differential features of various types of inflammation

	Catarrhal	**Serus**	**Fibrinous**	**Suppurative**	**Haemorr-hagic**	**Lymphocytic**	**Granulo-matous**	**Eosinophilic**
Macroscopic features	1. Congestion	1. Congestion	1. Organ becomes firm and tense.	1. Presence of pus in lesion	1. Colour of organ/tissue becomes red/ cyanotic.	1. No Characteristic gross lesion; Sometimes there is formation of Small modules on serosa of the Affected organ.	1. Presence of hard, tiny, nodules in the organ.	1. Congestion
	2. Presence of Increased amount of slimy, stringy mucin along with stool.	2. Watery exudate in cavity/vesicle / in Intercellular Spaces	2. Surface of organ lost its shine.	2. Pus is white yellow/ greenish, thin, watery or viscid/ material.	2. Exudate contains clot of blood.	2. Enlargement of Lymphnodes	2. Lungs become hard, patchy.	2. No characteristic gross lesion

	Catarrhal	Serus	Fibrinous	Suppurative	Haemorr-hagic	Lymphocytic	Granulo-matous	Eosinophilic
	3. Mucus Nasal discharge, if Respiratory mucosa is Involved	3. On rupture of vesicle clear fluid comes out	3. Produces adhesions in between two layers or two organs.	3. When pus present in a cavity it is known as abscess. While the presence of pus diffusely scattered Throughout the subcutaneous tissue is known as Phlegmon or cellulitis.	3. Petechial, echymotic haemorrhages on the surfaces of organs.	3. Presence of white/gray Lymphoid nodules in organ.	3. Lymphnodes become hard and fibrous.	
	4. Mucous Vaginal discharges, in Uterine disorders or As Physiological phenomenon.		4. False membrane/ Crupous membrane present, which can be Removed easily e.g. Fibrinous membrane over heart and liver due To Colisepticemi a in birds.		4. Mucous membranes become pale / anemic.		4. Later the affected organ calcified and gives cracking sound on cut.	

	Catarrhal	**Serus**	**Fibrinous**	**Suppurative**	**Haemorr-hagic**	**Lymphocytic**	**Granulo-matous**	**Eosinophilic**
	1. Increased number of goblet cells on mucous surface.	1. Congestion	1. Congestion	1. Congestion	1. Presence of erythrocytes out side the blood vessels in extracellular spaces along with neutrophils/ lymphocytes/ macrophage.	1. Presence of Lymphocytes in abundant number as Principal constituent of the exudate.	1. Presence of granuloma in the tissue/ organ.	1. Presence of eosinophils in Abundant Numbers
	2. Increased amount of mucin, which takes basic stain.	2. Presence of Serus exudate-acidophilic in tissue.	2. Presence of Fibrin Network (thread like) on the surface or in the organ.	2. Presence of neutrophils as Main constituent of the exudate.	2. Serus/ serofibrinous exudates.	2. Accumulation of Lymphocytes around the blood vessels, "Peri vascular cuffing"	2. Central caseative necrosis, surrounded by epithelioid cells, macrophages, lymphocytes, giant cells and covered by fibrous connective tissue capsule.	2. Congestion

	Catarrhal	Serus	Fibrinous	Suppurative	Haemorr-hagic	Lymphocytic	Granulo-matous	Eosinophilic
	3. Hyperplasia of epithelial cells on mucous surface.	3. Infiltration of neutrophils/ lymphocytes/ mononuclear Cells	3. Infiltration of Inflammatory cells like neutrophils, Lymphocytes and macrophages.	3. Liquifactive necrosis of the cells / tissue.		3. Aggregation of lymphocytes leading to lymphofollicu lar reaction.	3. Caseative area contains causative organisms also, which can be demonstrated by special staining e.g. Tuberculous organisms by Acid-fast staining.	
	4. Infiltration of neutrophils, Lymphocytes and macrophages.						4. Calcification of necrosed area at later stage looking black/ violet colour on H&E stain.	3. Accumula-tion of Eosinophils around the parasites and/ or blood vessels.

Eosinophilic Inflammation

It is characterized by the presence of eosinophils as the main constituents of the exudate (Figs. 6.40 & 6.41).

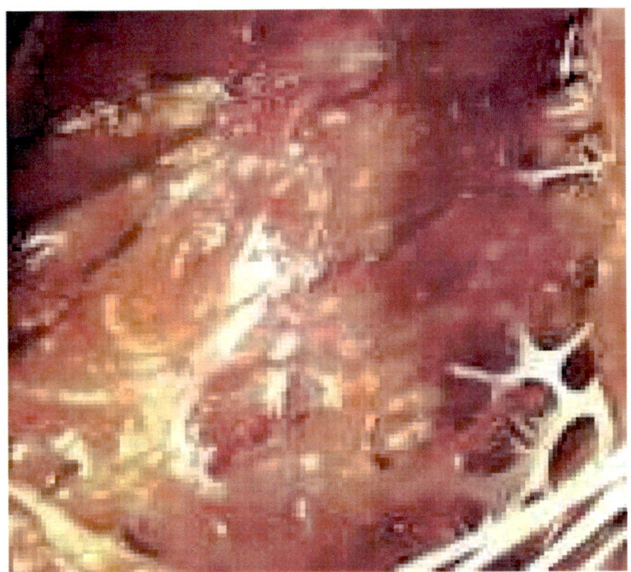

Fig. 6.40: Photograph of heart showing eosinophilic inflammation

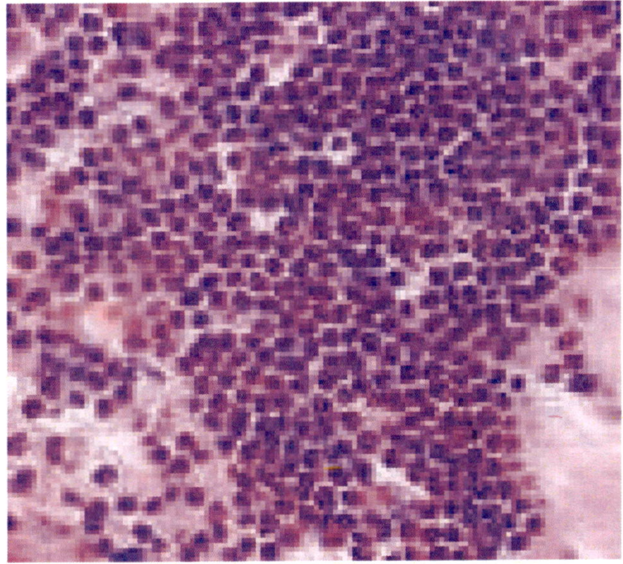

Fig. 6.41: Photomicrograph of heart showing eosinophilic inflammation

Etiology

- Allergy/ Hypersensitivity.
- Parasitic diseases.

Macroscopic features

- Congestion.
- No characteristic gross lesion.

Microscopic features

- Presence of eosinophils in abundant numbers
- Congestion.
- Accumulation of eosinophils around the parasites and/ or blood vessels.

Healing

Healing is characterized by the body response to injury in order to restore normal structure and function of the damaged organ/tissue. It is of two types (Figs. 6.42 to 6.45).

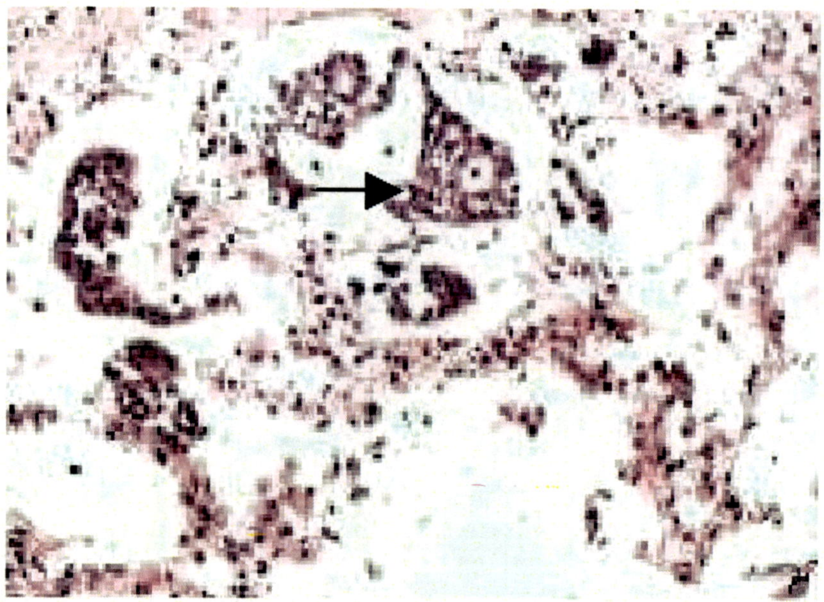

Fig. 6.42: Photomicrograph of lung showing regenerative changes

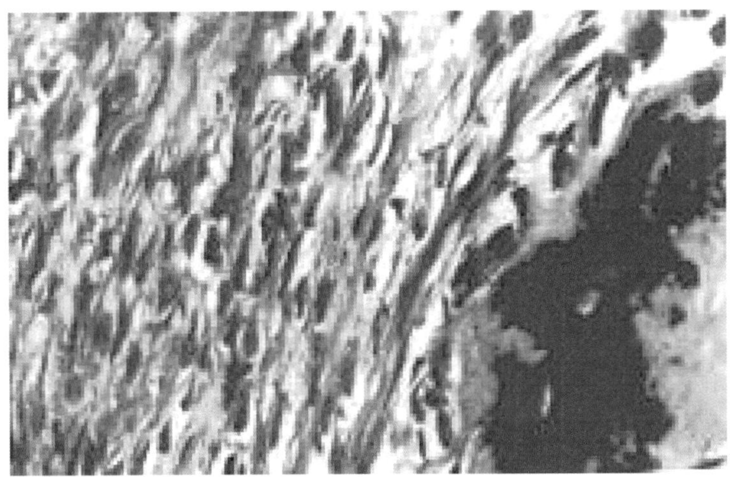

Fig 6.43: Photomicrograph of fracture showing healing

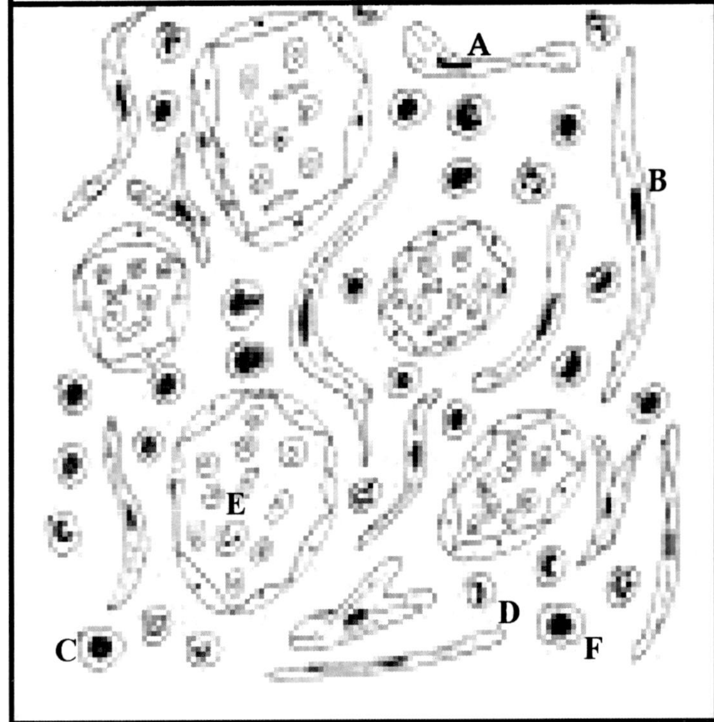

Fig. 6.44: Diagram showing granulation tissue in repair

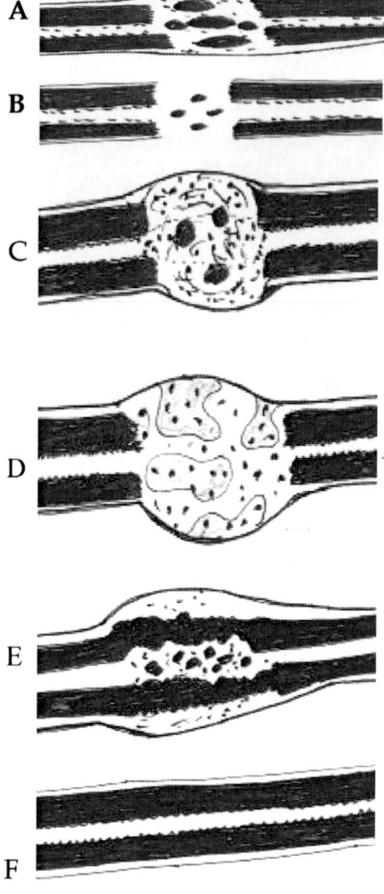

Fig. 6.45: Diagram showing fracture repair **A.** Hematoma **B.** Inflammatory reaction **C.** Growth of granulation tissue and formation of soft callus **D.** Formation of procallus **E.** Formation of osseous callus and **F.** Remodelled bone with complete healing

Regeneration

Healing is by proliferation of parenchymatous cells leading to complete restoration of the original tissue.

Macroscopic features

- No significant gross lesion.

Microscopic features

- Proliferation of parenchymal cells.
- Hyperplasia of the cells.

Repair

Repair is the replacement of injured tissue by proliferation of fibrous tissue.

Macroscopic features

- Pink/red granules (granulation tissue) appear on healing part. These are the indication of formation of new blood vessels.
- It can be seen just beneath the scab.

Microscopic features

- Formation of granulation tissue i.e. fibroblasts, angioblasts, histiocytes, macrophages and parenchymal cells of organ.
- Fibroblasts are elongated fibrillar cells with ovoid hyperchromatic nuclei.
- Mitosis is frequently observed.

7

Immunity and Immunopathology

Immunity

Immunity is the resistance of body against extraneous etiological factors of disease, which is afforded by the interaction of chemical, humoral and cellular reactions in body. This is an integral part of the body without, which one cannot think of life. During the process of evolution, nature has provided this defense mechanism in the bodies of all living creatures particularly of higher animals and man, that protects them from physical, chemical and biological threats. It can be classified as natural or paraspecific and acquired or specific immunity.

Natural/paraspecific immunity

There are some species which are resistant to particular diseases due to presence of natural resistance against them e.g. horse, pig, cat are resistant to canine distemper virus; dogs are resistant to feline panleucopenia virus, chickens are resistant to anthrax. Even within species, there is natural resistance that protects some individuals while others are susceptible e.g. Indian deshi cattle Zebu (Bos indicus) is quite resistant to piroplasmosis in comparison to Bos taurus. Besides, there are the mechanisms or barriers in body provided by nature. These are

- Skin and mucous membrane prevent organisms from gaining entrance in body.
- Mucous prevents from infections by trapping and keeping them away.
- Saliva, gastric juice and intestinal enzymes kill bacteria.
- Tears, nasal and GI tract secretions are bactericidal due to presence of lysozymes.
- Phagocytic cells such as neutrophils kill bacteria through phagocytosis.
- Macrophages kill organisms through phagocytosis.
- Natural antibodies act as opsonins and help in phagocytosis.

- Interferons have antimicrobial properties. They are host/species specific and arrest viral replication.
- Interleukins, cytotoxins and growth factors stimulate the immune reactions and inflammation.
- Natural killer cells kill targets coated with IgG.

Acquired/specific immunity

Acquired immunity develops in body as a result of prior stimulation through antigen. It is specific to a particular antigen against which it was developed. It can be restimulated on second or subsequent exposure with antigen and thus, it has memory for a particular antigen. It differs from natural immunity in respect of prior stimulation, specificity and memory. It can be classified as humoral and cell mediated immunity.

Humoral immunity

This is the immunity present in fluids of body mainly in blood. There are antibodies in serum of blood, which protect body from diseases. It is specific to particular antigen. Antibodies are formed in blood as a result of exposure of the foreign substances including bacteria, virus, parasite and other substances.

Antigen is foreign substance, which is able to stimulate the production of antibodies in body. They may be of high molecular weight protein, polysaccharides, and nucleic acids. Simple chemicals of low molecular weight are not able to induce immunity. However, they may be conjugated with large molecular weight molecules such as protein to become antigenic and induce antibody production, such substances are termed as haptens. Antibodies are protein in nature present in serum and produced as a result of antigen. Antibodies are specific to antigen. Most of the microorganisms have several antigenic determinants and antibodies are produced against each antigenic determinant specifically. The antibody response to antigen can be enhanced if the antigen is released slowly in body. There are several substances like oils, waxes, alum, aluminium hydroxide, which may be added with antigen so that it is released slowly in body to increase the antibody production. Such substances are known as adjuvants. Antibodies are also known as immunoglobulins as they are the part of globulins. They are glycoprotein in nature and are of 5 types IgG, IgA, IgM, IgD and IgE (Fig. 7.1).

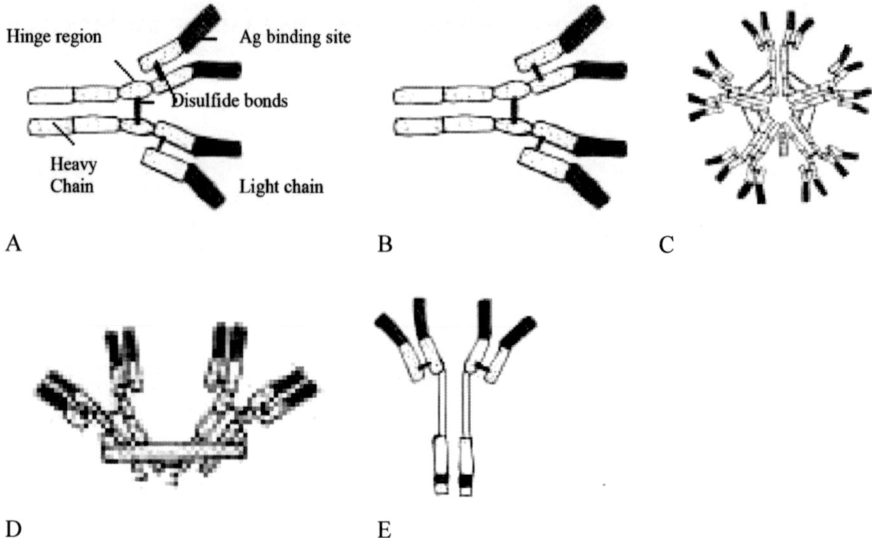

Fig. 7.1: Diagram showing **A.** Structure of antibody with its different parts **B.** Immunoglublin–G (IgG), **C.** Immunoglobulin-M (IgM), **D.** Immunoglobulin-A (IgA) and **E.** Immunoglobulin-E (IgE).

Immunoglobulin G (IgG)

It is the main antibody found in high concentration (75%) in serum with a mw 150 KD. It is produced by plasma cells in spleen, lymph nodes and bone marrow. It has two identical light chains and two gamma heavy chains. The light chains may be of kappa or lamda type. IgG is the smallest immunoglobulin which may pass through blood vessels with increased permeability. It has the capacity to quickly bind with foreign substances leading to opsonization. Its binding with antigen may also activate the complement.

Immunoglobulin M (IgM)

This is about 7% of total serum immunoglobulins. It is also produced by plasma cells in spleen, lymphnodes and bone marrow. It is pentamer, five molecules of conventional immunoglobulin with mw 900 KD. These five molecules are linked through disulfide bonds in a circular form. A cysteine rich polypetide of 15KD mw binds two of the units to complete circle and is known as 'J' chain. It is produced in body during primary immune response. It is considered to be more active than IgG for complement activation, neutralization of antigen, opsonization and agglutination. IgM molecules are confined to the blood and have no or little effect in tissue fluids, body secretions and in acute inflammation.

Immunoglobulin A (IgA)

It is secreted as dimmer (mw 300 KD) by plasma cells present under body surfaces like intestinal, respiratory and urinary system, mammary gland and skin. Its concentration is very little in blood. IgA produced in body surfaces is either secreted on surface through epithelial cells or diffuse in blood stream. IgA is transported through intestinal epithelial cells having a receptor of 71 KD which binds with the secretory component covalently to form a secretory IgA. This secretory component protects IgA in the intestinal tract from digestion. It cannot activate the complement and cannot perform the opsonization. IgA can neutralize the antigen and agglutinate the particulate antigen. IgA prevents adherence of foreign particles/antigen on the body surfaces and it can also act inside the cells. It is about 16% of total immunoglobulins present in serum.

Immunoglobulin E (IgE)

It is also present on body surfaces and produced by plasma cells located beneath the body surfaces. It is in very low concentration in serum. It can bind on receptors of mast cells and basophils. When any antigen binds to these molecules, it causes degranulation from mast cells leading to release of chemical mediators to cause acute inflammation. It mediates hypersensitivity type I reaction and is responsible to provide resistance against invading parasitic worms. It is of shortest half life (2-3 days) and thus is unstable and can be readily destroyed by mild heat treatment. It is 0.01% of total immunoglobulin in serum with 190 KD molecular weight.

Immunoglobulin D (IgD)

IgD is absent in most domestic animals. However, it is present in very minute amount in plasma of dog, non-human primates and rats. IgD can be detected in plasma. However, it cannot be found in serum due to lysis by proteases during clotting. It is only 0.2% of total immunoglobulin in serum with mw 160 KD.

On the basis of their function, antibodies are classified as:

Antitoxins have the property to bind with toxins and neutralise them.

Agglutinins are those antibodies, which can agglutinate the RBCs and/or particulate material such as bacterial cells.

Precipitins can precipitate the proteins by acting with antigen and inhibit their dissemination and chemical activity.

Lysins can lyse the cells or bacteria through complement.

Opsonins have the property to bind with foreign particles, non specifically leading to opsonization, making the foreign material palatable to phagocytic cells.

Complement fixing antibodies bind with antigen and fix the complement for its lysis.

Neutralizing antibodies are those, which specifically neutralize/destroy the target /antigen; merely binding with antigen cannot be considered as neutralizing antibodies.

Immune Response

When the antigen enters the body of an animal is trapped, processed and eliminated by several cells, including macrophages, dendritic cells and B-cells. There are two types of antigen in body i.e. exogenous and endogenous. The exogenous or extracellular antigens are present freely in circulation and are readily available for antigen processing cells.

The endogenous or intracellular antigens are not free and are always inside the cells such as viruses. But when these viruses synthesize new viral proteins using biosynthetic process of the host cells, these proteins also act as antigen and are termed as endogenous or intracellular antigens.

The processing of antigen by macrophages is comparatively less efficient as most of the antigen is destroyed by the lysosomal proteases. An alternate pathway of antigen processing involves antigen uptake by a specialized population of mononuclear cells known as dendritic cells located throughout the body specially in lymphoid organs. Such dendritic cells have many long filamentous cytoplasmic processes called dendrits and lobulated nuclei with clear cytoplasm containing characteristic granules (Fig. 7.2).

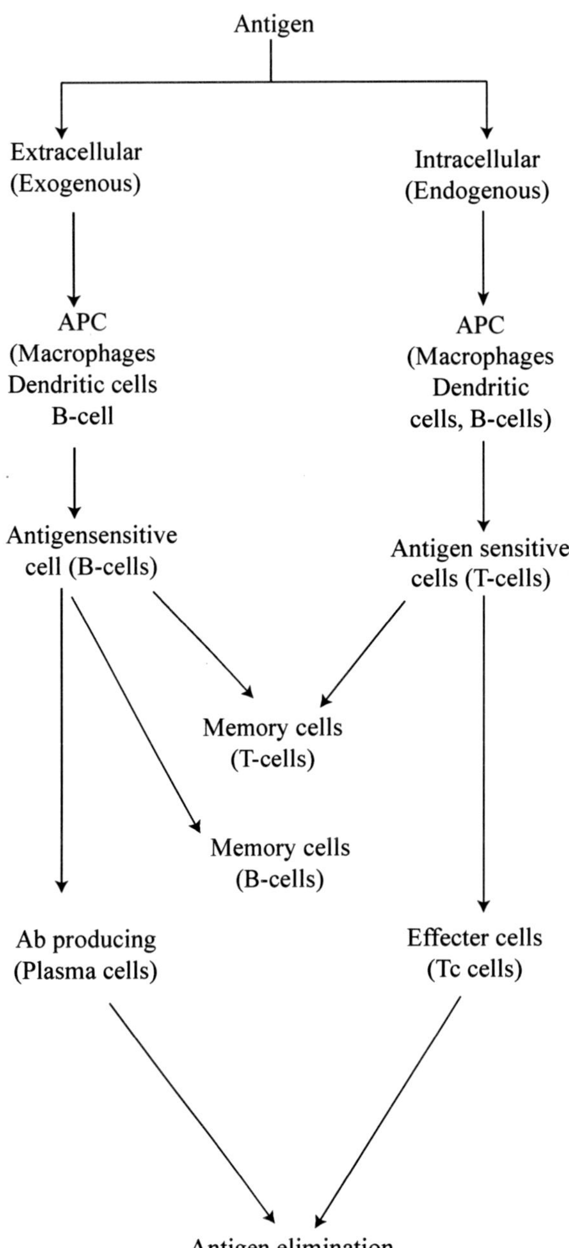
Antigen
Extracellular
(Exogenous)
Intracellular
(Endogenous)
APC
(Macrophages
Dendritic cells
B-cell
APC
(Macrophages
Dendritic
cells, B-cells)
Antigensensitive
cell (B-cells)
Antigen sensitive
cells (T-cells)
Memory cells
(T-cells)
Memory cells
(B-cells)
Ab producing
(Plasma cells)
Effecter cells
(Tc cells)
Antigen elimination

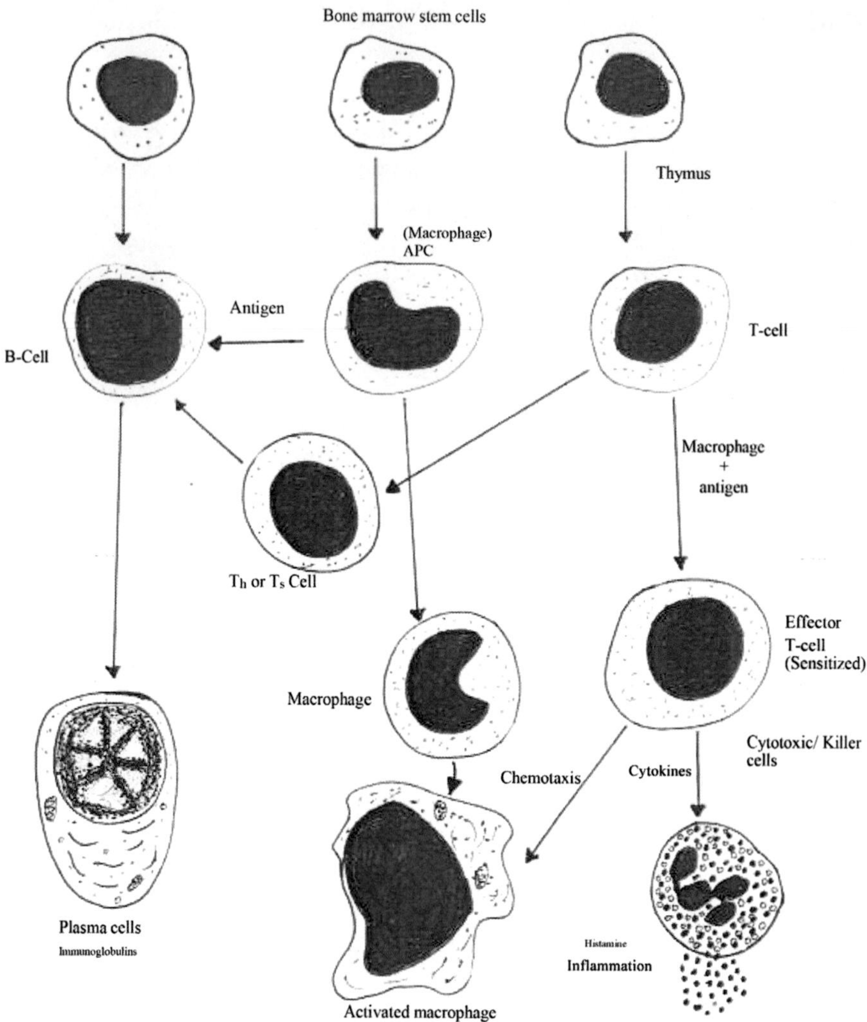

Fig. 7.2: Diagram showing mechanism of induction of immunity in body

Antigen presenting cells process the exogenous antigen and convert into fragments to bind with MHC class II molecules. Such processed antigen along with MHC class II molecule and certain cytokines such as IL-1 is presented to antigen recognizing cells (T-helper cells). Macrophages also regulate the dose of antigen to prevent inappropriate development of tolerance and provide a small dose of antigen to T- helper cells. However, if the antigen is presented to T-cells without MHC class II molecule, the T-cells are turned off resulting into tolerance. On an average, an antigen presenting cell possesses about $2x10^5$ MHC class II molecules. A T-cell requires activation by 200-300 peptide-

MHC class II molecules to trigger an immune response. Thus, it is estimated that an antigen-presenting cell may present several epitopes simultaneously to T-helper cells. A counterpart of T- helper cell also exists and is known as suppressor T-cell (T_s cell) which suppresses the immune response. The viral encoded proteins, endogenous antigens are handled in a different manner from exogenous antigens. Such antigens are bound to MHC class Ia molecules and transported to the cell surface. Such antigen and MHC class Ia molecule complex triggers a lymphocytic response i.e. T-cytotoxic cells (Tc-cells). These cytotoxic T-cells recognize and destroy virus infected cells. However, there is some cross priming leading to cell mediated immune response by exogenous antigens and humoral immune response by endogenous antigens. Some lymphocytes also function as memory cells to initiate secondary immune response.

On antigen exposure, there is a latent period of about four to six days and only after that serum antibodies are detectable. The peak of antibody titre is estimated around 2 weeks after exposure to antigen and then declines after about 3 weeks. During this primary immune response, majority antibodies are of IgM type whereas in secondary immune response, it is always predominated by IgG.

Immunopathology

Immunopathology includes the disorders of immune system characterized by increased response or hypersensitivity, response to self antigens (autoimmunity) and decreased responses (immunodeficiencies).

Hypersensitivity

It represents an accelerated immune response to an antigen (allergen), which is harmful to body rather than to provide protection or benefit to the body. Such violent reactions may lead to death. This condition is also known as allergy or atopy. The hypersensitive reactions can be classified into four classical forms including anaphylaxis (Type I), cytotoxic hypersensitivity (Type-II), Immune complex mediated hypersensitivity (Type III) and delayed type hypersensitivity (Type-IV) reaction.

Anaphylaxis or Type-I Hypersensitivity

Anaphylaxis or type I hypersensitivity reaction is rapidly developing immune response to an antigen characterized by humoral antibodies of IgE type (reagin). These reagins sensitize basophils/mast cells to release chemical mediators (Histamine, Serotonin, Prostaglandins, CFA for neutrophils and eosinophils) of inflammation leading to acute inflammatory reaction (Fig. 7.3).

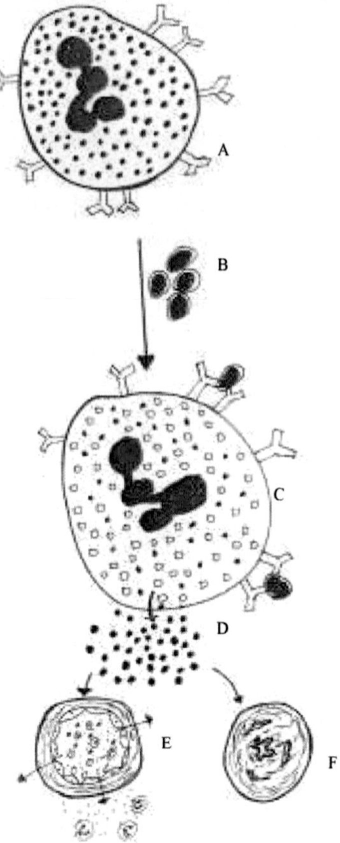

Fig. 7.3: Diagram showing IgE mediated Type-I hypersensitivity reaction **A.** Mast cell **B.** Allergen, **C.** Allergen binds with two IgE molecules **D.** Degranulation and release of histamine, serotonin, mediators of inflammation IL-2,3,4,5,6,7,13.,TN-α, LTB4, LTC4, PAF and PGD2 , **E.** Increased vascular permeability and **F.** Bronchoconstriction.

Etiology

Administration of drugs. Administration of serum. Bite of insects, bee etc.

Dust, pollens etc.

Macroscopic features

Bronchial asthma.

Wheel and flare reaction on skin.

Oedema, congestion, erythema, itching on skin.

Rhinitis.

Microscopic features

Congestion, pulmonary oedema, emphysema, constriction of bronchioles.

Oedema, congestion, haemorrhage on skin.

Cytotoxic or Type II Hypersensitivity Reaction

Cytotoxic reactions are characterized by lysis of cells due to antigen-antibody reaction on the surface of cells in the presence of complement.

Etiology/Occurrence

Blood transfusion. Hemolytic anemia.

Infections such as Equine infectious anemia, rickettsia, parasites (trypanosomiosis, babesiosis).

Thrombocytopenia.

Drugs such as penicillin, phenacetin, quinine cephalosporins.

Macroscopic features

Anemia. Jaundice.

Haemoglobinuria.

Microscopic features

Erythrophagocytosis.

Lysis of erythrocytes/agglutination of erythrocytes Hemolytic anemia (Fig. 7.4).

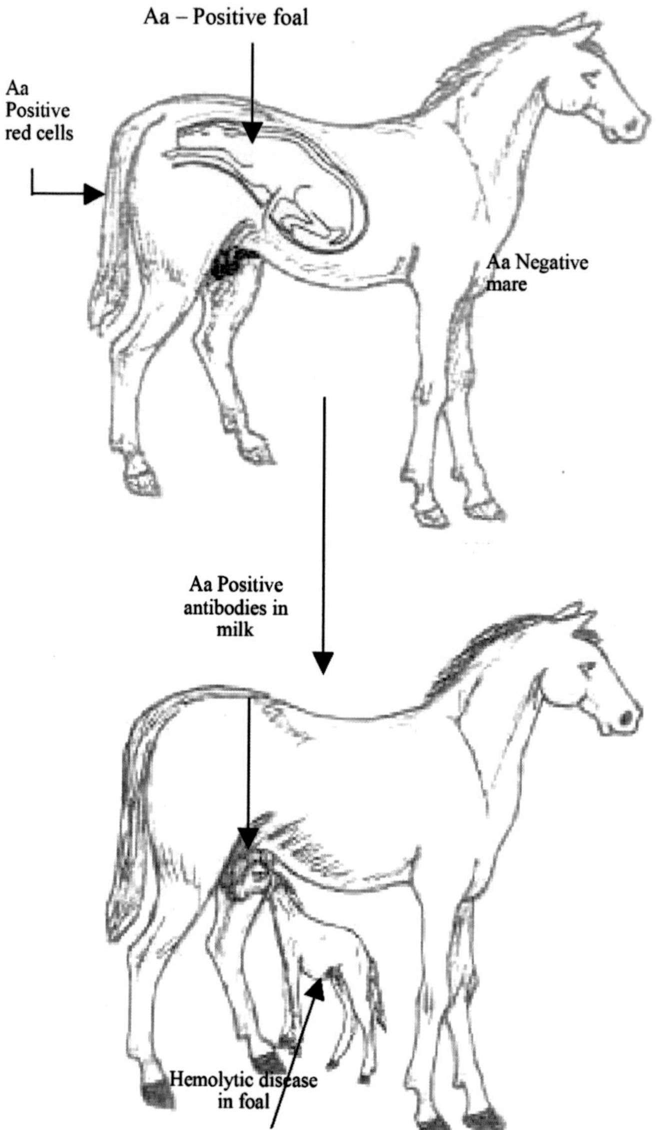

Fig. 7.4: Diagram showing type II hypersensitivity (hemolytic disease in foal)

Increased number of hemosiderin laden cells in spleen.

Immune Complex Mediated or Type-III Hypersensitivity Reaction

Type-III hypersensitivity reaction is characterized by the formation of immune complexes as a result of antigen-antibody reaction and their deposition in body tissues leading to inflammatory reaction (Fig. 7.5).

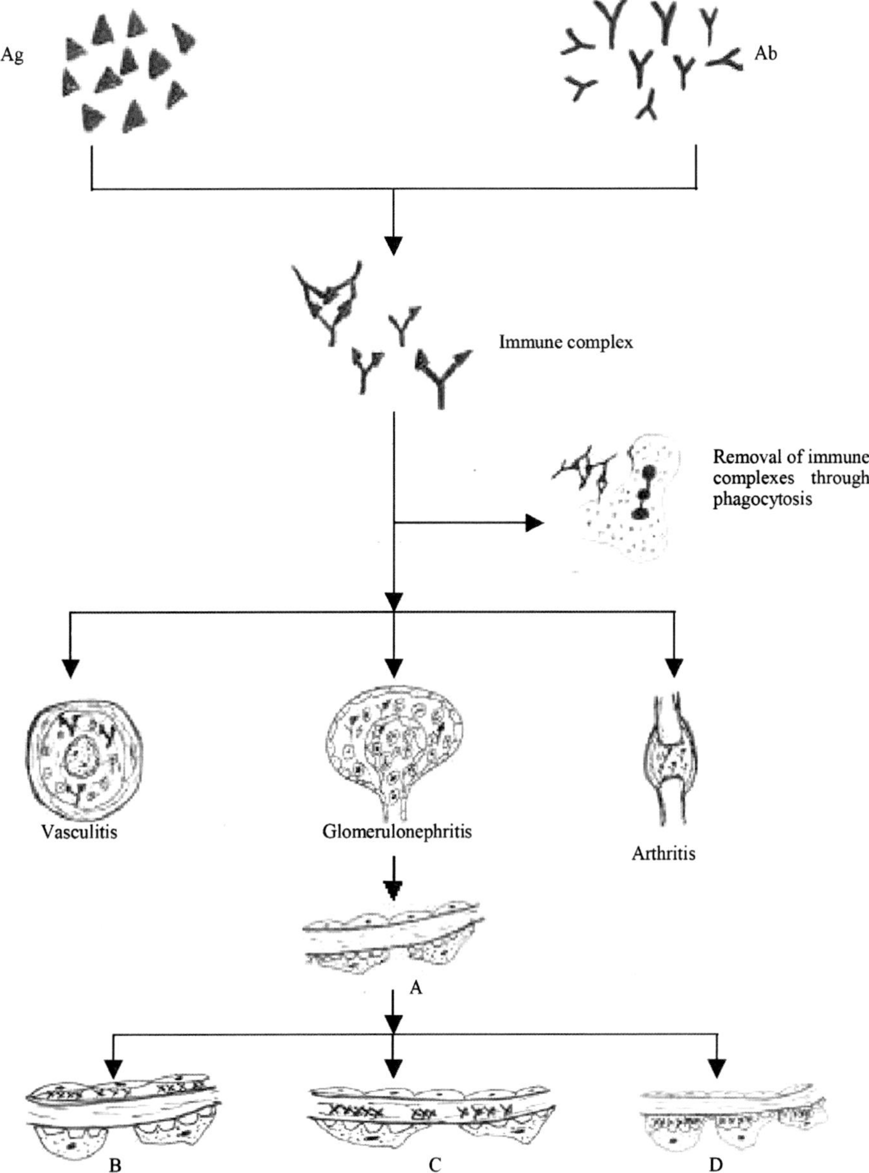

Fig. 7.5: Diagram showing Type-III hypersensitivity reaction. **A.** Normal architecture of glomeruli **B.** Type I, **C.** Type II and **D.** Type III Membrano proliferative glomerulonephritis (MPGN)

Etiology

Immunoglobulins.

Tumor antigens, nuclear antigens.

Environmental pollutants e.g. pesticides. Infections such as Leishmaniasis.

Macroscopic features

Arthus reaction is focal area of inflammation, necrosis at the site of infection.

Serum sickness is necrotizing vasculitis, endocarditis and glomerulonephritis.

Chronic immune complex disease is renal failure due to glomerulonephritis, vasculitis, chroiomeningitis and arthritis.

Microscopic features

Deposition of immune complexes in wall of blood vessels.

Deposition of immune complexes in glomeruli (Fig. 7.6).

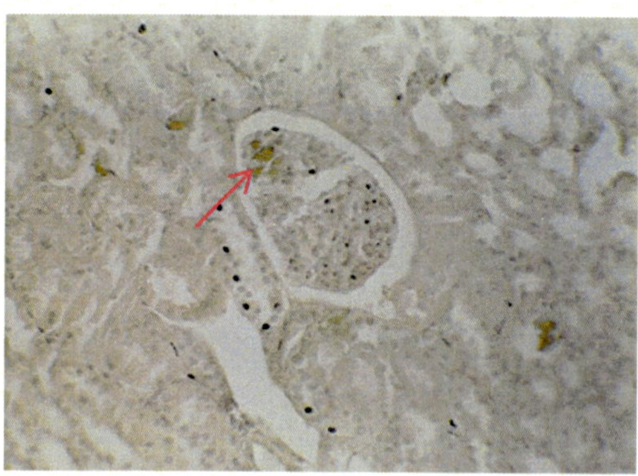

Fig. 7.6: Photomicrograph of immune complex mediated glomerulonephritis

Infiltration of inflammatory cells such as neutrophils, macrophages and lymphocytes.

Lesions of glomerulonephritis, polyarthritis.

Delayed Type Hypersensitivity (Dth) or Type IV Hypersensitivity Reaction

DTH reaction is mediated by sensitized T-lymphocytes and is the manifestation of cell-mediated immune response (Figs. 7.7 to 7.11).

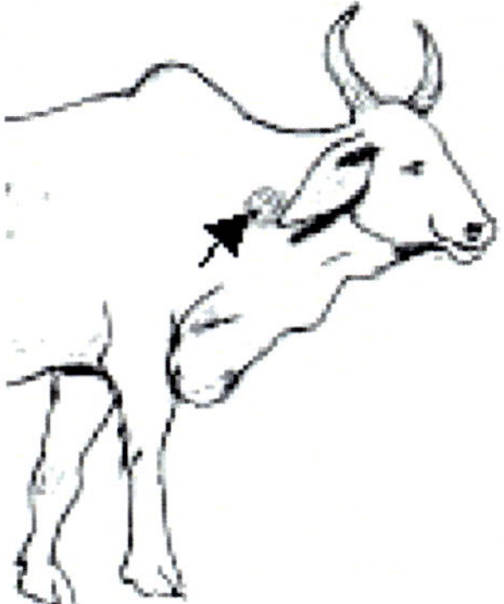

Fig. 7.7: Diagram showing of tuberculin reaction

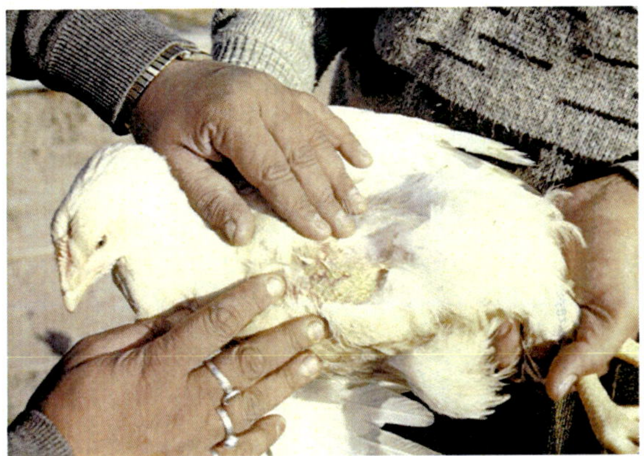

Fig. 7.8: Diagram showing DTH reaction of DNCB

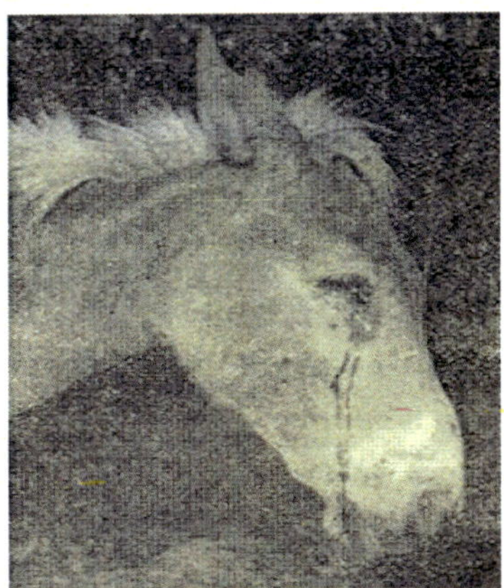

Fig. 7.9: Photograph showing mallein reaction

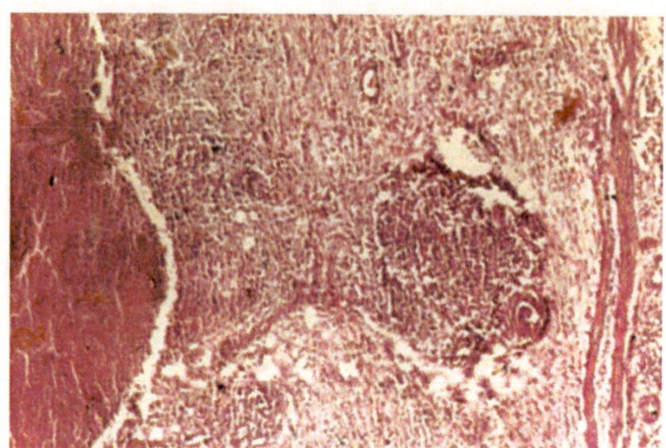

Fig. 7.10: Photomicrograph showing DTH reaction-lymphofollicular lesions

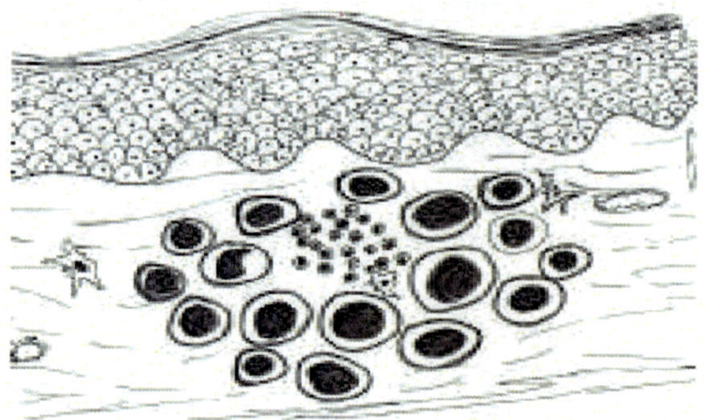

Fig. 7.11: Diagram showing microscopic picture of DTH reaction

Etiology

Tuberculin reaction.

Graft versus host reactions.

Granulomatous reaction.

Macroscopic

features

Formation of nodules, which are hard, painful to touch.

Rejection of transplants/grafts.

Microscopic

features

Heavy infiltrations of mononuclear cells

Particularly of T-lymphocytes macrophages.

Congestion and oedema.

Lymphocytic infiltration is more common around the blood vessels.

Lymphofollicular reaction.

Table 7.1: Differential features of various types of Hypersensitivity Reaction

	Anaphylaxis or Type-I Hypersensitivity Reaction	Cytotoxic or Type II Hypersensitivity Reaction	Immune Complex Mediated or Type-III Hypersensitivity Reaction	Delayed Type Hypersensitivity (DTH) or Type IV Hypersensitivity Reaction
Macrosc opic features	1. Bronchial asthma.	1. Anemia	1. Arthus reaction is focal area of inflammation, necrosis at the site of infection.	1. Formation of nodules, which are hard, painful to touch.
	2. Wheel and flare reaction on skin.	2. Jaundice	2. Serum sickness is necrotizing vasculitis, endocarditis and glomerulonephritis.	2. Rejection of transplants/ grafts.
	3. Oedema, congestion, erythema, itching on skin.	3. Haemoglobinuria	3. Chronic Immune complex disease is renal failure due to glomerulonephritis, vasculitis, chroiomeningitis and arthritis.	
	4. Rhinitis			
Microsc opic features	1. Congestion, pulmonary oedema, emphysema, constriction of bronchioles.	1. Erythrophago-cytosis	1. Deposition of immune complexes in wall of blood vessels.	1. Heavy infiltrations of mononuclear cells particularly of T- lymphocytes and macrophages.
	2. Oedema, congestion, haemorrhage on skin	2. Lysis of erythrocytes/ agglutination of erythrocytes.	2. Deposition of immune complexes in glomeruli	2. Congestion and oedema
		3. Increased number of hemosiderin laden cells in spleen.	3. Infiltration of inflammatory cells such as neutrophils, macrophages and lymphocytes.	3. Lymphocytic infiltration is more common around
			4. Lesions of glomerulonephritis, polyarthritis.	4. Lymphofollicular reaction.

Autoimmunity

In autoimmunity (auto=self) the immune response is generated against self antigens. It is an aberrant reaction that serves no useful purpose in body. Rather, the immunity developed against self antigens destroys the tissues of body and causes inflammation leading to death.

Etiology/Occurrence

Hidden antigens e.g. spermatozoa.

Alteration of antigens e.g. infections, mutations, chemicals bind with normal body proteins recognized as foreign (Fig. 7.12).

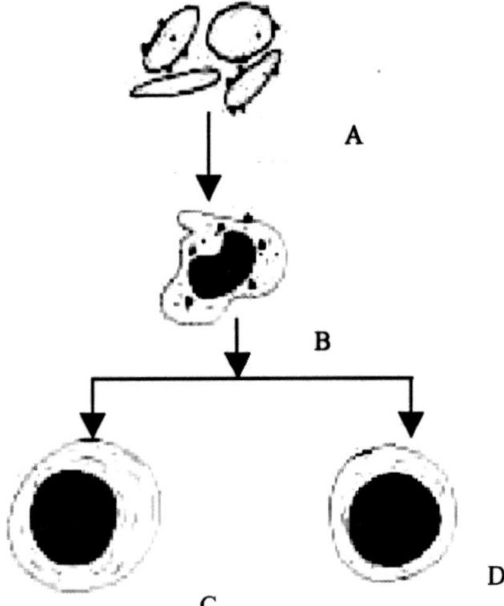

Fig. 7.12: Diagram Showing autoimmunity **A.** RBC showing presence of auto antigens **B.** Recognition of auto antigen by APC and their processing **C.** B-cells for antibody production and **D.** T-cells for cytotoxicity

Cross reaction between antigens of self and foreign nature.

Forbidden clones of immunocytes.

Macroscopic features

Autoimmune hemolytic anemia (Fig. 7.4).

Anti-glomerular basement membrane (GBM) nephritis.

Lymphocytic thyroditis.

Lupus erythematosus- antinuclear antibodies.

Microscopic features

Hemolytic anemia. Leukopenia.

Presence of antinuclear antibodies.

Infiltration of lymphocytes/ macrophages (Lymphocytic thryroditis).

In anti-GBM nephritis, there is immune complex mediated glomerulonephritis.

Immunodeficiency

The alterations in immune system, which decrease the effectiveness or destroy the capabilities of the system to respond to various antigens are designated as immunodeficiency. This precarious situation may be attributed to poorly developed immunocompetence or depressed immunity as a result of genetic and environmental factors.

Immunodeficiences are thus classified as congenital or primary and acquired or secondary.

Congenital immunodeficiency

In this type of immunodeficiency, the defect in immunity is genetically determined and is present in animals since their birth.

Etiology/Occurrence

Defect in basic cellular components e.g. stem cells.

Defective genes. Defect in enzymes.

Defective expression of cell components.

Types

Combined immunodeficiency syndrome (CIS)

Absence of stem cells of immunocytes. Agammaglobulinemia.

Absence of T and B cells in blood, leucopenia. Occurs due to autosomal recessive gene.

Aplasia or hypoplasia of thymus, lymphnodes, spleen.

Defects in T-lymphocytes

Thymic hypoplasia.

B-cells are normal and adequate amount of immunoglobulins present in blood.

Absence of T-dependent regions in lymphnodes.

In Danish cattle, exanthema, alopecia, parakeratosis occurs due to T-cell defect with A- 46 lethal trait gene.

Defects in B-lymphocytes

*I*n equines – equine agammaglobulinemia

Normal T-cell count, absence of B-cells, absence of all classes of immunoglobulins.

'X' linked defects in gene occurs in males.

Absence of primary lymphoid follicles in germinal centres in spleen and lymphnodes.

Selective IgA, IgM and IgG deficiency may also occur.

Transient hypogammaglobulinemia in new born calves.

Partial T and B cell defects

Partial presence of T and B lymphocytes. Recurrent infections, eczema, purpura.

Due to 'X' chromosome-linked genetic defect. Poor platelet aggregation.

Deficiency of complement

Rare, associated with abnormal regulation of immune responses leading to autoimmunity.

Complement component C_1 C_2 and C_3 are deficient and deficiency is associated with systemic lupus erythematosus, polyarteritis nodosa, glomerulonephritis, rheumatoid arthritis.

$C_{5,}$ $C_{6,}$ C_7 and C_8 deficiency leads to recurrent infections.

Absence or deficiency of C_3 makes animal susceptible to bacterial infections due to lack of opsonization, chemotaxis and phagocytosis.

Defects in phagocytosis

Neutropenia, leucopenia.

Defects in neutrophils, macrophages, platelets, melanocytes and eosinophils.

Defective chemotaxis, phagocytosis and bactericidal activity.

Persistent bacterial infections, pyogenic infections.

Associated with autosomal recessive gene defect and is also known as "Chediak Higashi syndrome".

Acquired or Secondary Immunodeficiency

An animal can acquire the suppression of immune system due to drugs, diseases, deficiency of nutrition, neoplasm or environmental pollution. This is clinically manifested by increased susceptibility to infections, vaccination failures, recurrent infections and occurrence of new diseases and neoplasms.

Etiology/ Occurrence

Drugs

Corticosteroids, azathioprines, alkalating agents, cyclophosphamide, cyclosporin A, antibiotics.

Azathioprines used to suppress graft rejection Cyclophosphamides and chlorambucil affect the DNA reduplication of T- and B-lymphocytes leading to immunosuppression with no affect on macrophages.

Cyclosporin A depresses CMI responses.

Aspirin decreases phagocytosis and lymphocyte functions.

Antibiotics like gentamicin, chloramphenicol, cephalosporin etc. cause decrease in immunity.

Infections

Bovine herpes virus-1 (BHV-1) decreases CD_4^+ and CD_8^+ cells in blood.

Equine herpes virus (EHV-1) causes reduction in T-cell functions.

Marek's disease virus acts as lymphocytolytic agent in lymphoid follicles of spleen, bursa and thymus.

Bovine viral diarrhoea virus reduces CD_4^+ and CD_8^+ T-lymphocytes, B-lymphocytes, neutrophils and IL- 2 in cattle.

Respiratory syncytial virus inhibits lymphoproliferative responses in sheep and cattle leading to increased susceptibility to

Pasteurella multocida infection.

Blue tongue virus infects CD_4^+ and CD_8^+ lymphocytes and causes their destruction.

Canine parvovirus causes depletion of lymphoid cells. Canine distemper virus activates the T-suppresser cells (T_s cells) leading to suppression of immunity.

Infectious bursal disease virus selectively affects B-lymphocytes leading to increased susceptibility of birds.

Infectious laryngotracheitis virus infects macrophages and causes their destruction.

Feline leukemia virus causes lymphoid depletion, glomerulonephritis, defects in macrophages and complement.

Feline immunodeficiency virus causes neutropenia, lymphopenia and inhibits the T-and B- cells' co-operation.

Bovine immunodeficiency virus replicates in macrophages and CD_4^+ lymphocytes leading to their destruction and immunosuppression. It also causes lymphadenopathy, lymphocytolysis, reduction in lymphokine production.

Trauma/surgery

Trauma or surgical interventions reduce specific immune responses and functional capacity of phagocytic cells.

Such defects are transient and may reverse after healing of trauma/ surgery.

Surgical operation/trauma increases the number of T- suppressor cells (T_s cells), which in turn depresses the immunity.

Environmental pollution (Fig. 7.13 to 7.16)

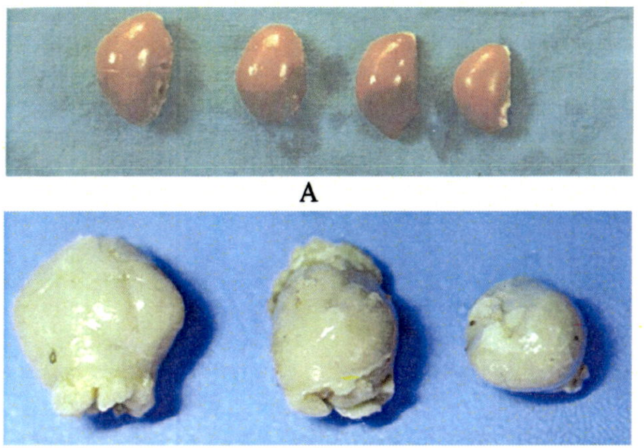

Fig. 7.13: Photograph showing atrophy of lymphoid organs due to **A.** Pesticide and **B.** heavy metals in birds

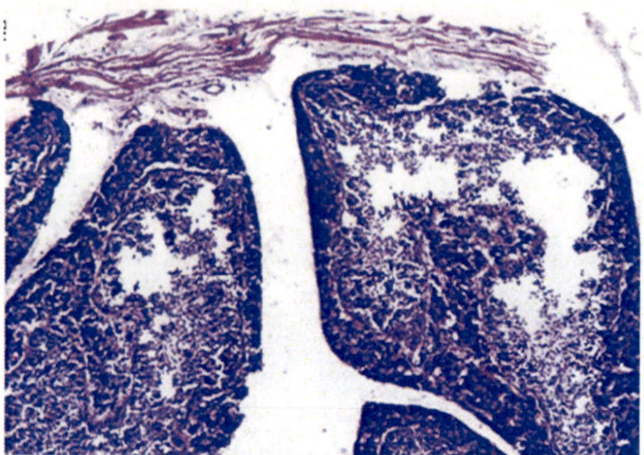

Fig. 7.14: Photomicrograph of bursa showing depletion of lymphoid tissue

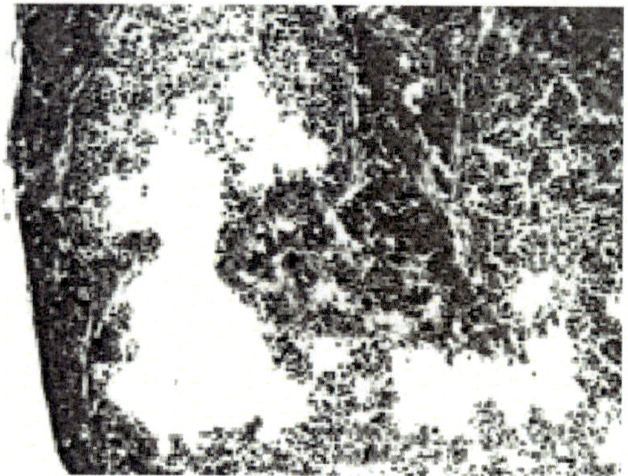

Fig. 7.15: Photomicrograph of thymus showing depletion of lymphoid tissue

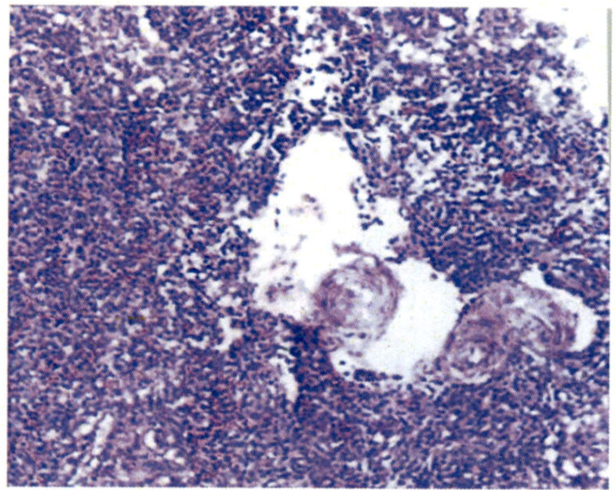

Fig. 7.16: Photomicrograph of spleen showing depletion of lymphoid tissue

Pesticides used in agriculture, animal husbandry and public health operations remain in ecosystem and food items for longer period and enter in body of animals and man through food, air, water and affect the immune system leading to its depression and increased susceptibility to infections.

Heavy metals are common contaminants of pesticides, fertilizers and are inadvertently accumulated in soil, plant, water, which enters directly or indirectly in the animal's body. These heavy metals (lead, mercury, cadmium) may exert their immunotoxic effects leading to immunosuppression.

Mycotoxins such as aflatoxin, ochratoxin, zearalenone etc. also affect the immune system of animals leading to its suppression resulting increased susceptibility to infectious diseases.

8

Disturbances in Calcification and Pigment Metabolism

Calcification

Calcification is the deposition of calcium phosphates and calcium carbonates in soft tissues other than bones and teeth. It may be classified as dystrophic and metastatic calcification.

Dystrophic Calcification

Dystrophic calcification is characterized by the deposits of calcium salts in necrosed tissue of any organ (Fig 8.1).

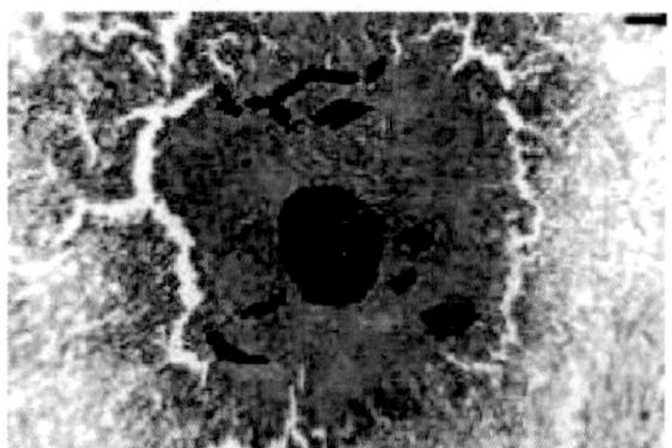

Fig. 8.1: Photomicrograph of lung showing dystrophic calcification in tuberculous granuloma

Etiology /Occurrence

- Necrosis.
- Parasitic infections.
- Tuberculous lesions.

Macroscopic features

- Organ becomes hard, nodular.
- Grey/white deposits in necrosed tissue looking like honey comb.
- Gritty sound on cutting.

Microscopic features

- Irregular deposits of calcium salts in necrosed tissue.
- Calcium takes black/purplish colour on H & E staining.

Metastatic Calcification

Metastatic calcification is characterized by deposition of calcium salts in soft tissue as a result of hypercalcemia (Fig. 8.2).

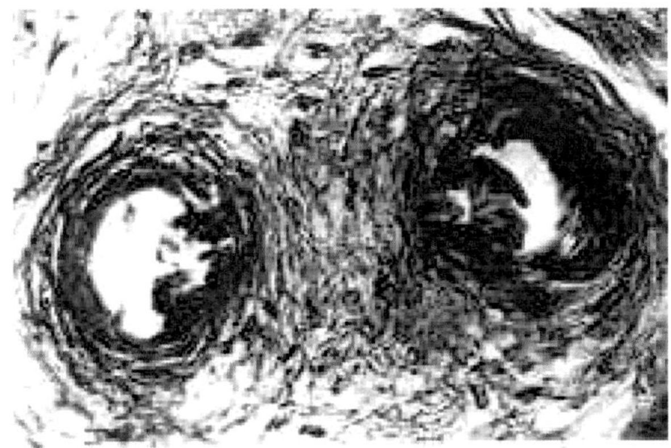

Fig. 8.2: Photomicrograph of arteries showing metastatic calcification

Etiology/ Occurrence

- Hyperparathyroidism.
- Renal failure.
- Excess of vitamin-D.
- Increased calcium intake.

Macroscopic features

- Organ becomes hard.
- Wall of arteries becomes hard due to calcium deposits.

Microscopic features

- Deposition of calcium in soft organs like myocardium, arteries, muscles, etc.
- Purplish/black colour calcium surrounded by comparatively normal tissue.

Melanosis

Melanosis is the deposition of melanin, a brown/ black pigments in various tissues/ organs specially in lung, blood vessels and brain (Figs. 8.3 to 8.5).

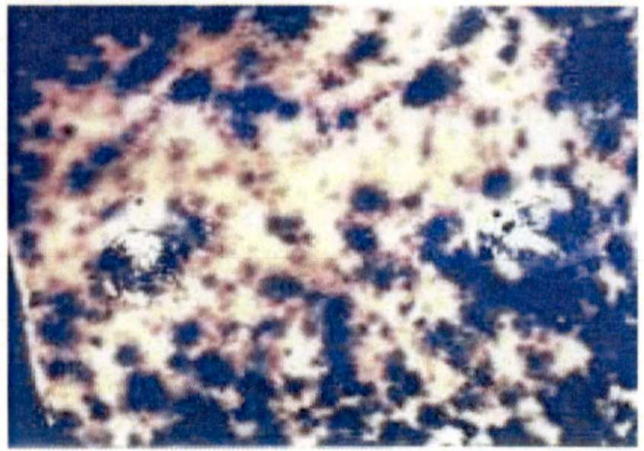

Fig. 8.3: Photograph showing melanosis

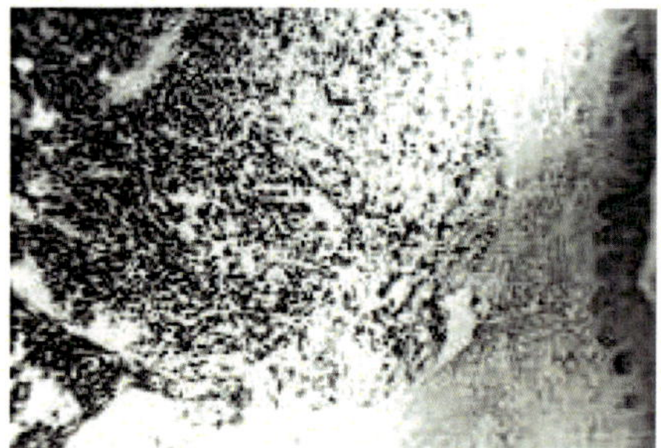

Fig. 8.4: Photomicrograph of skin showing melanosis

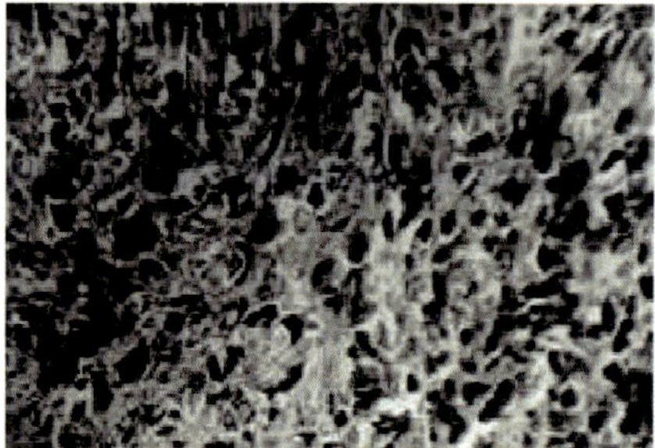

Fig. 8.5: Photomicrograph of skin showing melanosis.

Etiology/Occurrence

- Hyperadrenalism.
- Melanosarcoma.
- Melanoma.

Macroscopic features

- Organ/tissue involved becomes black in colour.
- Discolouration may be focal or diffused.

Microscopic features

- Brown/black colour pigment is seen in cells.
- The size, shape and amount of pigment vary.

Hemosiderosis

Hemosiderosis is characterized by deposition of hemosiderin pigment in spleen and other organs. Hemosiderin is a blood pigment with a shiny golden yellow colour and is usually found within the macrophages (Fig. 8.6).

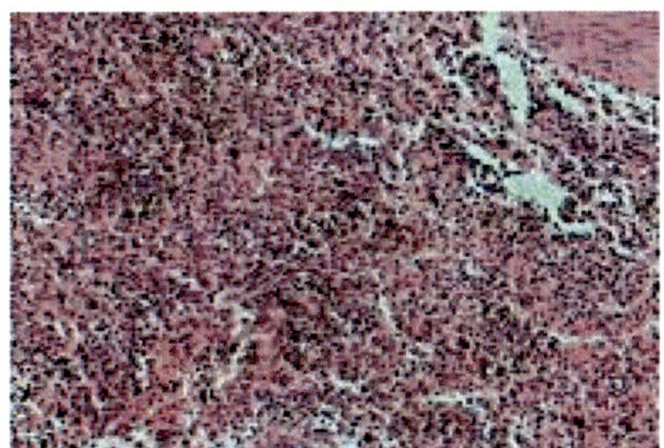

Fig. 8.6: Photomicrograph of spleen showing hemosiderosis

Etiology/ Occurrence

- Extensive lysis of erythrocytes.
- Haemorrhage.
- Hemolytic anemia.

Macroscopic features

- Colour of organ becomes brownish.
- Brown induration of lungs.

Microscopic features

- Presence of golden yellow/golden brown pigment in red pulp of spleen, lungs, liver and kidneys.
- In most of the cases, the pigment is found intracellularly in macrophages.

Bile Pigments

Bile pigments are derived from the breakdown of erythrocytes such as bilirubin and biliverdin. The icterus is hyperbilirubinemia as a result of either excessive lysis of erythrocytes or due to damage in liver or obstruction in the bile duct. The hemolysis results in iron, globin and porphyin; the latter being converted into biliverdin. Biliverdin is reduced to produce bilirubin, an orange-yellow pigment bound to albumin and transported by RE cells to liver. In hepatic cells, it is separated from albumin and conjugated with glucuronic acid and excreted in bile as bilirubin diglucuronide. In intestine, it is further reduced by bacteria to urobilinogen, which is reabsorbed into circulation and carried to liver for re-excretion in bile while a small amount enters in circulation and is excreted through urine. The unabsorbed urobilinogen is oxidized in lower intestine to form urobilin and stercobilin, which give normal pigment to faeces.

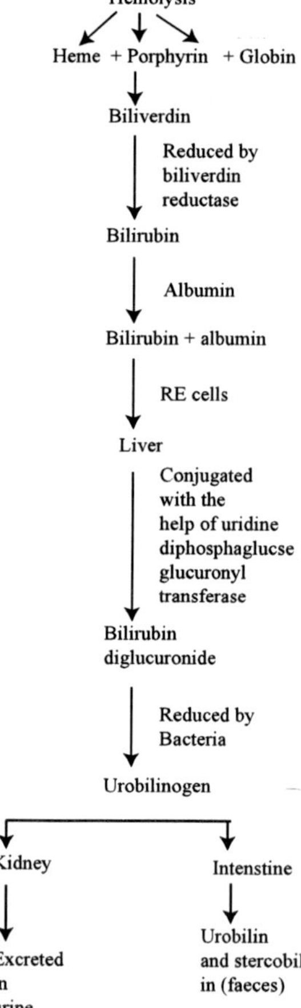

Icterus

Icterus is increased amount of bile pigments in blood and is often called as hyper- bilirubinemia or jaundice. It is of three types hemolytic, toxic and obstructive jaundice.

Hemolytic Jaundice

Hemolytic jaundice occurs as a result of excessive hemolysis in circulating blood. It is also known as pre-hepatic jaundice.

Etiology/ Occurrence

- Piroplasmosis (*Babesia bigemina*).
- Anaplasmosis (*Anaplasma marginale*).
- Leptospirosis (*Leptospira ictehaemmorrhagae*).
- Equine infectious anemia virus.
- Anthrax (*Bacillus anthracis*).
- Clostriduum hemolyticum.
- β- haemolytic streptococci.

Toxic Jaundice

Toxic jaundice occurs as a result of damage in liver leading to increased amount of unconjugated and conjugated bilirubin in blood. It is also known as hepatic jaundice.

Etiology

- Toxin/Poisons.
- Copper poisoning.
- Leptospirosis.

Obstructive Jaundice

Obstructive jaundice occurs as a result of obstruction in bile duct causing hindrance in normal flow of bile. It is also known as post-hepatic jundice.

Etiology

- Blocking of bile canaliculi by swollen hepatocytes
- Obstruction in bile duct (Liver flukes, tapeworms and ascaris).

- Biliary cirrhosis, Cholangitis and Cholelithiasis.
- Pressure on bile duct due to abscess, neoplasm.
- Inflammation and swelling at duct opening in duodenum.

Macroscopic features

- Mucous membrane yellow in colour.
- Omentum, mesentry, fat become yellow.
- Increased yellow colour in urine.
- Conjunctiva becomes yellow.

Microscopic features

- Brownish pigment in tubules of kidney.
- Bile pigments in spleen.
- Hemolysis, erythrophagocytosis.
- Hepatitis.

Diagnosis

- Van-den-Bergh reaction.
- Direct reaction detects bilirubin diglucuronide (Obstructive jaundice).
- Indirect reaction detects hemobilirubin (Hemolytic jaundice).
- Both reaction (Toxic jaundice).

Table 8.1: Differential features of various types of Jaundice

	Hemolytic (Prehepatic)	**Toxic (Hepatic)**	**Obstructive (Post hepatic)**
Etiology	1. Piroplasmosis (Babesia bigemina)	1. Toxin/Poisons 2. Copper poisoning	1. Blocking of bile canaliculi by swollen hepatocytes
	2. Anaplasmosis (Anaplasma marginale)	2. Copper	2. Obstruction in bile duct (Liver flukes, tapeworms and ascaris)
	3. Leptospirosis (Leptospira ictehaemmorrhagae)	3. Leptospirosis	3. Biliary cirrhosis, Cholangitis and Cholelithiasis
	4. Equine infectious anemia virus		4. Pressure on bile duct due to abscess, neoplasm.
	5. Anthrax (Bacillus anthracis)		5. Inflammation and swelling at duct opening in duodenum.

	Hemolytic (Prehepatic)	**Toxic (Hepatic)**	**Obstructive (Post hepatic)**
	6. Clostriduum hemolyticum		
	7. β- haemolytic streptococci		
Vanden Berg's Reaction Direct Indirect	Negative Positive	Positive Positive	Positive Negative

Table 8.2: Vanden Berg's reaction

	Type of reaction	**Type of jaundice**	**Type of Pigment**
1.	Direct reaction (+)	Obstructive	Cholibilirubin
2.	Indirect reaction (+)	Hemolytic	Hemobilirubin
3.	Biphasic reaction (+)	Toxic/Hepato-cellular	Both present

Pneumoconiasis

Pneumoconiasis is the deposition of dust/carbon particles in lungs through air inhalation. It is also known as anthracosis (carbon), silicosis (silica) or asbestoses (asbestos) (Fig 8.7).

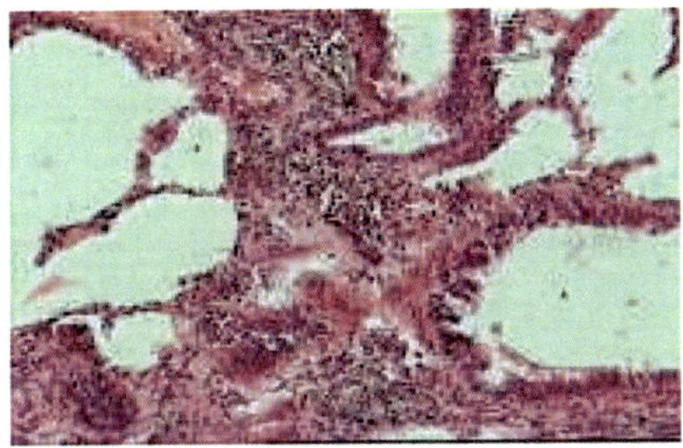

Fig. 8.7: Photomicrograph of lung showing pneumoconiasis

Etiology/ Occurrence

- Dusty air containing carbon/silica/asbestos
- Near factory/coal mines.

Macroscopic features

- Hard nodules in lungs.
- Nodules may have black /brown /grey colour
- Nodules may produce cracking sounds on cut.

Microscopic features

- Presence of carbon/other exogenous pigment in intercellular spaces or in cytoplasm of alveolar cells and macrophages.
- Formation of granuloma around the foreign particles including the infiltration of macrophages, lymphocytes, giant cells and fibrous tissue proliferation.

Crystals

Deposition of different kinds of crystals in tissues like uric acid, sulfonamides and oxalates etc. The uric acid and urates when deposited in tissues are known as gout.

Gout (Urates & Uric Acids)

Gout is a disease condition in which urates and uric acid are deposited in tissues and is characterized by intense pain and acute inflammation (Figs. 8.8 to 8.10).

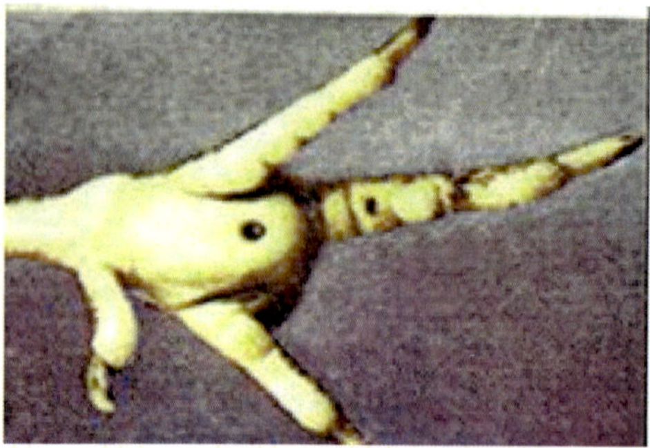

Fig. 8.8: Photograph of foot pad of a bird showing gout

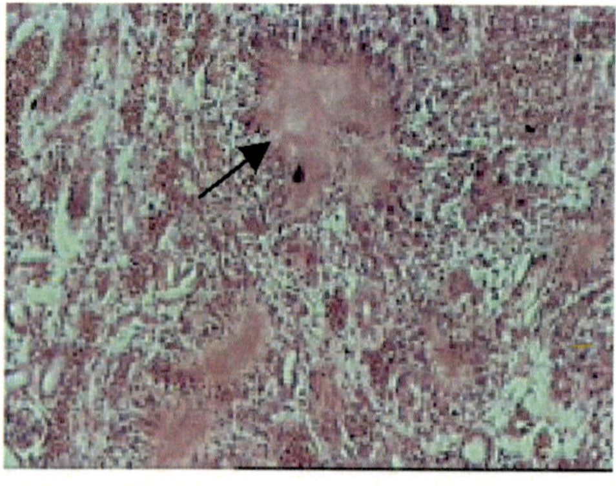

Fig. 8.9: Photomicrograph of kidney showing urates (gout)

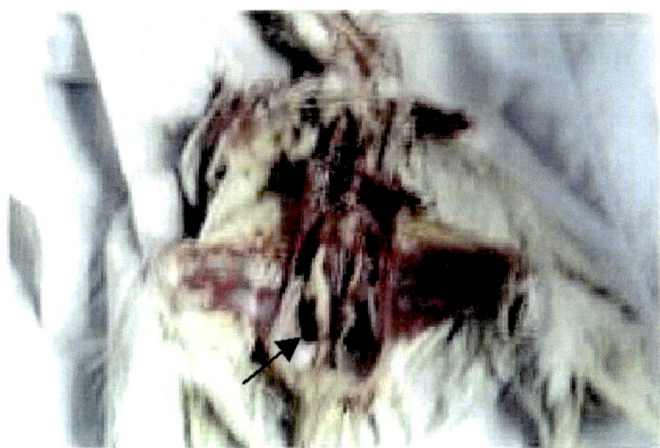

Fig. 8.10: Photograph of a bird showing deposition of urates and uric acid in ureter (gout)

Etiology/Occurrence

- Common in poultry due to deficiency of uricase enzyme.
- Deficiency of vitamin A.
- Absence or inadequate amount of uricase.

Macroscopic features

- White chalky mass of urates and uric acid.
- Deposition of urates/uric acid on pericardium, kidneys etc.
- Dialation of ureter due to excessive accumulation of urates.

Microscopic features

- Presence of sharp crystals in tissue.
- Crystals are surrounded by inflammatory cells including macrophages, giant cells and lymphocytes.

9

Disturbances in Growth

Aplasia/Agenesis

Aplasia or agenesis is absence of any organ (Fig. 9.1).

Hypoplasia

Hypoplasia is failure of an organ/tissue to attain its full size (Fig. 9.1).

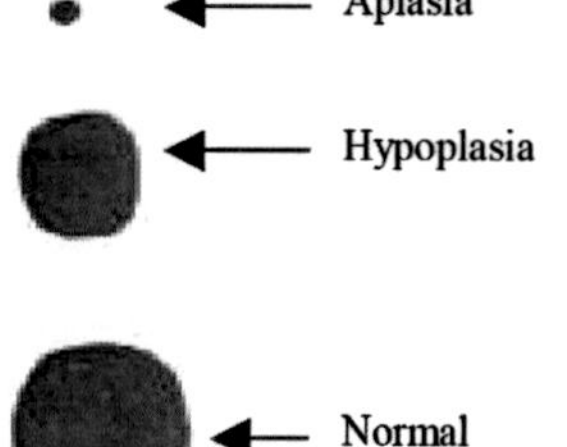

Fig. 9.1: Diagram showing Aplasia and Hypoplasia

Etiology

- Congenital anomalies e.g. hypoplasia of kidneys in calves.
- Inadequate innervation.
- Inadequate blood supply.
- Malnutrition.
- Infections e.g. cerebral hypoplasia in bovine viral diarrhoea.

Macroscopic features

- Organ size, weight, volume reduced

Microscopic features

- Reduced size of cells.

- Reduced number of cells.
- Connective tissue and fat is more.

Atrophy

Atrophy is decrease in size of an organ that has reached its full size (Figs. 9.2 & 9.3).

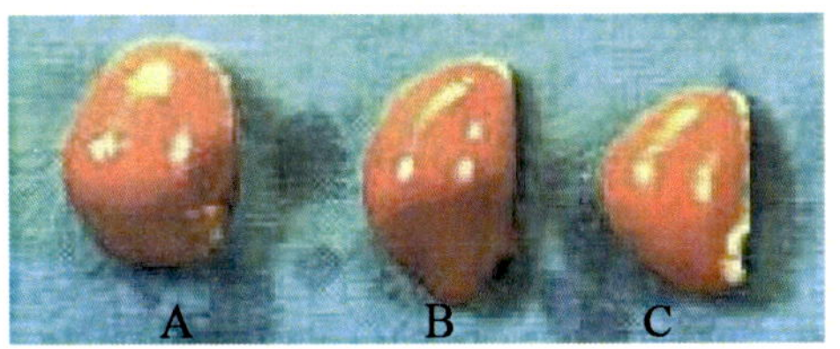

Fig. 9.2: Photograph of spleen showing atrophy (c)

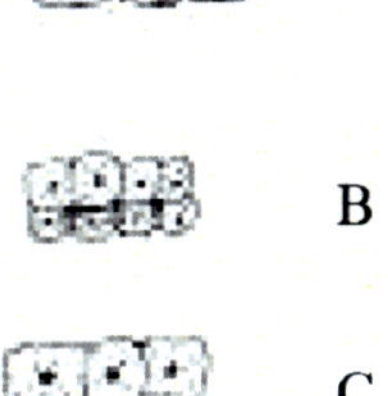

Fig. 9.3: Diagram showing atrophy (a) normal (b) decrease in size and (c) decrease in number of cells

Etiology

- Physiological e.g. senile atrophy.
- Pressure atrophy.
- Disuse atrophy e.g. atrophy of immobilized legs.
- Endocrine atrophy e.g. atrophy of testicles.
- Environmental pollution e.g. atrophy of lymphoid organs.
- Inflammation/ fibrosis.

Macroscopic features

- Size, weight, volume of organ decreased.

- Wrinkles in capsule of organ.

Microscopic features

- Size of cell is smaller.
- Cell number is less.
- Fat and connective tissue cells are more.

Hypertrophy

Hypertrophy is increase in size of cells leading to increase in size of organ/ tissue without increase in the number of cells (Fig. 9.4).

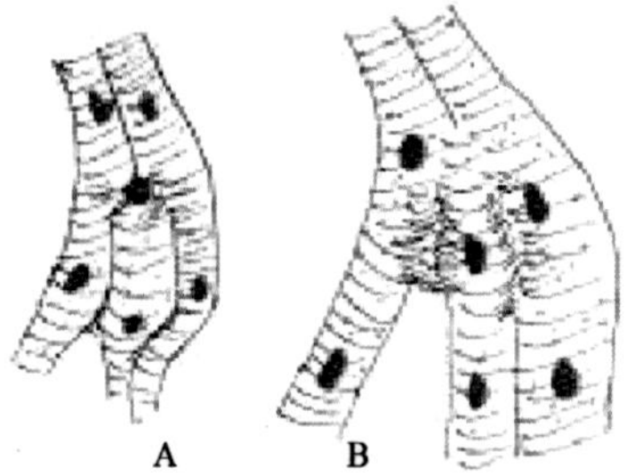

Fig. 9.4: Diagram showing hypertrophy (a) Normal (b) Hypertrophy

Etiology

- Increase in metabolic activity e.g. myometrium during pregnancy.
- Compensatory e.g. if one kidney is removed, another becomes hypertrophied due to compensatory effect.

Macroscopic features

- Organ becomes large in size.
- Organ weight increases.

Microscopic features

- Size of cells increases.

Hyperplasia

Hyperplasia is increase in number of cells leading to increase in size of organ/ tissue (Fig. 9.5).

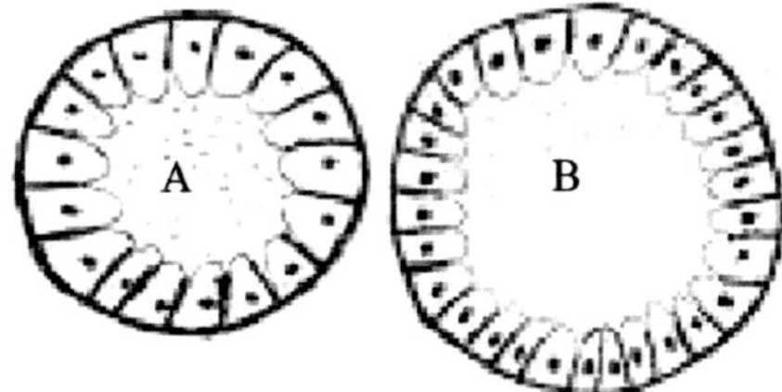

Fig. 9.5: Diagram showing hyperplasia (a) Normal (b) hyperplasia

Etiology

- Prolonged irritation e.g. fibrosis/nodules in hands, pads.
- Nutritional disorders e.g. iodine deficiency.
- Infections e.g. pox.
- Endocrine disorders e.g. prostate hyperplasia.

Macroscopic features

- Increase in size, weight of organ.
- Nodular enlargement of organ.

Microscopic features

- Increased number of cells.
- Displacement of adjacent tissue.
- Lumen of ducts/ tubules obstructed.

Metaplasia

Metaplasia is defined as transformation of one type of cells to another type of cells (Fig. 9.6 & 9.7).

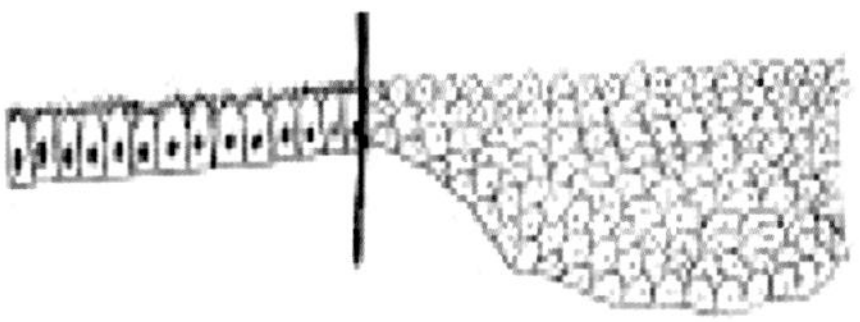

Fig. 9.6: Diagram showing Metaplasia

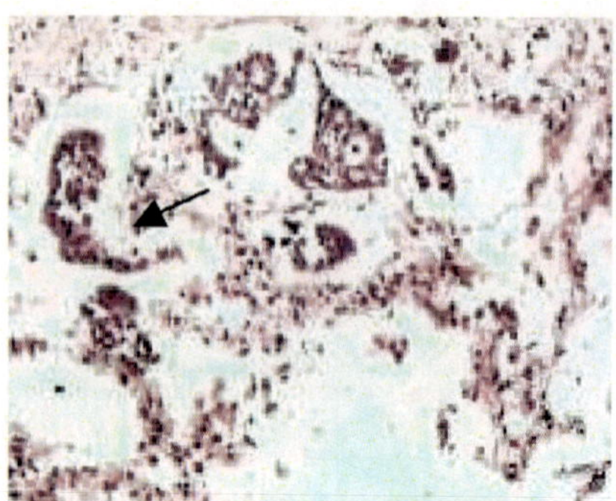

Fig. 9.7: Photograph showing Metaplasia

Etiology

- Prolonged irritation e.g. gall stones cause metaplasia of columnar cells to stratified squamous epithelial cells in wall of gall bladder.
- Endocrine disturbances e.g. in dog, columnar epithelium of prostate changes into squamous epithelium.
- Nutritional deficiency e.g. nutritional roup. In poultry, cuboidal/ columnar epithelium of oesophageal glands change into stratified squamous epithelium.
- Infections e.g. pulmonary adenomatosis

Macroscopic features

- Mucous membrane becomes dry in squamous metaplasia.
- Presence of nodular glands on oesophageal mucous membrane due to vitamin A deficiency in chickens also known as Nutritional roup.

Microscopic features

- Change of one type of cells to another type.
- In place of columnar cells, there are squamous epithelial cells.
- In place of endothelial cells, cuboidal or columnar cells in alveoli giving it glandular shape. e.g. pulmonary adenomatosis.

Anaplasia

Anaplasia is defined as reversion of cells to a more embryonic and less differentiated type. It is a feature in neoplasia. Neoplasia is uncontrolled new growth that serves no useful purpose, has no orderly structural arrangement and is undifferentiated or less differentiated in nature with more embryonic characters of the cells (Fig. 9.8 and 9.9).

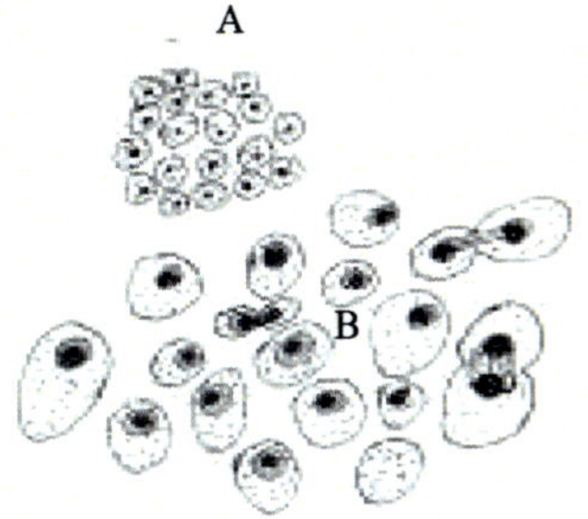

Fig. 9.8: Diagram showing anaplasia (a) Normal (b) Anaplastic cells

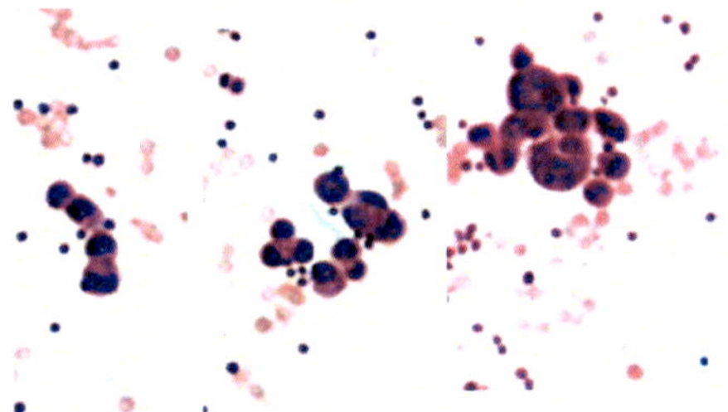

Fig. 9.9: FNAC of peritoneal fluid showing anaplastic cells

Etiology

- Chemicals.
- Radiation.
- Viruses e.g. oncogenic viruses.

Macroscopic features

- Enlargement of organ/ tissue.
- Nodular growth of tissue, hard to touch.

Microscopic features

- Presence of pleomorphic cells and less or undifferentiated cells.
- **Hyperchromasia.**
- Size of cells increases.
- Size of nucleus and nucleolus increases.

- Presence of many mitotic figures.
- Seen in neoplastic conditions.

Dysplasia

Abnormal development of cells/tissues which are improperly arranged. It is the malformation of tissue during maturation (Fig. 9.10).

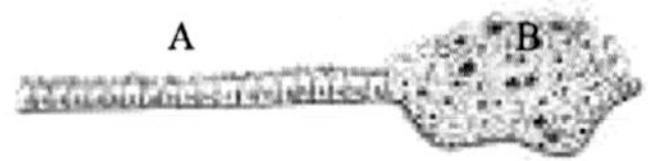

Fig. 9.10: Diagram showing dysplasia (a). Normal (b) Dysplasia

1. Spermatozoa head and tailpiece are structurally abnormal or aligned in improper way.
2. Fibrous dysplasia in bones.
3. In gastrointestinal tract, disruption of cellular orientation, variation in size and shape of cells, increase in nuclear and cytoplasmic ratio and increased mitotic activity.

10

Concretions

Concretions

Concretions are solid, compact mass of material, endogenous or exogenous in origin, found in tissues, body cavities, ducts or in hollow organs. Concretions are stone-like bodies commonly occur in urinary system, gall bladder and gastrointestinal tract. Concretions of endogenous origin are known as calculi while those formed from exogenous material are known as piliconcretion (Hair), phytoconcretion (plant fibres) and polyconcretion (polythenes).

Calculi

Calculi are formed due to deposition of salts around the nucleus/nidus consisting of either fibrin, mucus, desquamated epithelial cells or clumps of bacteria. Due to the gradual and repeated precipitation of salts, calculi become laminated. In the process of calculi formation, the inner structural arrangement gets shrink, producing a rough superficial surface. Calculi formation is more common in urinary system and in gall bladder of man and animals; however, they may also occur in salivary gland, pancreas and intestines.

Urinary Calculi

Urinary calculi are formed in renal tubules, pelvis or in urinary bladder which may be carried away by urine and may cause obstruction in ureter or urethra. Urinary calculi is also known as urolith and the process of formation of calculi is termed as urolithiasis (Figs. 10.1 & 10.2).

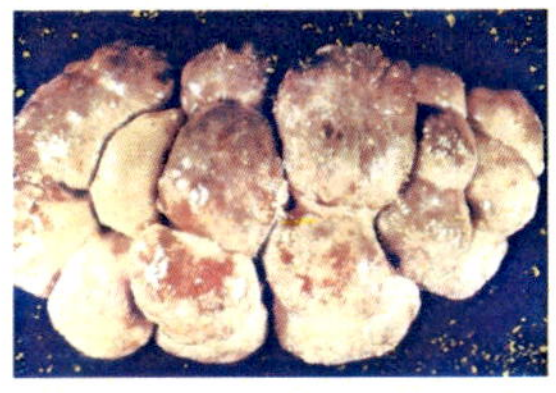

A

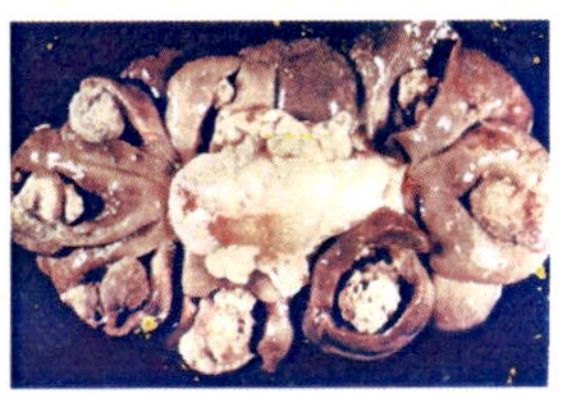

B

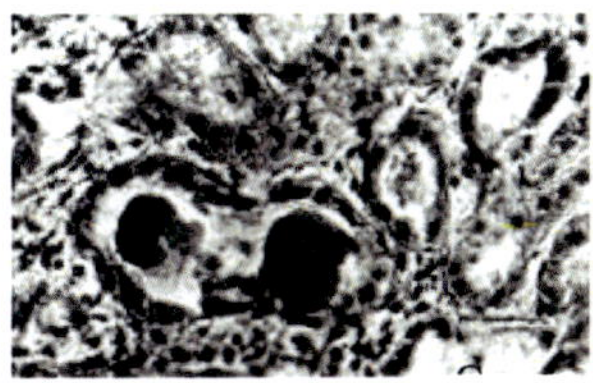

C

Fig. 10.1. Photograph of kidney of bullock showing presence of calculi **A.** Gross intact kidney **B.** Cross section of kidney and **C.** Microscopic structure of kidney having concretion.

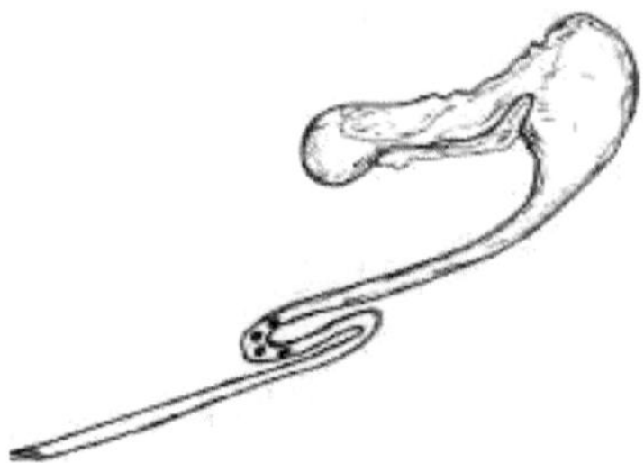

Fig. 10.2: Diagram showing predilection site of calculi in sigmoid flexure of urethra in bullocks

Etiology

- Vit A deficiency.
- Bacterial infection e.g. E. coli, Micrococci, Streptococci.
- Sulfonamide therapy.
- Hormonal therapy.
- Hyperparathyroidism.

Macroscopic features

- May vary in size from 1 mm to several mm.
- Mostly rounded, pearl-like, laminated.
- Brown, grey and yellowish in colour.
- Enlargement and fibrosis of kidneys.

Microscopic features

- In kidney sections tiny, laminated bodies of concretion.
- Hydronephrosis.
- Chemical composition of urinary calculi may vary in various species of animals.
- Horse:- Calcium carbonate, calcium phosphate, magnesium carbonate.
- Ruminants:- Calcium phosphate, magnesium phosphate, aluminium phosphate, calcium oxalate.
- Pigs:- Ammonium phosphate, magnesium phosphate, calcium carbonate, magnesium carbonate, magnesium phosphate, magnesium oxalate.

- Dogs:- Calcium carbonate, calcium phosphate, sodium urate, ammonium urate.

Biliary Calculi

Biliary calculi are formed in gall bladder and bile ducts and are also known as cholelith. These are common in man; however, in cattle and pigs gall stones are also seen. They are semisolids but become hard and brittle on drying.

Etiology

- Bacteria.
- Sand particles.
- Particles of ingesta / intestinal contents.
- Desquamated epithelium.

Macroscopic features

- In gall bladder and bile duct.
- 1 mm to 3-4 cm in diameter.
- Numbers vary from 1 to many.
- Obstructive jaundice.
- Cholecystitis and cholangitis.

Microscopic features

- In sections, concentric layers of cholesterin, bilirubin, calcium carbonate and coagulated material.
- Cholecystitis, cholangitis.

Salivary Calculi

Salivary calculi are formed in excretory ducts of the parotid, sublingual and submaxillary salivary glands. Size of such calculi vary upto 25-30 mm diameter. They are made up of salts like calcium carbonate, calcium phosphate, magnesium carbonate, sodium carbonate, around the plant fibres. Salivary calculi also known as sialolith.

Pancreatic Calculi

Pancreatic calculi or pancrealolith are rare in occurrence in animals but may be found in cattle. Pancreatic calculi are grey in colour with size up to few centimeter. They are made up of calcium carbonate, calcium oxalate and calcium phosphate around a nidus of cholesterol or fatty acids.

Enteric Calculi

Enteric calculi or enterolith are common in horses, and occur mostly in large intestine 'colon'. In horse, a nidus is surrounded by wheat and rye bran containing magnesium phosphate. The nidus may be a piece of metal or sand on which concentric layers are deposited. They may look like a ball of round or oval in shape (Fig. 10.3). Colour of enterolith may vary from greyish to dark brown. In dogs, bone in diet may provide a nidus and such concretions are known as coproliths.

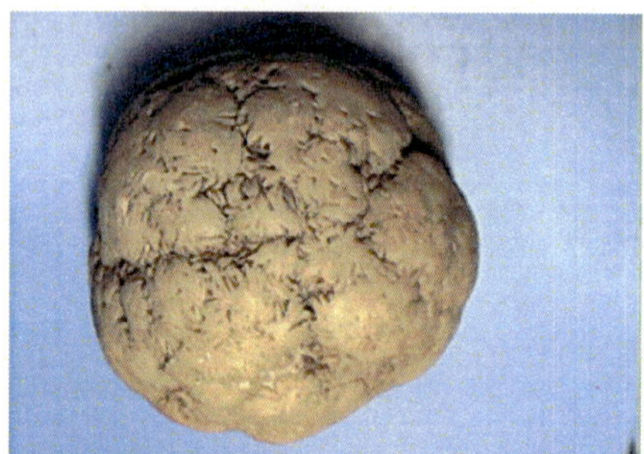

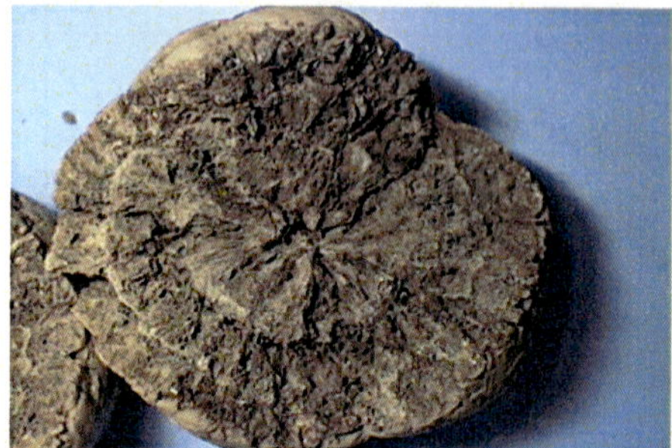

Fig. 10.3: Photograph of enterolith **A.** Intact **B.** Cross section of enterolith

Piliconcretions

Piliconcretions are hair balls, that occur in calves or in adults due to excessive licking of skin. Due to licking, animals swallow large amount of hairs which take the shape of ball due to movements of stomach. Mostly, the hair balls are found in stomach or in colon (Fig. 10.4).

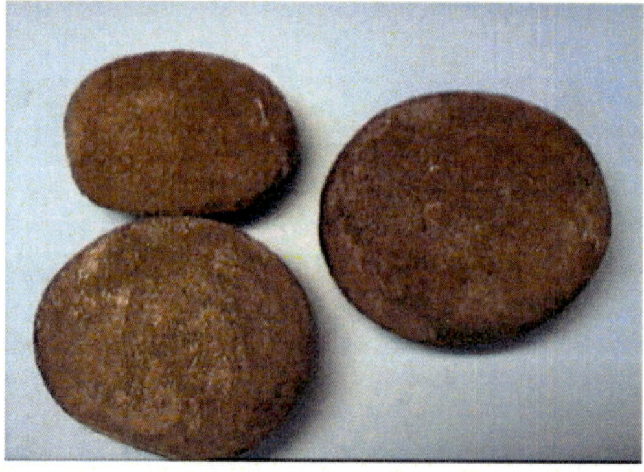

Fig. 10.4: Photograph of Piliconcretion

Phytoconcretions

Phytoconcretions are formed around the food materials and may occur in stomach and intestine of animals and in crop of poultry. They may cause obstruction of bowel. They are also known as phytobezoars.

Polyconcretions

They are made up of polythenes and excessive deposition of salts around them. They may vary in size from a few centimeters to several centimeters and weigh upto kilograms. They cause obstruction leading to death of animals (Fig. 10.5).

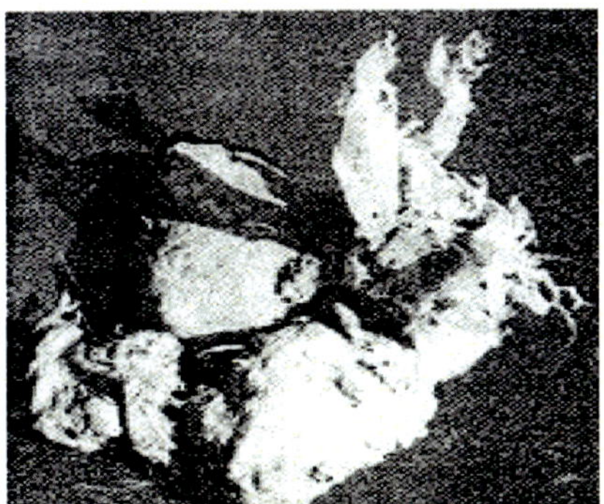

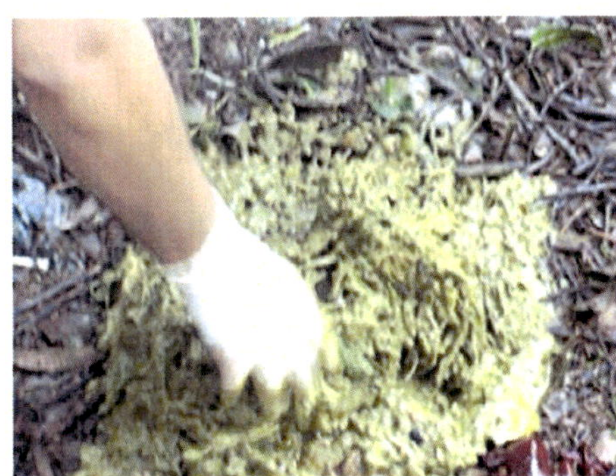

Fig. 10.5: Photograph of Polyconcretion

Such concretions are observed in cattle wandering on street in cities and in zoo animals. The polythene containing vegetable waste or green leaves and food materials are thrown away on roads, and are easily available to the animals. Polythene is not degraded in stomach and remains there to form a nidus, around which the salts are deposited and take the shape of calculi leading to obstruction of digestive tract passage.

11

Animal Oncology

- Neoplasm General
- Neoplasm in cattle and buffaloes
- Neoplasm in sheep and goat
- Neoplasm in equines, swine and camels
- Neoplasms in pet animals
- Neoplasms in poultry
- Neoplasms in wild animals
- Neoplasms in laboratory animals

General Considerations

The word neoplasm has been derived from Greek language means "New formations or new growth" (Neo=new, plasm=growth). Thus, the neoplasm can be defined as **"*A mass of tissue formed as a result of abnormal, excessive, uncoordinated, autonomous and purpose less proliferation of cells*"**. The oncology is branch of science which deals with the study of tumours (Oncos=tumour, logos=study). The neoplasm is a new growth of cells that proliferate continuously without control, have resemblance to their embryonic stages and without any orderly arrangement and that serves no useful function of body. The growth of tumour persists in the same excess even after cessation of the stimuli / etiology. A neoplasm is thus, characterized by the following key points.

1. Continuous growth
2. Resemblance to embryonic cells
3. No structural arrangement
4. No useful function
5. No clear etiology

The historical moments in the oncology are given in Table 11.1.

Table 11.1: Historical milestones in neoplasms

Sl. No.	Year	Name of Scientist & Country	Development in area of neoplasms
	500BC	Jeevak (India)	Surgical removal of intestinal tumour
	1838	Moller (Germany)	Cellular nature of neoplasms
	1858	Leblane (France)	Animal tumours have similar cellular composition
	1858	R. Virchow	Cellular characteristics of tumours
	1876	Novinsky (Russia)	Transplantability of canine venereal tumour
	1889	Hardley	Transplantation of neoplasm from one rat to another
	1903	Jenson (Denmark)	Reproduction of mouse mammary gland tumour through serial passage.
	1905	Bombay Veterinary College Scientists	Horn Cancer in bullocks
	1907	Tyzzer	Genetic relatedness of tumours in inbred mice
	1908	Ellerman and Bang (Denmark)	Transmissibility of avian lymphoid tumours
	1910	Rous	Transmission of Rous sarcoma of chicken by cell-free suspensions
	1910	Clunev (France)	Tumours experimentally produced by X-radiation
	1912	Murphy	Growth of rat tumours on chicken chorioallantoic membrane
	1914	Yamagiwa (Japan)	Carcinogenicity of coal tar by long-term application to skin of rabbits
	1924	Little and Strong	Development of inbred strains of mice for genetic analysis of tumours
	1932	Shope	Viral etiology of rabbit papilloma
	1933	Warburg	High rate of anaerobic glycolysis in tumour cells
	1936	Lucke	Virus induced renal carcinoma of frog
	1936	Bittner	Viral agent in milk causing mammary gland carcinoma of mice
	1943	Gross	Tumour specific antigens
	1947	Berenblum	Two stages in chemical carcinogenesis: initiation and promotion
	1951	Gross	Virus etiology of mouse lymphoma
	1962	Epstein and Barr	Herpes virus from Burkitt's lymphoma
	1964	Jarrett	Retrovirus as etiology of feline lymphosarcoma
	1969	Friedrich-Freksa	Chemical carcinogenesis induced altered enzyme patterns in liver
	1973	CM Singh (India)	Bovine lymphosarcoma/leukemia in buffaloes

The tumours are reported even thousand years B.C. in the records of India and Egypt but Johannes Muller in the year 1838 was first to demonstrate that the tumour is composed of cells. In 1858, R. Virchow described cellular characteristics and in 1889 Hardley transplanted a neoplasm from one rat to another. Tyzzer established the genetic relatedness of tumours in inbred mice in 1907 while in 1914 Yamagiwa found tar as one of the important cause of cancer in rabbits. Rous in the year 1910 described Rouse Sarcoma in fowls with a viral etiology. In 1932 Shope described papilloma due to transmissible viral agents while in 1936 Bittner's milk factor was associated with transplanted cancer in baby mice.

To understand the neoplasms, their characteristics and pathology, it is advisable to have a general idea about the growth disturbances. The neoplasm is also one of the growth disturbances or development related diseases. In brief, the important growth disturbances (Fig. 11.1) are defined as follows:

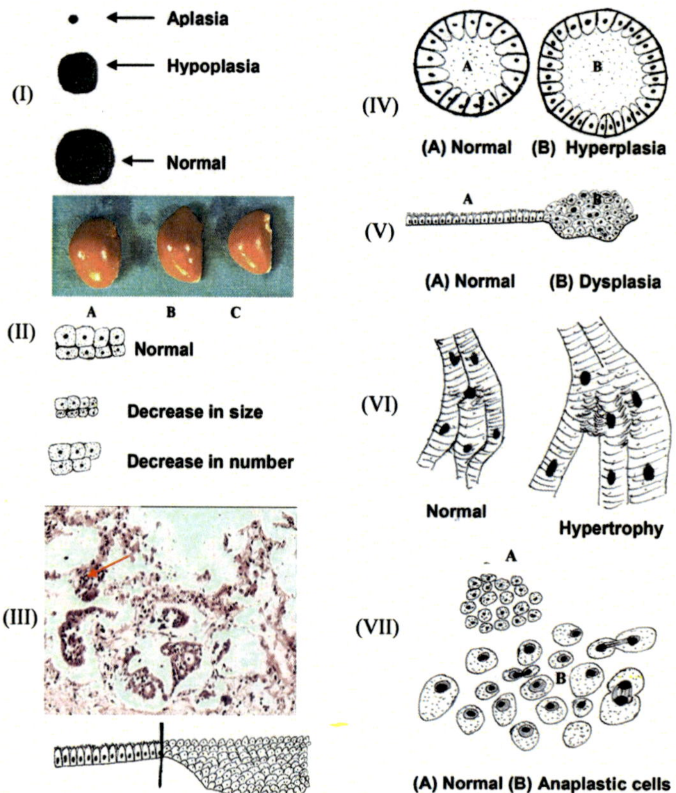

Fig. 11.1: Growth disturbances (I) Aplasia and Hypoplasia, (II) Atrophy of spleen- (A) Normal, (B)&(C) Atrophied, (III) Metaplasia, (IV) Hyperplasia, (V) Dysplasia, (VI) Hypertrophy and (VII) Anaplasia

Agenesis: Complete absence of growth of an organ/tissue.

Aplasia: Congenital disturbance with complete failure of development of an organ or tissue. Only primitive structure or rudimentary structure is present.

Hypoplasia: Failure of an organ to develop to its normal size.

Atrophy: Reduction in size of an organ/tissue less than its former normal size. The reduction of size is either due to decrease in number or size of cells of an organ.

Hypertrophy: Increase in size of an organ or tissue due to increase in the size of cells of that organ.

Hyperplasia: Increase in size of an organ or tissue due to increase in the number of cells of that organ.

Metaplasia: Substitution of one cell type by another type of cells. *e.g.* Squamous metaplasia of oesophageal glands of poultry in Vitamin A deficiency (nutritional roup).

Dysplasia: Abnormal development of cells in a tissue/organ.

Anaplasia: Reversion of cells to a more primitive or embryonic and less differentiated type.

In comparison to tissue growth as in case of hyperplasia or hypertrophy, a neoplastic growth does not obey the laws of the healing or normal tissue growth. The cells of a neoplasm continue to multiply indefinitely irrespective of any structural or functional requirements and form an ever increasing mass of tissue.

The macroscopic appearance of tumours is characterized by different size, shape, colour and consistency which depends on many factors such as location, type of tumour, blood supply, rate of growth and length of time tumour present in body. The size of a tumour varies from one mm to several centimeter diameter. The common warts/papilloma over skin have smaller size while certain tumours have many centi meter diameter such as uterine tumours etc. The weight of tumour also varies from few milli gram to several kg. A tumour of 48 kg was removed from uterus of a cow. The different shape of tumours are given in Fig. 11.2, which included as round, spherical, elliptical or multi lobulated. Some tumours have crab like structures which formed as a result of its invasion to the surrounding tissue. The colour of tumours may be grayish white, yellow, red, brown or black. If tumour has fatty tissue it looks like yellow in colour while haemorrhage or congestion may give the pink or red colour to tumour; melanoma or melanosarcoma are characterized by black colour. The disintegration of haemoglobin gives brown colour to tumour due to presence of haemosiderin. The consistency of a tumour depends on the type of tissue involved. The tumour of bone is hard while connective tissue tumours are firm and dense or sclerotic. Brain tumours are mostly soft. If there is necrosis in mass of tumour it becomes soft and liquefied. In certain tumours, there are oedematous fluid which gives it watery consistency. Some tumours have mucin leading to its slimy consistency.

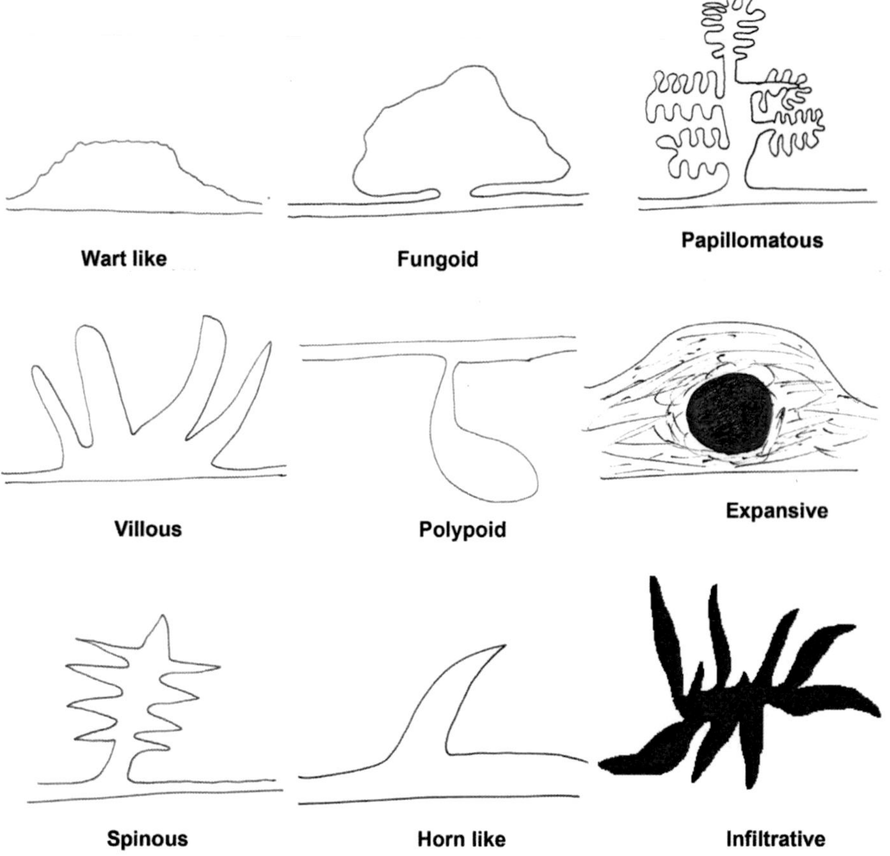

Fig. 11.2: Shape of tumours

Microscopically, the tumour is composed of cells which resembles the type of tissue/organ involved. The appearance of cells vary on degree of malignancy. ***In benign tumours, the cells are of adult type while in malignant tumours these cells are having characteristics of embryonic stages***. This reversion towards embryonic type is also known as ***anaplasia***. The more anaplastic cells we see in a tumour more malignancy will be there. However, it will depend on the degree of anaplasia which have following characteristics:

1. **Enlargement of nucleus:** The nucleus of tumour cell is enlarged which is indicative of a rapid cell growth and towards embryonic stage of the cell.
2. **Multiple nuclei in a cell:** The tumour cells having multiple nucleus are indicative of rapid cell division and such cells are known as ***tumour giant cells***. Such cells are formed because of the fact that nucleus is dividing more rapidly than cytoplasm.
3. **Enlargement of nucleolus:** The increased size of nucleolus is also an indication of rapid cell growth; sometimes it becomes 2-3 times larger in size than normal.
4. **Increase number of mitotic figures:** If one finds more number of mitotic figures in a field under microscope, it is an indication of malignancy. More number of mitotic figures, the more severe malignancy will be there.
5. **Hyperchromasia of the cell:** The neoplastic cell takes intense colour and if it is more embryonic, it takes more intense colour and nucleus stains dark with hematoxylin.
6. **Embryonic type cells:** The neoplastic cell loses its resemblance to adult cells. The cell growth is not under control.

Classification, difference between benign and malignant neoplasms

The classification of neoplasms is summarized in Table 11.2 and Table 11.3.

1. Benign
2. Malignant (cancer)
3. Preneoplastic conditions
4. Neoplastic like malformations

Table 11.2: Classification of benign and malignant neoplasms

	Tissue of origin	Benign	Malignant
I *Neoplasms of one parencymal cell type*			
(i) *Epithelial neoplasms*			
1.	Squamous epithelium	Papilloma	Squamous cell carcinoma
2.	Transitional epithelium	Papilloma	Transitional cell carcinoma
3.	Glandular epithelium	Adenoma	Adenocarcinoma
4.	Basal cell layer	-	Basal cell carcinoma
5.	Melanoblasts	Melanoma	Melanocarcinoma
6.	Hepatocytes	Liver cell adenoma	Hypatocellularcarcinoma
7.	Placenta	-	Choriocarcinoma
(ii) *Non-epithelial neoplasms (mesenchymal)*			
1.	Adipose tissue	Lipoma	Liposarcoma
2.	Fibrous tissue (adult)	Fibroma	Fibrosarcoma
3.	Fibrous tissue (embryonic)	Myxoma	Myxosarcoma
4.	Bone	Osteoma	Osteosarcoma
5.	Cartilage	Chondroma	Chondrosarcoma
6.	Smooth muscle	Leiomyoma	Leiomyosarcoma
7.	Skeletal muscle	Rhabdomyoma	Rhabdomyosarcoma
8.	Blood vessels	Hemangioma	Hemangiosarcoma
9.	Lymph vessels	Lymphangioma	Lymphangiosarcoma
10.	Meninges	Meningioma	Invasive meningioma
11.	Lymphoid tissue	Lymphoma	Malignant lymphoma
12.	Brain nerve sheath	Neurofibroma	Neurogenic sarcoma
13.	Brain nerve cell	Ganglioneuroma	Neuroblastoma
14.	Blood cells (lymphocytes)	-	Leukemia
15.	Mesothelium	-	Mesothelioma
II. *Mixed neoplasms*			
	Salivary gland	Mixed salivary neoplasm	Malignant mixed salivary neoplasm
III. *Neoplasms of more than one germ layer*			
	Gonads	Mature teratoma	Immature teratoma

Table 11.3: Difference between benign and malignant tumours

Sl.No.	Characteristics	Benign	Malignant
1.	Growth rate	Slow	Rapid
2.	Growth limits	Circumscribed/covered	Unrestricted
3.	Mode of growth	Expansion	Invasion
4.	Differentiation	Good	Anaplasia
5.	Metastasis	Absent	Frequent
6.	Recurrence on surgery	Rare	Frequent
7.	Microscopic features	Resembles with tissue of origin	Poor resemblance with tissue of origin

Sl.No.	Characteristics	Benign	Malignant
8.	Basal polarity	Retained	Often lost
9.	Pleomorphism	Absent	Present
10.	Tumour giant cells	Absent	Present
11.	Anaplastic	Often absent	Present

1. Benign neoplasms

Neoplasms that are well differentiated, grow slowly by expansion and do not invade below basement membrane are called as benign neoplasms. They remain localized, encapsulated and can be removed by surgery. They are classified with addition of a ***suffix-oma*** to the cell type. *e.g.* Fibroma, Chondroma, Adenoma, Papilloma.

2. Malignant neoplasms

Neoplasms whose cells are anaplastic, metastasize and invade the adjacent tissues and destroy normal tissue. They are also called as ***cancer*** "like crab". They can adhere to any part of body. They are classified with suffix as carcinoma or sarcoma. Ectodermal origin- Carcinoma, Mesodermal origin- Sarcoma. *e.g.* Lymphosarcoma, Adenocarcinoma, Squamous cell carcinoma.

Some tumours are highly undifferentiated they are referred as "undifferentiated malignant tumours".

3. Preneoplastic conditions

There are some preneoplastic lesions which predisposes the subsequent development of cancer. These are as follows

a. *Chronic inflammatory conditions of liver* of old dogs have multiple nodules which are considered preneoplastic nodules and neoplastic cells do arise from such nodules. Such dogs have higher incidence of hepatocellular carcinoma.

b. *Intraepithelial neoplasia* are restricted to the epithelium only without infiltration in adjacent tissue. On cytology there are malignant features of the cells but with no invasion and they remain confined to epithelium. *e.g.* Uterine cervix, Solar keratosis, Bowen's disease of skin, Oral leucoplakia

c. *Role of pre neoplastic lesions* in squamous cell carcinoma, transitional cell carcinoma of bladder and malignant melanomas of skin and oral cavity is well established.

d. *Some benign tumours* like multiple adenoma of large intestine becomes malignant (adenocarcinoma) after sometime.

4. Neoplasia like malformations

A ***hamartia*** is a tissue defect of cells normally found in a particular area. ***Hamartoma*** is a tumour characterized by excessive focal overgrowth of mature cells in an organ. ***Chorista*** is a tissue defect of structures not found normally in that area. ***Choriostoma*** is tumour of such structures. ***Teratoma*** are made up of a number of parenchymal cell types arising from more than one germ layer.

Etiology

1. Instrisic or predisposing factors

(i) ***Heredity:*** Some chicken are susceptible for leucosis whole others are resistant for leucosis.

(ii) ***Age:*** Neoplasms are more common in old age.

(iii) ***Pigmentation:*** In white horses Melenosarcoma is common. Squamous cell carcinoma is common in hereford cattle.

(iv) ***Sex:*** No difference, tumours of genital tract are common in females.

2. Extrinsic factors

(i) Physical factors

Radium or UV-rays, X-rays, ionizing radiation

(ii) Chemical factors

A. Initiators

1. Coal-tar
2. Naturally occurring products e.g. Aflatoxins, Actinomycin D, Mitomycine, Safrole
3. Alkalating agents e.g. cyclophosphamide, chlorambucil, nitrosourea.
4. Polycyclic aromatic hydrocarbons- Tobacco, smoke, pollutants, methylcholanthrene, banzapyrene, benzanthracene
5. Aromatic amines- b-naphthylamine bezidine
6. Azodyes

7. Acylating agents- acetyl imidazole
8. Vinyl chloride monomer
9. Arsenic
10. Metals- Nickel, lead, cobalt, chromium
11. Insecticides- Aldrin, Dieldrin, Chlordane

B. Promoters

1. Phenols
2. Hormones- Estrogen
3. Drugs- Phenobarbital
4. Artificial sweetners- Saccharine
5. Colouring/flavouring agents, preservatives

(iii) Virus

1. Papilloma virus
2. Polyoma virus
3. Adeno virus - Hamsters- Sarcoma
4. Poxvirus- Rabbit- Myxomatosis
5. Hepdna virus- Hepatitis B virus
6. Retrovirus
7. Herpes virus

Neoplastic Cell Genesis (Carcinogenesis)

Cell differentiation

Specialized cells derived from less specialized cells (embryonic cells) is controlled by specific gene. Cells become differentiated so that the genes that control embryonic characters are switched off and genes for more differentiated characters are activated. In neoplastic cells, the presence of abnormal genes (genetic mechanisms) or normal genes expressed at abnormal level (epigenetic mechanism) favour proliferation over differentiation.

Genetic mechanisms

Mutation in a somatic cell nucleic acid occurs to provide a stable and monoclonal population of cells.

Epigenetic mechanism

Genome is normal in cancer cell but transcription and translation is abnormal which is responsible for abnormal growth of cells.

In most tumours genetic mutation or genetic rearrangement occurs like DNA transcribe to mRNA and mRNA translated to protein (enzymes) which direct cells for proliferation. Changes occur in DNA as a result of direct chemical or radiation damage or there is insertion of viral genes to host DNA that induces cell proliferation through neutralizing normal growth controlling gene.

Tumours do not arise from completely differentiated cells such as neurons or keratinized epithelial cells, but stem cells (pluripotential) must be present for the growth of tumour. Neoplastic cells do not "dedifferentiate" but fail to respond to normal signals for differentiation.

Viral Oncogenesis

Oncogenes are the transforming genes present in host tumour cells of animal and man. It is also present in certain viruses. Experimentally, when they are incorporated in cells in culture it transforms the cells to multiply. When such genes are present in normal cells that are known as ***cellular oncogenes (c-oncs)*** or ***proto-oncogenes***, which are present in a wide range of cells and has a physiological role of proliferation of cells through protein product.

Proto-oncogenes are converted into active oncogenes through following mechanisms

1. **Point mutation:** Change in a single base pair of the nucleic acid.
2. **Translocation:** Transfer of one segment of chromosome to another chromosome.
3. **Gene amplification:** Extra copies of ***c-oncs*** are inserted leading to increased number of oncogenes.
4. **Inappropriate expression of proto-oncogenes:** When the expression of oncogenes is not in proper way and it gives rise to the products responsible for formation of tumours.

5. **Integration of viral DNA into host cell DNA:** Integration of viral DNA into host cell DNA causes adjacent gene activated for growth of the cell without control.

Cellular oncogenes of host cell can transcribe its copies in viral genome (retroviruses) and then it is known as *v-oncogenes* (*v-oncs*). So *c-oncs* or *v-oncs* are closely related genes and have high degree of homology.

Antioncogenes

Antioncogenes are genes that suppresses the cellular proliferation. By inactivating antioncogene we can produce cancers. So neoplastic growth occurs either as a result of activation of oncogene or due to inactivation of antioncogene.

How the viruses cause cancers

1. A direct effect of gene (*v-oncs*).
2. A viral factor that affects a host gene (*c-oncs*).
3. A factor that inactivates the antioncogene.
4. Genes that do not affect the cell growth but influence the expansion/ metastasis.

There are many RNA and DNA viruses which can cause cancers.

1. Retrovirus

It produces cancers through 3 mechanisms.

i. RNA of Rous Sarcoma Virus utilizing reverse transcriptase converts into DNA (proviral DNA) which incorporated in host cell DNA. The *src* gene of the virus is thus responsible for transformation of the cells.

ii. Proviral DNA of avian leucosis virus has no oncogenes. However, it carries a viral RNA segment known as "Long Terminal Repeat (LTR)" present at the end of viral genome. This LTR has segments of promoters and enhancers, which activate transcription of viral genome to mRNA and activates the adjacent normal cell gene for growth and production of slow tumours. Gene (myc) of ALC virus is amplified and plays a role is transforming the cells.

iii. Some virus has a protein that transactivate the gene of proliferation and thus it increases the proliferation of gene to divide the cells.

2. Papova virus

These are the DNA viruses having two main genera Papilloma and Polyoma. Papilloma virus has *src, raf, myc* oncogene which produces warts/ benign tumours. These warts regress through cell mediated immune response. Polyoma produces multiple nodules in body.

3. Hepadna virus

Hepadna virus has *hap* oncogene causing hepatocellular carcinoma. It includes hepatitis-B virus and duck hepatitis virus.

4. Herpesvirus

DNA virus *e.g.* Marek's disease virus which causes polyneuritis and malignant lymphoma in poultry. This is the only virus for which a vaccine is available to control cancer.

Possible Viral Induced Tumours

1. Pulmonary adenomatosis of sheep

It is progressive respiratory distress characterized by emaciation and proliferation of glandular cells. In this the squamous epithelium becomes metaplastic to cuboidal or columnar. Metastasis occurs in lymph nodes, skeletal muscles, kidneys and peritoneum.

2. Nasal adenocarcinoma of sheep.

3. Equine cutaneous histiocytoma

The *src* gene product of rouse sarcoma virus synthesizes protein kinase (60 kd) enzyme which stimulates DNA synthesis leading to mitosis. All vertebrate possess a cell gene related to *src* gene; which also produce similar protein kinase.

Over 20 retroviral oncogenes (*v-oncs*) have been identified. All have relatives in normal cells (proto oncogenes).

Some of the oncogenes are

1. Rous Sarcoma Virus – *src*
2. Avian Leucosis Virus – *myc, myb, erb-B, erb-A*
3. Feline Leukemia Virus – *pim-1, myc*
4. Papilloma virus- *src,raf,myc*

5. Hepadna virus- *hap*
6. Reticuloendotheliosis- *rel*
7. Avian sarcoma virus- *yes, ros*
8. Feline sarcoma virus- *fes, fms*

Neoplastic Cell Metabolism

Normal regulation of programmed protein synthesis is lost in neoplastic cells. Gene expression and mRNA translation is being directed towards:

1. Purine synthesis to meet the requirement of mitosis
2. Defective sodium pump (ATPase) due to abnormal receptor molecules and surface glycoproteins on neoplastic cells.
3. Increased glycolysis
   a. Increased glycolysis may occur due to damage in self replicating DNA of mitochondira. *e.g.* Carcinogenic metabolite of benzopyrene have affinity to mitochondrial DNA.
   b. Enhanced glycolysis is also related to over production of inorganic phosphorus due to high rate of ATP hydrolysis. Inorganic phosphorus is required to phosphorylate glucose to glucose-6-phosphate.

      ATP---------> ADP + Pi -----> Stimulate glycolysis

      Hydrolysis
   c. Abnormal enzymes on cell surface may promote glycolysis. ATPase (Sodium pump, Na-K-dependent ATPase) is inefficient in cancer cells. Additional ATPs are required to pump out Na^+ which produces ADP and inorganic phosphorus that further stimulates glycolysis.

Neoplastic Cell Structure

1. **Anaplasia:** Neoplastic cells are having anaplastic characters. More anaplasia represents more undifferentiated neoplasm.
2. **Loss of contact:** Neoplastic cells loss contact with neighbouring cells due to decreased adhesiveness. It helps in invasion and metastasis. Such cells bear more negative charge on surface, decrease in calcium content and presence of abnormal glycoprotein and glycolipids. Fibrinolectin is present on normal cell surface but it is absent or decreased in neoplastic cells. Fibrinolectin forms matrix for stabilization of cells and absence of

matrix destabilizes tumour cells. Fibrinolectin suppresses invasiveness, absence of which increases invasiveness.

3. **Neoplastic cell lack contact inhibition**: Normally cell growth is inhibited after the fulfillment of function i.e. healing of wound due to contact and exchange of information which establishes check on cell growth. But in cancer cell such contact does not work because of absence of gap junctions. Vitamin A promotes proliferation of gap junctions and thus this vitamin helps in checking the growth/spread of tumours.

4. **Abnormal cytoskeleton of cells**: Abnormal microfilament leads to defective actin polymerization while abnormal microtubules causes abnormal polymerization of tubulins leading to abnormal shape. Besides, unstable chromosome movements cause abnormality in cytoskeleton.

5. **Chromosomal defects:** Malignant cells are usually aneuploid i.e. cells having more or less than diploid number of chromosomes. This gives a pathologic karyotype in the form of chromosomal breaks or translocations. *e.g.* Plasmacytoma (tumour of B-lymphocytes) in which translocation of segments of chromosome 15 occurs to chromosome 12. This translocate carries the gene for production of monoclonal antibody in mice.

Thus gene for antibody production can be transported to chromosomes with gene of growth. The process of ***monoclonal antibody*** production is based on this principle.

Spread of Neoplasms

I. Expansion

Benign tumours are encapsulated and surrounded by fibrous tissue and hence they do not infiltrate in neighbouring tissue. However, they expand as their growth increases.

II. Distant spread/metastasis

Metastasis is the spread of tumours by invasion in such a way that detached tumour mass may form secondary tumour at the site of lodgment. Most of the malignant tumours metastasize except malignant tumour of central nervous system and basal cell carcinoma of skin. There are several methods of metastasis, which are as under:

1. **Infiltration:** Neoplastic cells infiltrate or invade the surrounding tissue. Various factors responsible for invasion are:

1. Growth of new cells so as to increase the size.
2. Lack of contact inhibition in malignant tumour cells.
3. Motility of malignant cells.
4. Secretion of lytic enzymes by some malignant cells.
5. Role of chemotactic factors and activation of complement.

2. **Lymphatic spread:** In general, epithelial tumours like carcinomas spread through lymphatic route. Cancer cells invade the wall of lymphatics which is known as lymphatic permeation (Fig. 11.3) and form tumour emboli. These cells are lodged in sub capsular sinus of lymph node and may grow. Nearest lymph node initially act as barrier filter and kill the tumour cells but later it provides fertile environment for growth of tumour cells. Sometimes lymphatic metastasis do not develop due to obliteration of lymphatics by inflammation; this is known as ***skip metastasis***. Obstruction of lymphatics by tumour cells also disturbs the lymphatic flow and is responsible for metastasis at unusual sites. This is termed as ***retrograde metastasis***. *e.g.* 1. Carcinoma of prostate to supra clavicular lymph node, 2. Metastasis in adrenals from lung cancer.

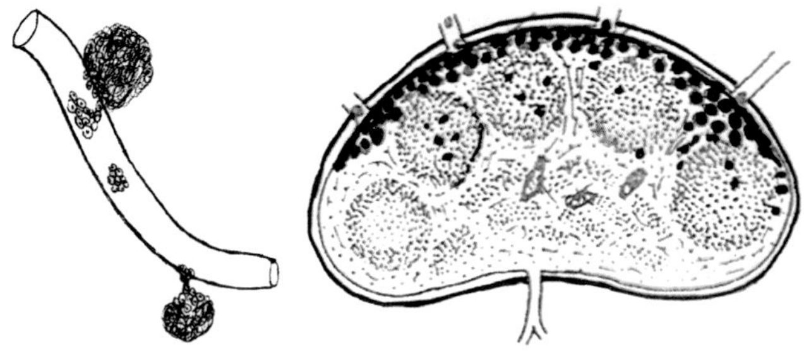

Fig. 11.3. Metastasis of neoplasm- (A) Lymphatic spread, (B) Lodgement of neoplastic cells in lymph node

3. **Hematogenous spread:** Metastasis through blood is common route for most of the sarcomas (connective tissue tumours). However, some carcinomas (lung, mammary gland, thyroid, kidney) may spread through blood. Common sites of lodgment of tumour cells are liver, lungs, kidneys, brain and bones. Cancer cell invade the wall of capillaries to form tumour emboli. Blood borne metastasis appear as multiple and rounded nodules scattered in the organ.

4. **Transcoelomic spread:** The tumour cells invade serosal wall and enters in coelomic cavity and then tumour cells implant at another place. *e.g.* Peritoneal cavity- carcinoma of stomach/ovary.

5. **Spread along epithelial lined surfaces:** Intact epithelium and mucous coat are quite resistant to penetration by tumour cells. The neoplasms of epithelium spread along the line of basement membrane without damaging it. *e.g.* 1. Spread of tumour through fallowpian tube from ovaries to endometrium, 2. Spread of tumour through bronchus to alveoli.

6. **Spread via Cerebrospinal Fluid (CSF):** Tumour of meninges may spread through cerebrospinal fluid as the detached tumour cells metastasize at other sites in central nervous system through CSF.

7. **Implantation:** It is very rare method of spread of tumours. In this the tumour cells are implanted at another site inadvertently. *e.g.* 1. Surgeon's scalpel, needle, sutures may transfer tumour cells from one to another place in body. 2. Cancer of lower lip may metastasize to upper lip.

Process of metastasis

The process of metastasis includes 5 steps.

1. **Penetration (Invasion):** The tumour cells penetrate or infiltrate in the adjoining tissue particularly in vascular space/cavity.

2. **Separation:** A group of tumour cells separate from primary tumour due to their lack of adhesiveness.

3. **Dissemination:** The separated cells reach at distant places through stream of blood/lymph or in cavity through amoeboid movement with a speed of 6.2 μm/min.

4. **Establishment:** At new site the tumour cells adapt in new environment for lodgment.

5. **Subsequent Proliferation:** As the tumour cells lodge and adapt in new environment, it starts unrestricted growth at new site and forms secondary tumours.

Tumour immunology

In some animals growth of neoplasm is very fast that leads to early death. In others, tumour growth is slow and the animal may survive several years. When malignant tumour is clinically manifested it takes 6 month to 1 year to cause death.

There are many systems/functions in the body which works together to fight with neoplastic cells. These are described as under:

1. Nonspecific lysis and phagocytosis

Most tumour cells are phagocytosed by polymorphonuclear cells and macrophages. On contact, macrophages insert cytoplasmic processes into the tumour cells and transfer lysosomal enzymes into the cytoplasm of cancer cell leading to death of cell. Because in cancer cell decreased catalase and glutathione contents makes them susceptible to oxidative injury by macrophages. On the contrary reactive oxygen metabolites of neutrophils "respiratory burst" are mutagenic and may act as tumour promoter.

Natural killer cell: A population of immature lymphocytes which bears Fc receptor that causes lysis of neoplastic cells or virus infected cells.

Antibodies: Antibodies against tumour antigens also restrain the growth of tumour.

Escape of neoplastic cells from immunological destruction

1. **Delayed immunostimulation:** The tumour antigens appear late on the anaplastic/neoplastic cell surface causing delayed immune response.
2. **Antigenic modulation:** Frequent change in antigenic determinants over neoplastic cell surface may escape the cell from immune response.
3. **Antigenic overload:** There are too many antigenic determinants on the neoplastic cell surface that leads to immune tolerance.
4. **General Immunodeficiency:** Neoplasia, in general, causes immunosuppression in body.
5. **Specific immunodeficiency:** There is lack of recognition of tumour antigens on neoplastic cells by the immunocytes that leads to suppression of specific immune response.
6. **Humoral antibodies:** Antibodies binds with tumour antigens and blocks the effect of more potent anti neoplastic action by another source.

Tumour antigens

Tumour cells develop certain biochemical alterations on their surface (protein change) that makes the "tumour" antigens". Tumour antigens are useful in differentiating between neoplastic or pre neoplastic cell. These tumour antigens may evoke immune response in body by humoral or cell mediated mechanism which may inhibit the tumour cell growth.

Types of tumour antigens

1. Fetal antigens and alpha fetoproteins produced by embryonic cells.
2. It is produced by liver cells but after birth it's production is stopped normally.
3. Differentiation antigen as in normal cells.
4. Viral antigens on cell surface. *e.g.* Retrovirus

Tumour antigens induced selective CMI response which destroys the malignant cells. During cytological or histological examination of biopsy material, if one finds lymphocytes along with cancer cells, the prognosis is considered as good.

Propionibacterium acnes (*Corynebacterium parvum)*, BCG and filterate of G^- bacterial cultures are used to stimulate the reticulo-endothelial system against tumours. Macrophages attract and attach on tumour growth and remove it through phagocytosis. *e.g.* In ocular squamous cell carcinoma, intra tumour injection of BCG reduces growth by 71%.

In early tumour growth, tumour cells excrete some products that inhibits the macrophages. *e.g.* Macrophages also release certain soluble factors that are having anti tumour activities, such as tumour necrosis factor (TNF) which causes necrosis of tumour cells. It needs to be activated by *P.acnes* or LPS of G^- bacteria. It affects subcutaneous transplantation of tumour.

Beneficial Effects of Neoplastic Cells

1. Monoclonal antibody production

Antibody production is done by B-cells but they have short life span. If fusion/hybrids are produced between B-cells and myeloma cells(neoplastic B-cells) then this hybrid cells are capable of multiplying indefinitely and produce antibody indefinitely. After fusion they are kept in HAT medium (Hypoxanthine, aminopterin, thymidine)- either B or myeloma cell cannot survive, only clones will survive. Myeloma cells are from BALB/C mice. The clone will grow as tumour in peritoneal cavity; i/p fluid or ascites fluid have a good concentration of antibodies which are monoclonal in nature.

Advantages

1. High titre of monoclonal antibody.
2. Mono specificity.
3. Immortal clones may produce more quantity of antibody.

4. On mass scale in culture media one can produce even up to 1000 liters of antibody.
5. Monoclnal antibody is used for confirmatory diagnosis of diseases.

2. Cell culture

Cancerous cells are used for virus culture as cell lines specific for different organ/cell. Such cell lines are serving very useful purpose as they are used in isolation, identification and characterization of viruses. Vaccines can be prepared from viruses using cell culture.

Epidemiology of Neoplasms

Horn caner is commonest neoplasm of cattle in India; however, it may also occur is buffaloes and sheep. This neoplasm was first reported in 1905 from Bombay Veterinary College and since then it has been recorded from every part of the country. Adult cattle of 5-10 years of age are mostly suffer from horn cancer. It has been recorded in long horned animals with white coat. The prevalence of horn cancer was found highest in Kankrej 8.24% followed by in Gir (7.33%), Malvi (6.99%), Khillari (2.96) and others (1.11%). Working bullocks are comparatively more susceptible to horn cancer. In a study of 968430 cattle and buffaloes during 1966-70, neoplasm of horn has been recorded in 2652 animals including 2268 cattle and 384 buffaloes. More than 90% of affected animals were in the age group of 5-10 years.

A survey was carried out from 1995 to 1982 (17 years) on neoplasms in cattle and buffaloes and the prevalence of different neoplasms was recorded as squamous cell carcinoma (48.4%), fibroma (19.61%), melanoma (6.5%), lymphosarcoma (4.5%) and papilloma (4.2%) (Fig. 11.4 & 11.5). The occurrence of neoplasms in different animals were as 62.3% in bullocks, 19.4% in cows, 16% in buffaloes and 2.3% in bulls.

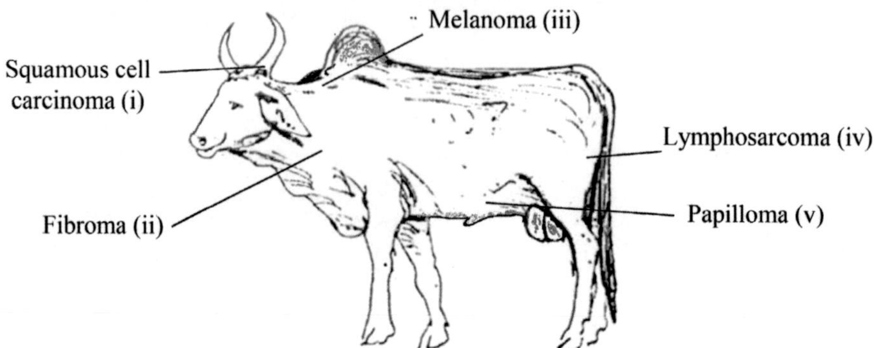

Fig. 11.4: Common neoplasms of cattle- most common (i) descending to (v)

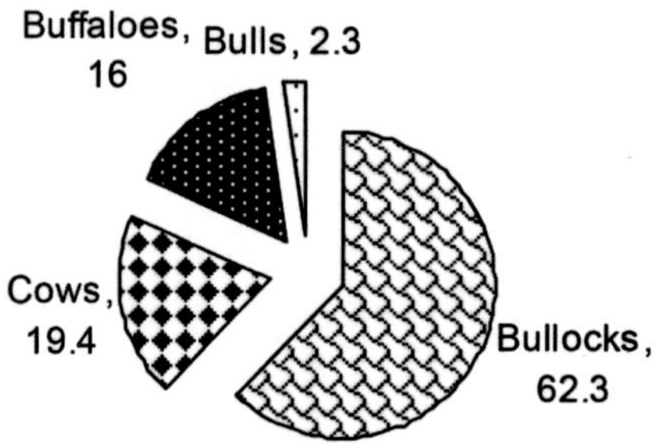

Fig. 11.5: Occurrence (in percent) of neoplasms in cattle and buffaloes

In dogs, a survey was conducted from (1940 – 1951) at Madras and 325 (13.5%) dogs were found to suffer from venereal tumour. Among various neoplasms diagnosed in dogs in Hisar (Haryana) are venereal neoplasm, papilloma, round cell sarcoma, adenocarcinoma, adenoma and lymphosarcoma. Canine venereal tumour was found more during summer (57.9%) as compared to winter (42.1%). The age group mainly involved was 1-5 years. Sex wise prevalence was 68.5% in females and 31.5% in males. In another survey, the frequency of different neoplasms in dogs was recorded as 42.2% of skin, 20.6% of mammary gland, 23.5% of genitalia and 13.2% of other organs (Fig. 11.6 & 11.7).

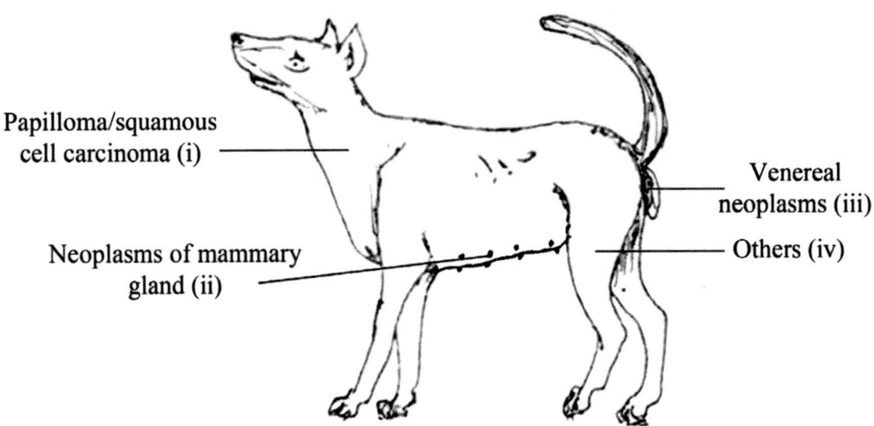

Fig. 11.6: Common neoplasms of dogs- most common (i) descending to (iv)

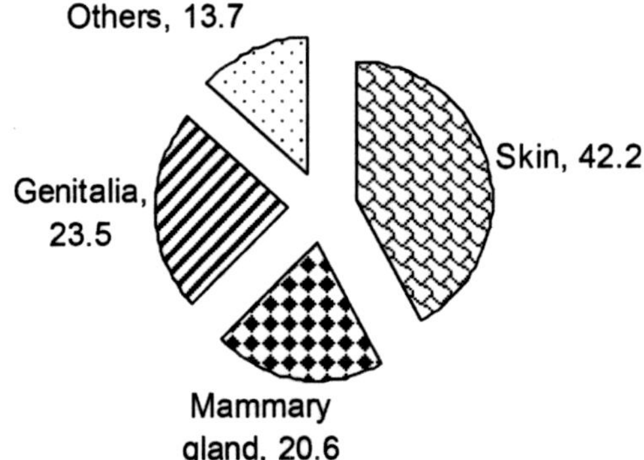

Fig. 11.7: Occurrence (in percent) of common neoplasms in dogs

A screening was conducted on neoplasms of equines from 1952 to 1973 in southern India, in which 69 horses and one donkey was found to be affected with neoplasms of skin and glands. Another survey conducted at Hisar from 1980-1988 suggested sarcoid as main tumour of horses. In Gujrat, a study of tumours in horses revealed 30% fibroma, 25% squamaous cell carcinoma, 16% fibrosarcoma, 6% papilloma and 6% melanoma (Fig. 11.8 & 11.19).

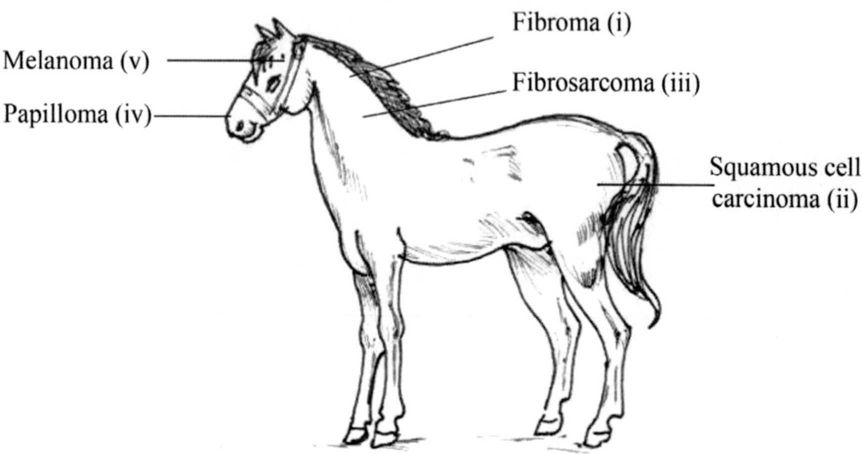

Fig. 11.8: Common neoplasms of horse- most common (i) descending to (iv)

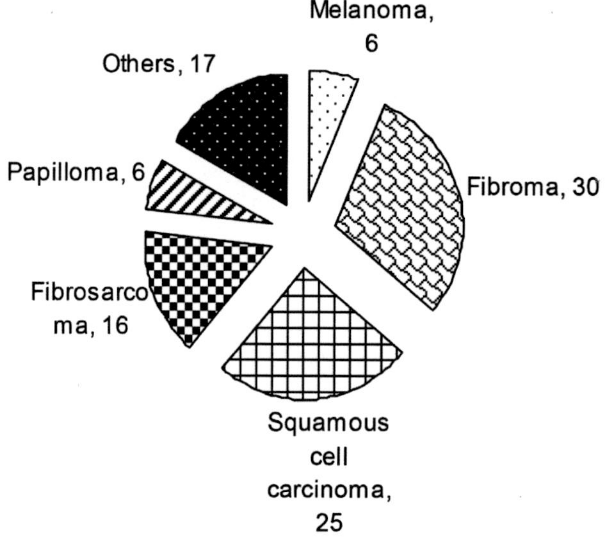

Fig. 11.9: Occurrence (in percent) of common neoplasms of horse

Clinicopathological Effects of Neoplasms

Malignant neoplastic cells kill animals through many effects which are categorized into local and systemic effects.

1. Local effects

The main local effect is pressure on surrounding tissue. The tumour causes pain, ischemia, oedema and lymphatic blockade in surrounding tissue. The lumen of ducts are obstructed due to pressure from outside tumours. *e.g.* Squamous cell carcinoma of respiratory tract causes dyspnoea and hypoxia due to obstruction in pharynx. Tumors which cause obstruction in urinary tract or obstruction in bile ducts may lead to death.

2. Systemic effects

a. **Cachexia:** Cachexia is main characteristic feature of malignant tumours. In later stages, anorexia occurs in animals leading to loss of weight and lethargRiness. Anorexia occurs due to depression of appetite centre in brain. A humoral factor is released by tumour cells that causes suppression of appetite centre in brain. Cytokines secreted by tumour cells or by altered macrophages (affected by neoplastic cell) are known as ***cachectin*** which causes suppression of gene that produces lipogenic enzymes responsible for fat deposition. Neoplastic cells act as amino acid trap and thus, drain out the essential amino acids leading to regression of skeletal muscles, liver, pancreas and other organs. Hepatocytes become atrophied.

b. **Hypoglycemia**: Hypoglycemia is characteristic feature of tumours of pancreas and other epithelial tumours. It is characterized by restlessness, weakness, tremors, episodes of collapse and seizures.

c. **Anemia:** Anemia is a common feature in all metastatic tumours. It is caused by:

   i. Haemorrhage through invasion by cancer cells.

   ii. Decreased erythropoiesis due to invasion of tumour cells in bone marrow.

   iii. Increased erythrocyte fragmentation as many blood vessels pass though tumours. In highly vascular tumour, there are more chances of anemia.

   iv. In hyperspleenism, there is spleenomegaly due to excessive removal of RBC from circulation.

   v. Iron deficiency due to tumour may leads to anemia.

   vi. Due to anticancer therapy there is non regeneration of stem cells. It causes death of stem cells or dividing cells of bone marrow leading to anemia.

vii. Autoimmune anemia occurs in lymphoid neoplasms.

viii. Suppression of erythropoitin by kidneys.

c. **Thrombocytopenia:** In tumour patients thrombocyte production is reduced. *e.g.* In viral leukemia, platelet survival rate is reduced from 40-80% in dogs.

d. **Thrombosis:** Tumour cells produce procoagulants which are responsible for intra vascular coagulation and thrombi formation.

e. **Hypercalcemia:** In most of the malignant neoplasms, hypercalcemia occurs through 2 mechanism:

i. In solid tumours due to osteolytic metastasis excessive bone resorption occurs leading to calcium release that results in hypercalcemia.

ii. Tumour cell secrete proteins that increases parathyroid hormone leading to increase in calcium level in blood. Pseudohyperparathyroidism is associated with mammary gland cancer, fibrosarcoma, lymphosarcoma and adenocarcinoma in dogs and gastric carcinoma in horses.

f. **Diarrhoea**: Prolonged diarrhoea occurs in malignant neoplasms which is unresponsive to therapy and non associated with microorganisms. Neoplastic cell secretes vasoactive intestinal peptides that cause diarrhoea leading to death of the animal.

g. **Fever:** Some tumour cells release pyrogens that increases body temperature which is anti neoplastic in nature. In late stage of metastatic tumours fever is a characteristic feature.

Diagnosis of Neoplasms

- Symptoms and lesions
- Clinicopathological effects
- Immunological methods by using tumour markers
- Gross and microscopic features (histopathological examination)

Prognosis of Neoplasms

Grading of neoplasms

Grading and staging are two systems used to determine the prognosis and choice of treatment. Grading is defined as the macroscopic and microscopic degree of differentiation of tumour. Broder's grading is as under:

Grade I: Well differentiated tumour (less than 25% anaplastic cells)

Grade II: Moderately differentiated tumour (25-50% anaplastic cells)

Grade III: Low differentiated tumour (50-75% anaplastic cells)

Grade IV: Poorly differentiated tumour (more than 75% anaplastic cells)

Sometimes it is very difficult to identify the origin of tumour due to its poor differentiation. In such cases the common practice is to classify such tumours as under:

- Well differentiated
- Undifferentiated
- Keratinizing
- Non-keratinizing

Staging of neoplasms

Staging means extent of spread of tumour. Solid tumours are classified for the purpose of surgery. Various methods of staging of neoplasms are as under:

(i) TNM System

T (primary tumour)

T_0 = No evidence of tumour

T_1 = Tumour confined to primary site

T_2 = Tumour invades adjacent tissue

Lymph node (penetration/metastasis)

(N = local lymph node)

N_0 = No evidence of tumour

N_1 = Regional node involvement

N_2 = Distant node involvement

Metastasis

(M = distal lymph node)

M_0 = No evidence of metastasis

M_1 = In same cavity/place as primary tumour

M_2 = Distant metastasis

Stage I = T_1, N_0, M_0

Stage II = T_1, N_0, /N_1, M_1

Stage III = T_2, N_1/N_2, M_2

(ii) American Joint Committee (AJC) Staging

It divides all cancers into stage 0 to IV taking into account 3 components: 1) Primary tumour, 2) Nodal involvement and 3) Distant metastasis

(iii) ABC Staging System

This system is mostly used to intestinal tumours. *e.g.* colon cancers. It was proposed by Duke's and thus also known as Duke's system. This system is helpful for surgical removal of cancer.

Stage A: When tumour is confined to sub mucosa and muscle and has a cure rate 100%.

Stage B: When tumour has penetrated the entire thickness of the wall into peri colic tissue and cure rate is 70%.

Stage C: It is characterized by lymph node metastasis and reduces the cure rate to 30%.

Animal tumours are classified as epithelial and non epithelial (Connective tissue tumours).

Epithelial Tumours

Papilloma

Papilloma is a benign tumour from a epithelial surface and involves squamous, transitional or columnar epithelium depending on the tissue of origin (Fig. 11.10).

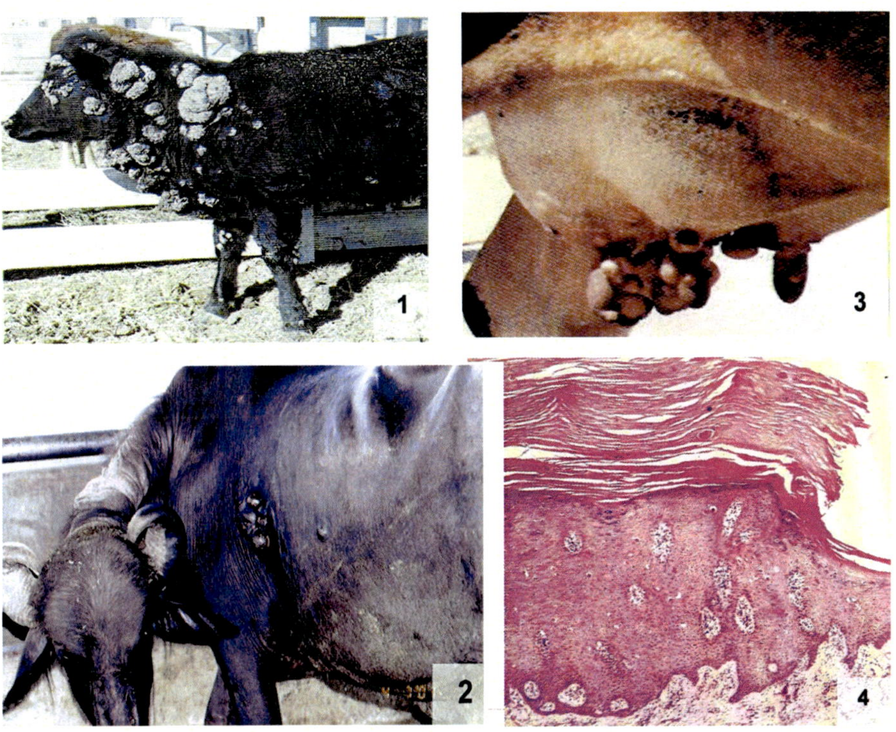

Fig. 11.10: Papilloma on skin of **(1)** Neck and face, **(2)** Shoulder, **(3)** Teats and **(4)** Microscopic features of papilloma

Etiology

- Papilloma virus of papovaviridae family.

Macroscopic features

- Size small from few mm to 10 cm diameter from skin
- Peduculated or broad based (urinary bladder).
- Surface may be smooth or horny.
- Some times finger like projections.

Microscopic features

- Thick layers of epithelium.
- Layer of connective tissue present.
- Epithelium irregularly arranged.

Diagnosis

- Symptoms and lesions
- Histopathological examination

Squamous Cell Carcinoma

Squamous cell carcinoma is a malignant tumour of squamous stratified epithelium. It is a common tumour of cattle in India; horn cancer is mostly seen in bullocks (Fig. 11.11).

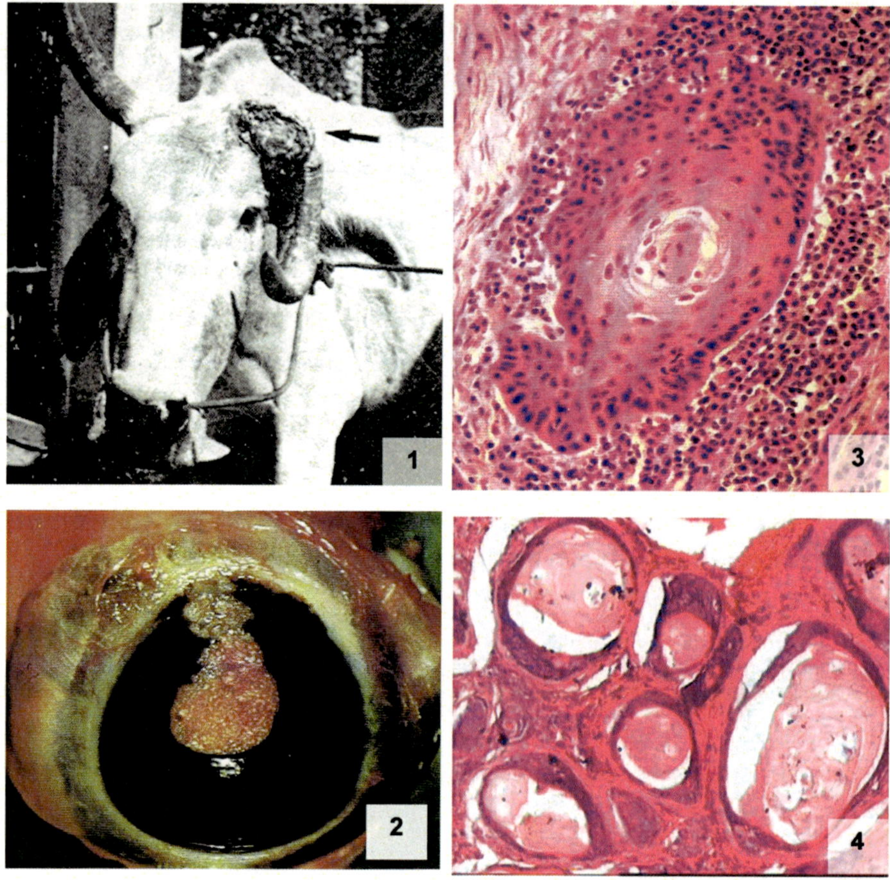

Fig. 11.11: Squamous cell carcinoma of (1) Horn (horn cancer) and (2) Eye (eye cancer), (3) Microscopic features of squamous cell carcinoma early state of epithelial pearl (4) Fully developed epithelial pearl

Etiology

- Exactly not known
- Possibly a virus
- Chronic irritation, trauma, paints, solar radiation
- Hormonal imbalances- Horn cancer, mostly occur in castrated animals

Macroscopic features

- Papillary projections or cauliflower like growth.
- Broad base
- Soft and grey or pink in colour
- Horn cancer invade the frontal sinuses
- Eye cancer arises from nictitating membrane of cornea

Microscopic features

- Stratum germinativum proliferate
- Concentric layers of keratin forms pearls ***'Epithelial pearls'***
- Mitotic figures seen
- Thickening of prickle cell layer

Diagnosis

- Symptoms and lesions
- Histopathological examination

Basal Cell Carcinoma

Basal cell carcinoma is a malignant tumour of basal cells of Malpigian layer of epidermis or hair matrix. They are also known ***hair cell carcinoma*** and are not invasive locally with no metastasis.

Etiology

- Not known
- Common in dogs, horses, cats.

Macroscopic features

- May occur singly and has broad base
- It is subcutaneous, rounded and encapsulated
- Firm in consistency
- Such skin shows alopecia and ulceration.

Microscopic features

- Pleomorphic cells- round or cigar shaped
- Hyperchromatic nuclei
- Cells arranged in columns descended to dermis
- Prickle cells are not observed
- No hair, mitotic figures seen.

Diagnosis

- Symptoms and lesions
- Histopathological examination

Adenoma and Adenocarcinoma

Adenoma is benign and adenocarcinoma is malignant tumour of glandular epithelium. They may arise from any gland of the body (Fig. 11.12).

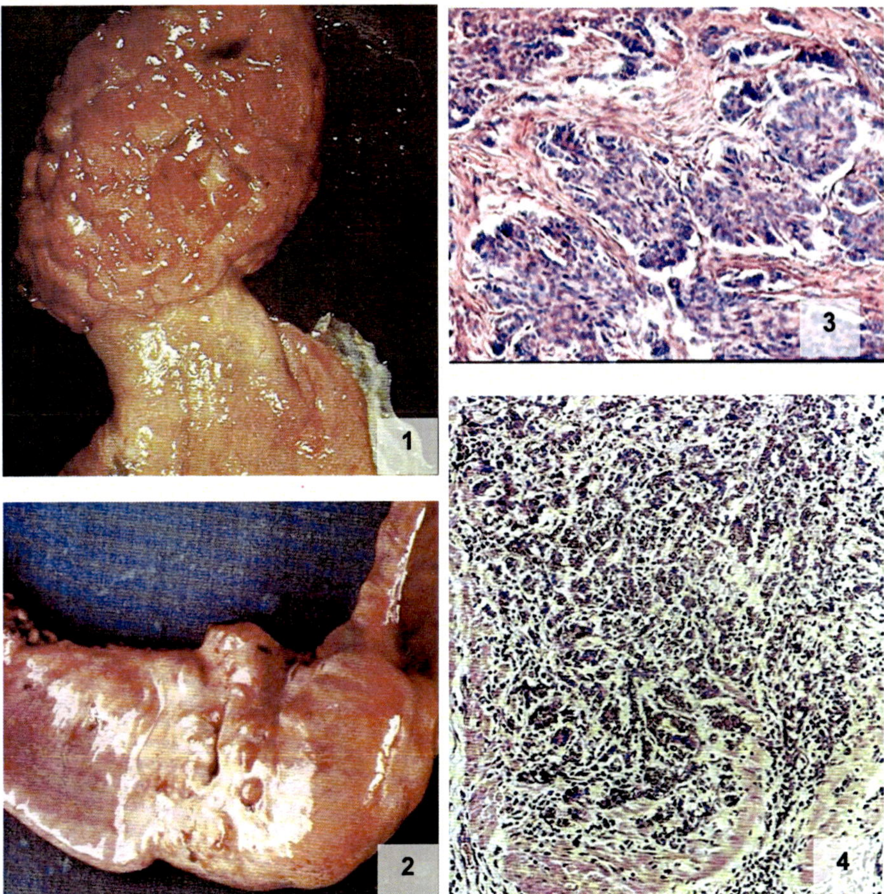

Fig. 11.12: (1) Adenoma in gall bladder, **(2)** Adenocarcinoma of intestine, **(3)** and **(4)** Microscopic features of adenocarcinoma

Etiology

- Not known

Macroscopic features

- Adenomas are nodular and encapsulated
- Clearly demarcated from surrounded tissues
- Pink in colour
- Polypoid in shape, may occlude gland or lumen of hollow organ.

Microscopic features

- Adenomas are having single layer of columnar or cuboidal epithelial cells
- Such cells show papillary projections in adenocarcinoma
- Pleomorphic cells, mitotic figures seen
- Small nucleus, with fine chromatin and fine nucleoli
- Such cells grouped into masses and invasive to basement membrane.

Diagnosis

- Symptoms and lesions
- Histopathological examination

Sebaceous Gland Adenoma

This is a benign tumour of sebaceous gland in skin and commonly observed in dogs at head, neck, eyelids, prepuce, tail and back.

Etiology

- Not known

Macroscopic features

- Small tumours, lobulated
- Grayish yellow in colour
- Tumours are greasy in touch.

Microscopic features

- Large polyhedral cells
- Fat droplets in cytoplasm
- Nucleus small and round with fine chromatin
- Cells are grouped in masses separated by connective tissue stroma.

Diagnosis

- Symptoms and lesions
- Histopathological examination

Perianal Adenoma of Dog

Perianal adenoma is modified benign tumour of sebaceous glands located at anal ring. These are commonly seen in dogs.

Etiology

- Not known

Macroscopic features

- Single or multilobular / nodular
- Firm, encapsulated
- Situated laterally or above the anus.

Microscopic features

- Epithelial cells arranged in lobules
- Polyhedral with giant granular acidophilic cytoplasm
- Cells are large and rounded
- Malignant tumours characterized by mitotic figures and anaplasia of the cells.

Diagnosis

- Symptoms and lesions
- Histopathological examination

Sweat Gland Adenoma

Sweat gland adenoma is benign tumour of sweat glands of skin of face and is common in dogs.

Etiology

- Not known

Macroscopic features

- Solid nodules small in size
- Hard to touch
- Grey in colour.

Microscopic features

- There may be columnar or cuboidal cells arranged in glandular fashion
- Acinis may have lumen or solid
- Cells have acidophilic and faintly granular cytoplasm
- Nucleus round or oval
- Secretion accumulated, then cyst adenocarcinoma/cystadenoma.

Diagnosis

- Symptoms and lesions
- Histopathological examination

Cholangiocellular Carcinoma

Cholangiocellular carcinoma is the tumour of bile duct commonly occurs in cattle and sheep (Fig. 11.13).

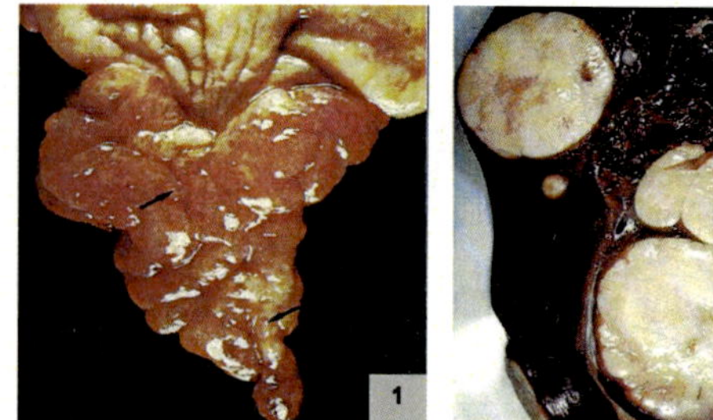

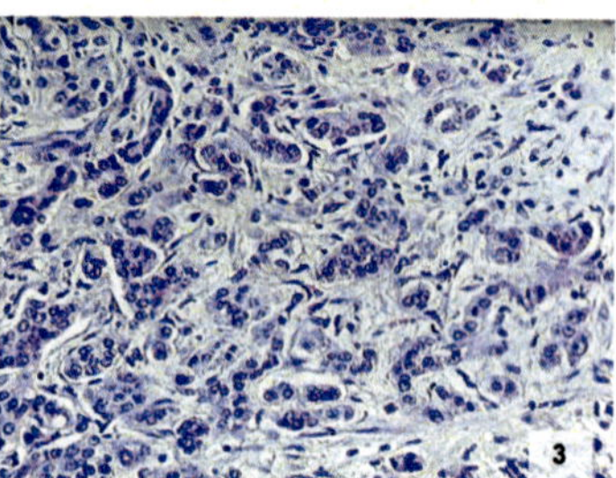

Fig. 11.13: Cholangiocellular **(1)** Adenoma of gall bladder and **(2)** Adenocarcinoma of bile duct. **(3)** Microscopic features of adenocarcinoma of bile duct

Etiology

- Not known
- More common in liver fluke infected animals
- Aflatoxins

Macroscopic features

- Small in size and multiple
- Round and encapsulated
- Yellowish white in colour

Microscopic features

- Consist acinis lined by columnar cells containing mucin
- Cyst like spaces filled with neoplastic cells
- Nucleus located at the base of cells
- Cells are surrounded by collagenous stroma.

Diagnosis

- Symptoms and lesions
- Histopathological examination

Hepatocellular carcinoma

Hepatocellular carcinoma is tumour of hepatic ells and observed in cattle and sheep (Fig. 11.14).

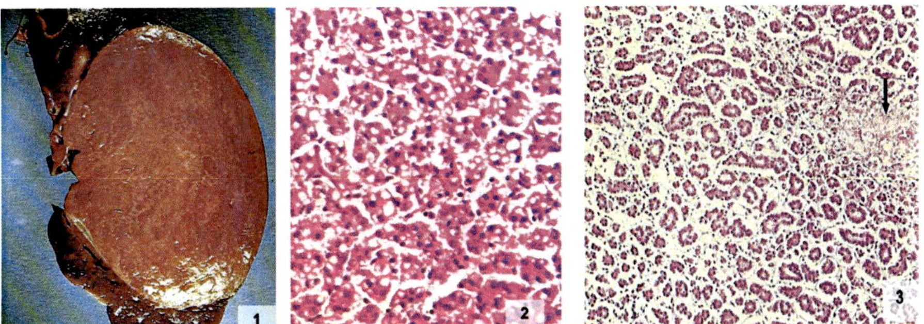

Fig. 11.14. (1) Hepatocellular carcinoma of sheep, (2) and (3) Microscopic features of hepatocellular carcinoma showing area of necrosis (arrow)

Etiology

- Not known
- Aflatoxin
- Liver fluke infection.

Macroscopic features

- Single, projected as brownish or greenish nodule
- Round or ovoid

Microscopic features

- Hepatic cells arranged in columns
- Cells are large and polyhedral with acidophilic granular cytoplasm
- Nucleus is very large, central and pale staining
- Numerous mitotic figures
- Tumour giant cells are seen
- Divided by connective tissue stroma.

Diagnosis

- Symptoms and lesions
- Histopathological examination

Papilloma / Malignant duct papilloma of Mammary gland

Papilloma or malignant duct papilloma is a tumour of duct epithelium of teat canal commonly seen in bitches (Fig. 11.15).

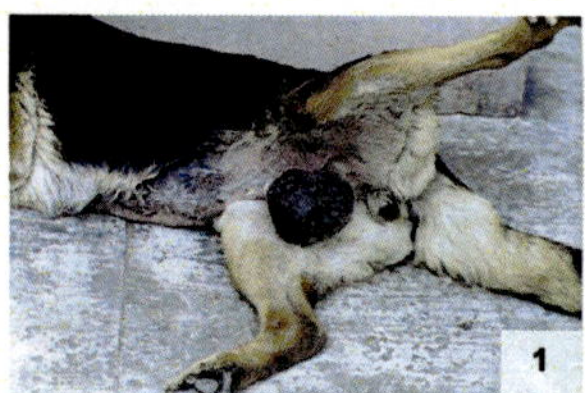

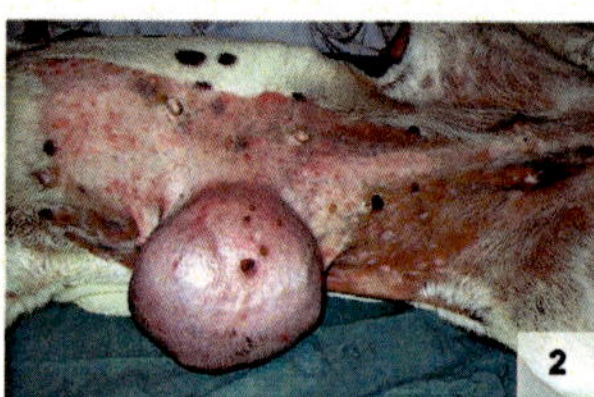

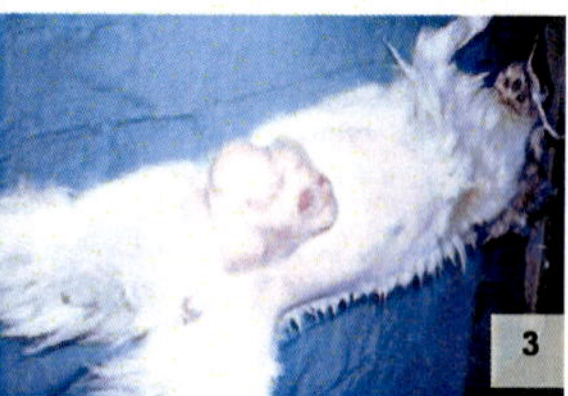

Fig. 11.15: (1) Papilloma and **(2&3)** Malignant duct papilloma of mammary gland in bitch.

Etiology

- Not known

Macroscopic features

- Tumours are soft or hard, cystic
- Grayish white in colour
- Enlarged teats
- Hard swelling

Microscopic features

- Tumour arises from lining epithelium of teat canal
- May be single

- Cells are cuboidal / columnar forms papillary projections
- Cells contain eosinophilic material
- Anaplastic cells have hyperchromasia
- Cells arranged in acinar or multi acinar form in malignant papilloma.

Diagnosis

- Symptoms and lesions
- Histopathological examination

Adenoma and Adenocarcinoma of thyroid

Adenoma of thyroid is common in horses. It is the benign tumour of thyroid. Adenocarcinoma is malignant tumour of thyroid commonly seen in old dogs.

Etiology

- Goiter
- Iodine deficiency may predispose.

Macroscopic features

- Small, rounded and encapsulated tumour
- Adenoma may cause pressure atrophy on rest of the gland
- Adenocarcinoma is multiple, unilateral, solid or cystic and highly invasive.

Microscopic features

- Formation of acini
- Columnar or cuboidal cells forms solid mass
- Nucleus oval, hyperchromatic
- Mitotic figures are common.

Diagnosis

- Symptoms and lesions
- Histopathological examination

Granulosa Cell Tumour of Ovary

Granulosa cell tumour arises from ovary mesenchyma and common in cattle. These tumours are seen in younger animals (Fig. 11.16).

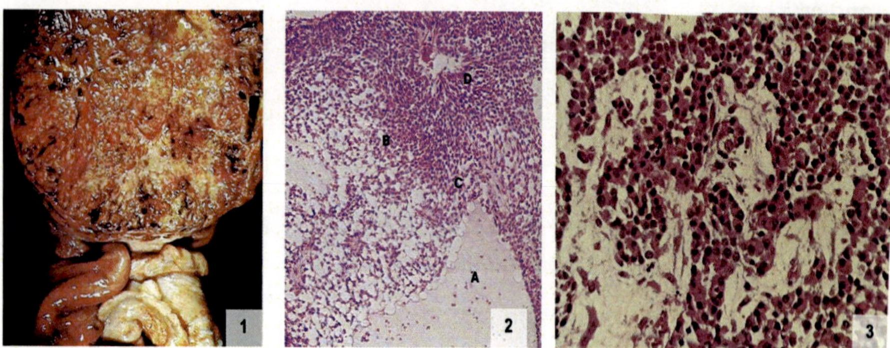

Fig. 11.16: Granulosa cell tumour of ovary- **(1)** Gross and **(2&3)** Microscopic features showing **A.** Cyst formation **B.** Typical granulosa cells, **C.** Granulosa cells arranged at right angle of cyst and **D.** Granulosa cells arranged at right angle of blood vessels.

Etiology

- Not known

Macroscopic features

- Single, very large even up to 20 cm diameter
- Rounded, lobulated projected on the surface of ovary
- Yellow in colour.

Microscopic features

- Tumour cells are arranged in columns, clusters or compact alveoli as irregular mass or pseudo glands
- In lumen, hyaline acidophilic material
- Several mitotic figures are seen.

Diagnosis

- Symptoms and lesions
- Histopathological examination

Seminoma

Seminoma is a malignant tumour of epithelium of seminiferous tubules of testes. It is common in dogs and bulls. It is more commonly seen in castrated and cryptorchid animals (Fig. 11.17).

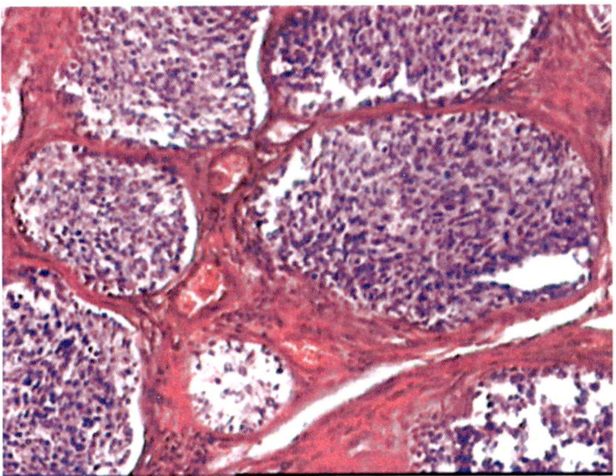

Fig. 11.17: Seminoma

Etiology

- Castration or cryptorchidism may predispose.

Macroscopic features

- White or grey in colour
- Lobulated as bulging from testes
- Areas of necrosis may be seen.

Microscopic features

- Epithelial cells are arranged as sheets or islands separated by thin strands of fibrous tissue
- Cells are round, large, uniform in size with acidophilic and granular cytoplasm
- Mitosis are numerous.

Diagnosis

- Symptoms and lesions
- Histopathological examination

Melanoma and Malignant Melanoma

Melanoma arises from melanoblasts situated in stratum germinativum of epidermis. Common in animals specially in old grey or white horses (Fig. 11.18).

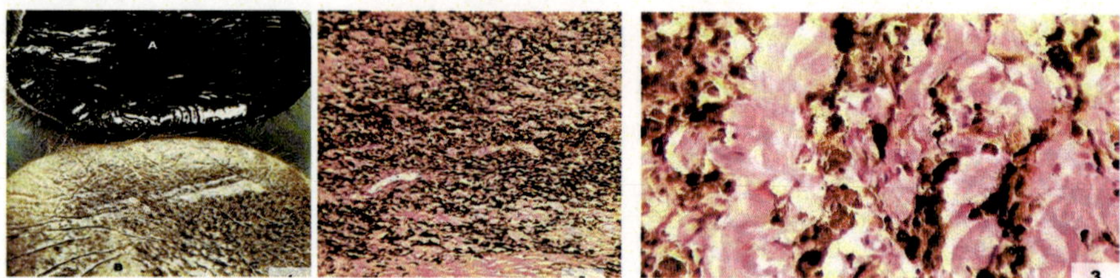

Fig. 11.18: Melanoma of skin **(1)** Gross **(2&3)** Microscopic features

Etiology

- Not known
- Mostly seen in dark coloured cattle, buffalo, sheep and goats

Macroscopic features

- Vary in size few mm diameter to several cm diameter
- Black or brown in colour
- Rounded, nodular, flat and pedunculated
- Firm and smooth
- On section, shiny black surface is seen
- Malignant melanomas are soft.

Microscopic features

- Collection of pigment laden cells covered by fibrous tissue
- Cells are polyhedral or oval or elongated
- In malignant melanomas, cells are anaplastic and may not have melanin
- Nucleus is large and vesicular
- Several mitotic figures are seen

Diagnosis

- Symptoms and lesions
- Histopathological examination

Venereal Lymphosarcoma

It is a transmissible venereal tumour in bitches or dogs seen at glans penis or vagina. Histogenic classification is not clear but may be a reticuloendothelial in origin (Fig. 11.19).

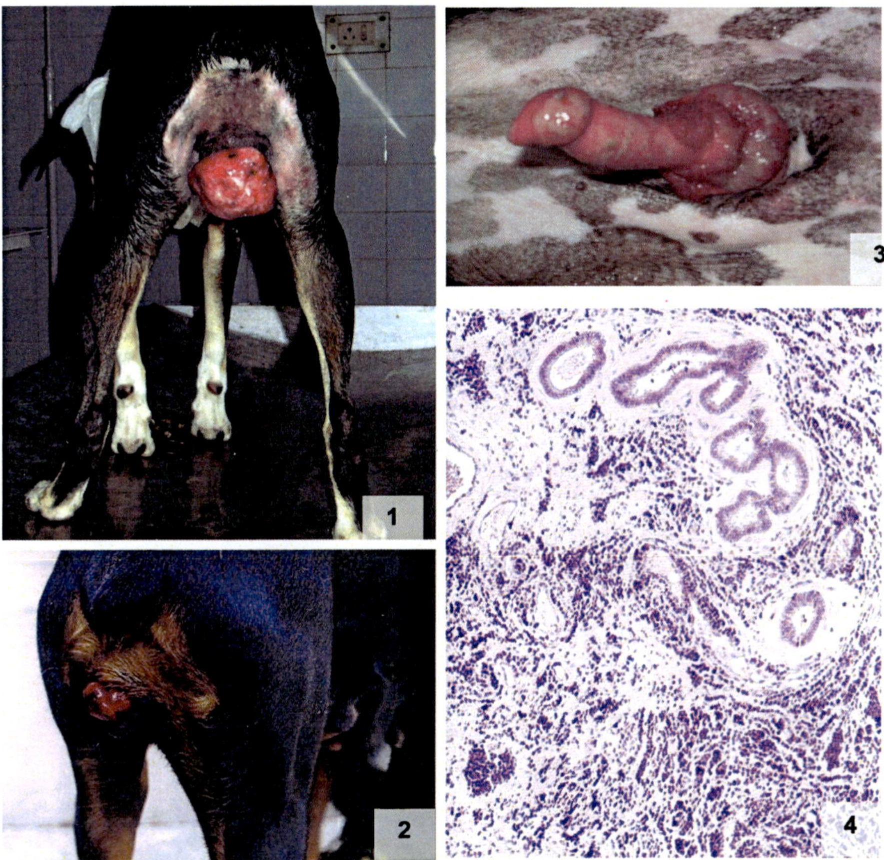

Fig. 11.19: Venereal lymphosarcoma in- **(1&2)** Bitch **(3)** Dog and **(4)** Microscopic features of lymphosarcoma

Etiology

- Not known. But it is transmissible in abraded mucous membrane through coitus

Macroscopic features

- Solitary/multiple
- Spreads like a cauliflower

- Pink in colour
- Soft in consistency
- Ulcerated and blood stained discharge.

Microscopic features

- Cellular mass, uniform in size and shape
- Round and polyhedral cells
- Finely granular acidophilic cytoplasm
- Numerous mitotic figures
- Nucleus large, round and central hyperchromatic.

Diagnosis

- Symptoms and lesions
- Histopathological examination

Adamantinoma

Adamantinomas are tumours arising from enamel organ. It is more common in cattle.

Etiology

- Not known

Macroscopic features

- Arises from alveolar border of maxilla or mandible
- Soft nodule
- Round or lobulated

Microscopic features

- Dense fibrous stroma having epithelial neoplastic ameloblasts
- Arranged in cyst or solid masses.
- Columnar epithelial cells with a giant basophilic cytoplasm
- Cells arranged in the form of a cyst
- Cyst may contain acidophilic debris.

Diagnosis

- Symptoms and lesions
- Histopathological examination

Connective Tissue Tumours

(Non-Epithelial Tumours)

Fibroma and Fibrosarcoma

Fibroma is a benign and fibrosarcoma is malignant tumour of fibrous connective tissue.

Etiology

- Not known
- 20% of skin tumours are fibropapilloma of gum, vagina, rectum or glans penis origin (Fig. 11.20).

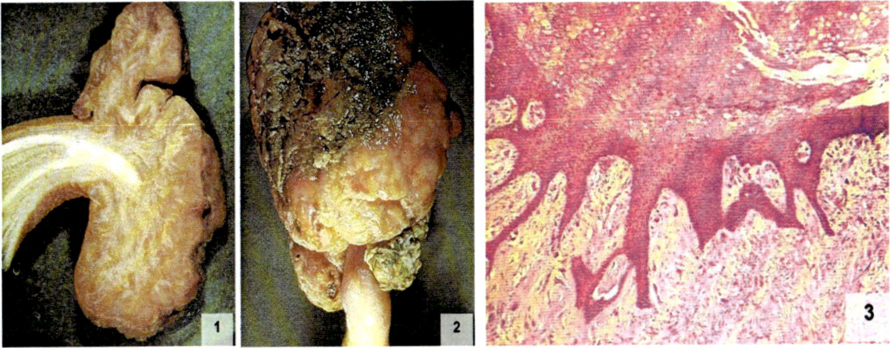

Fig. 11.20: Fibropapilloma in (1&2) Glans penis and (3) Microscopic features.

Macroscopic features

- Hard
- Common in horse, dogs
- Size from tiny nodules to large even up to several cm diameter
- Congestion

Microscopic features

- Interlacing bundles of fibrous connective tissue
- Nuclei of such cells are spindle shape
- Blood vessels, lymphocytes and monocytes are seen
- Increased number of mitotic figures (Malignant giant cells) in fibrosarcoma.

Diagnosis

- Symptoms and lesions
- Histopathological examination

Myxoma and Myxosarcoma

Myxoma is tumour of fibrous tissue capable of producing mucin and anaplasia. These are observed mostly on subcutaneous, subserous and submucous surfaces.

Etiology

- Unknown
- Myxomatosis virus in rabbits

Macroscopic features

- Rounded, bunch of grapes like structures
- Slimy in touch due to mucin content
- Present on subcutaneous, subserous or submucosal surfaces.

Microscopic features

- Spindle shaped cells
- Cells lying in basophilic mucinous matrix
- Pleomorphism
- Several mitotic figures
- Infiltration of inflammatory cells.

Diagnosis

- Symptoms and lesions
- Histopathological examination

Lipoma and Liposarcoma

Lipoma is a tumour of fat cells and seen in subcutaneous, subserosa, mesentery or submucosa. Lipoma is common in old aged animals while liposarcoma, the malignant tumour of fat cells is very rare (Fig. 11.21).

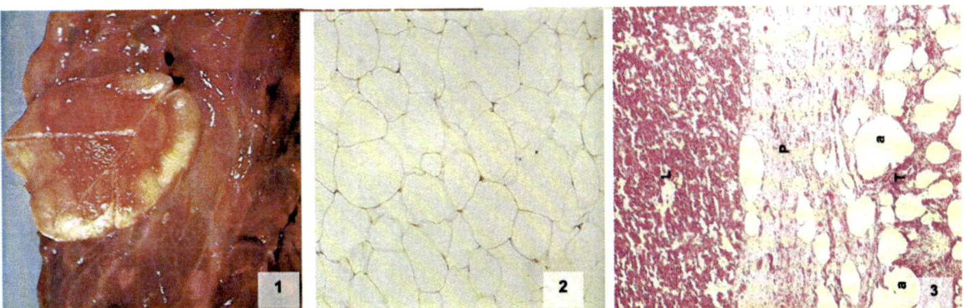

Fig. 11.21: Lipoma on pleura- **(1)** Gross, **(2 & 3)** Microscopic features.

Etiology

- Unknown

Macroscopic features

- Size vary from small nodule (1-2 mm dia) to large big mass (several cm diameter)
- Mostly spherical and lobulated
- On section, cut surface is oily
- Yellow in colour

Microscopic features

- Polyhedral cells may have a large fat globule or several small ones with marginal nucleus.
- Connective tissue divides the mass into lobules
- In malignancy, anaplastic cells have little fat.

Diagnosis

- Symptoms and lesions
- Histopathological examination

Chondroma and Chondrosarcoma

Chondroma is a benign and chondrosarcoma is malignant tumour of cartilage cells. These are rare in animals. In dogs, chondroma are reported in mammary gland (Fig. 11.22).

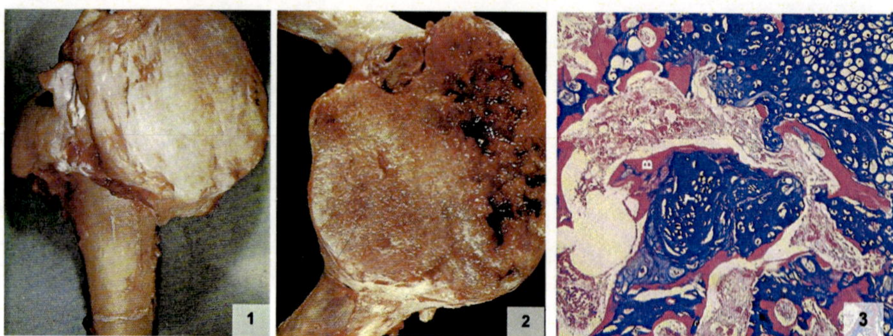

Fig. 11.22: (1) Chondroma of epiphyseal region of femur, (2) Chondrosarcoma in the distal end of radius and (3) Microscopic features of chondrosarcoma.

Etiology

- Not known
- Common in sheep, arises from osteochondral junction of scapula, ribs, humerus and femur

Macroscopic features

- Chondromas are multinodular
- Encapsulated and rounded
- Bluish white in colour
- Section shows translucent appearance
- Calcification may be observed

Microscopic features

- Rounded or ovoid cells in bluish matrix
- Cells are arranged mostly as single.
- Strands of fibrous connective tissue forms lobules
- Chondrosarcoma cells are pleomorphic
- Several mitotic figures

Diagnosis

- Symptoms and lesions
- Histopathological examination

Osteoma and Osteosarcoma

Osteoma is benign and osteosarcoma is malignant and hard tumour of bone. This is rarely seen in animals. On skull, scapula or pelvic bones, they are known as ***compact osteoma*** while on long bones they are called as ***spongy osteoma*** (Fig. 11.23).

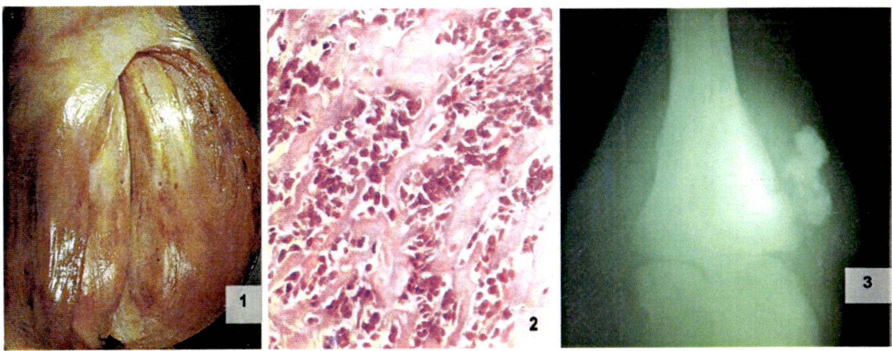

Fig. 11.23: (1) Osteoma of premaxilla (2) Osteosarcoma of femur and (3) Osteoma of femur (X-ray picture).

Etiology

- Not known
- Rare in occurrence

Macroscopic features

- Nodular, encapsulated
- Found on skull, scapula, pelvic bones or head of long bones.
- Round or ovoid in shape
- White, yellow or pink in colour.

Microscopic features

- Osteoid tissue with lamellar arrangement
- Confused with exostosis
- Osteosarcoma have pleomorphic cells

- Tumour giant cells
- Several mitotic figures
- Several new blood vessels

Diagnosis

- Symptoms and lesions
- Histopathological examination

Leiomyoma and Leiomyosarcoma

Leiomyoma is a benign tumour of smooth muscle found in different organs like uterus, vagina, stomach, intestines, urinary bladder, esophagus etc. Such tumours are commonly seen in cow, dog and poultry. Leiomyosarcoma is malignant neoplasm of smooth muscles (Fig. 11.24).

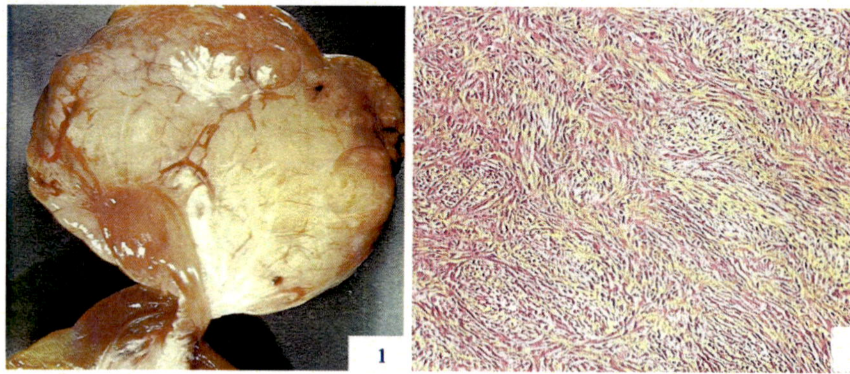

Fig. 11.24: Leiomyoma of (a) Mesentery and intestine and (2) Microscopic features of leiomyoma

Etiology

- Not known

Macroscopic features

- Small size tumours with broad base
- Firm, lobulated and pink in colour.

Microscopic features

- Muscle bundles arranged in all directions and planes
- Muscle bundles separated by fibrous tissue with blood vessels

- Nucleus becomes cigar shaped and contain filamentus chromatin
- Leiomyosarcoma have anaplastic cells with shorter chromatin
- Mitotic figures are common.
- Such tumours are invasive to adjacent tissues.

Diagnosis

- Symptoms and lesions
- Histopathological examination

Rhabdomyoma and Rhabdomysarcoma

Rhabdomyoma is a benign and rhabdomyosarcoma is malignant tumour of skeletal and cardiac muscles and are rare in animals (Fig. 11.25).

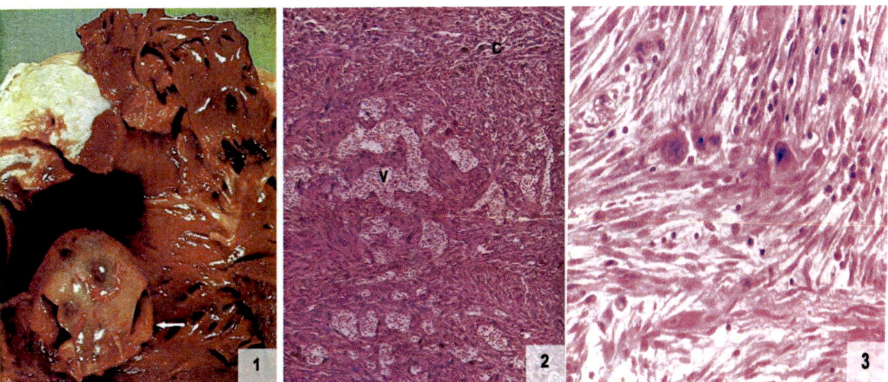

Fig. 11.25: (1) Rhadomyosarcoma of heart muscles (2) Microscopic features- V. Vasuclar and C. Cellular parts of the rhabdomyosarcoma and (3) Anaphastic features of tumor.

Etiology

- Not known

Macroscopic features

- Found in tongue, chest, sternal muscles, neck region, cardiac muscles
- Broad based.

Microscopic features

- Striated muscles grow on different directions
- Fibrous tissue divides the muscle bundles into lobules

- In Rhabdomyosarcoma, the anaplastic cells are pleomorphic, polyhedral and spindle shaped.
- Presence of tumour giant cells.

Diagnosis

- Symptoms and lesions
- Histopathological examination

Haemangioma and Haemangiosarcoma

Haemangioma is benign while haemangiosarcoma is malignant tumour of blood vessels (Fig. 11.26).

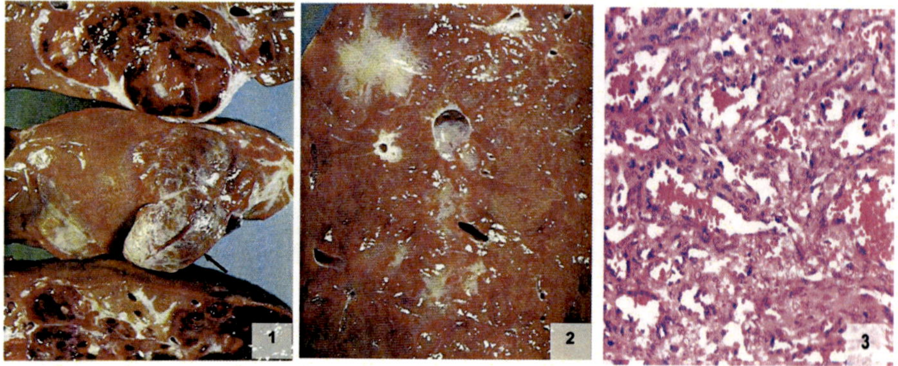

Fig. 11.26: Haemangiosarcoma (1&2) Liver and (3) Microscopic features in spleen.

Etiology

- Not known

Macroscopic features

- Usually single
- Vary in size few mm diameter to several cm diameter.
- Dark red in colour and confused with haematoma
- Bleeding is severe on rupture or injury.

Microscopic features

- Many capillaries are seen
- Usually single cell lined capillaries
- Lumen filled with newly formed endothelial cells
- Pleomorphism in endothelial cells
- Such cells grouped into masses in malignant tumours
- Numerous mitotic figures are seen.

Diagnosis

- Symptoms and lesions
- Histopathological examination

Mesothelioma

Mesothelioma is a tumour of mesothelial lining cells of serous cavities specially of peritoneum and pleura. Such tumours are found in thorax and abdomen (Fig. 11.27).

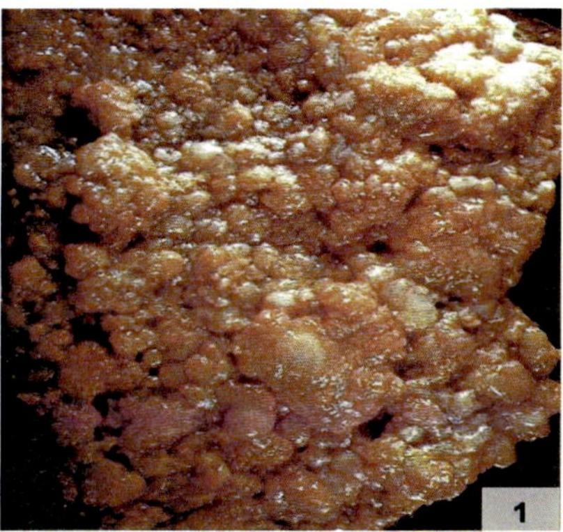

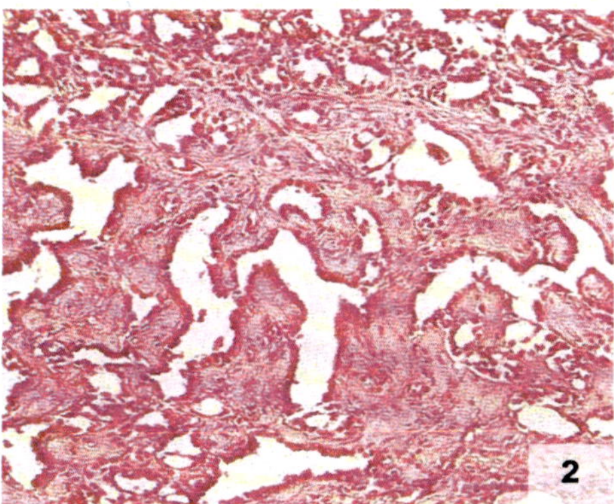

Fig. 11.27: Mesothelioma of peritoneum- (1) Gross and (2) Microscopic features having low columnar epithelium supported by connective tissue stroma.

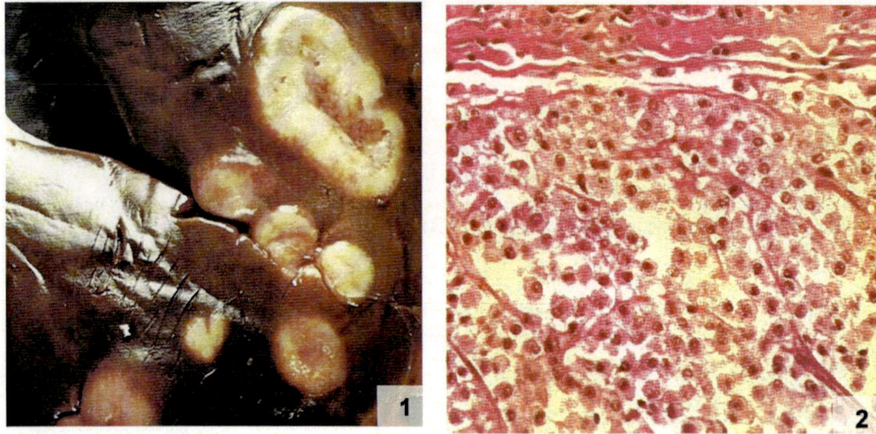

Fig. 11.28: Myelosarcoma in liver- (1) Gross and (2) Microscopic features of basophilic myelosarcoma in lungs.

Etiology

- Not known

Macroscopic features

- Pink in colour and hard
- Multiple, nodular and scattered in cavity
- Found in thorax and/or abdominal cavity.

Microscopic features

- Collection of cells resembling epithelial cells
- Cells have acidophilic granular cytoplasm and large vesicular nucleus
- Numerous blood vessels in tumour
- A core of fibrous tissue present
- Mitotic figures may be seen.

Diagnosis

- Symptoms and lesions
- Histopathological examination

Mastocytoma

Mastocytoma is a tumour of mast cells commonly seen in dogs in subcutaneous tissue of hind legs.

Etiology

- Not known

Macroscopic features

- Usually single and have a size of about 8-12 cm diameter.
- Nodular, pedunculated
- Hard, pink or grey in colour
- Ulceration over tumour is common.

Microscopic features

- Pleomorphic mast cells
- Inflammatory cells like neutrophils and lymphocytes are also seen
- Darkly stained cells
- Cytoplasm is more than in lymphocytes
- No or little cytoplasmic granules
- Few mitotic figures

Diagnosis

- Symptoms and lesions
- Histopathological examination

Lymphoma and Lymphosarcoma

Lymphoma is a benign and lymphosarcoma is a malignant neoplasm of lymphoid cells primarily found in lymph nodes (Fig. 11.29).

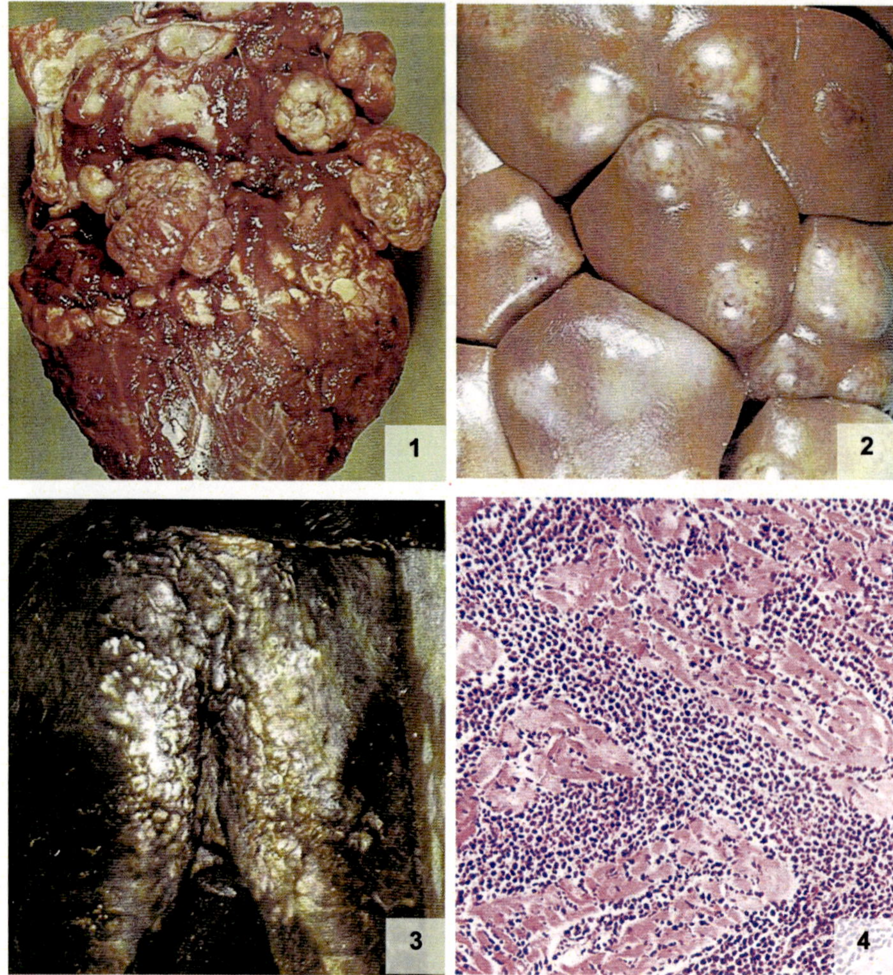

Fig. 11.29: Lymphosarcoma of **(1)** Heart **(2)** Kidney and **(3)** Skin and **(4)** Microscopic features of lymphosarcoma in heart.

Etiology

- Not known
- Possibly a retrovirus

Macroscopic features

- Tumours in several lymph nodes and spleen.

- Obliteration of lymph vessels / blood vessels.
- Common in dogs (canine venereal tumour), cat and cattle.
- Enlargement of lymph nodes.
- Spleen is enlarged, soft and friable.
- Liver enlarged and pale.

Microscopic features

- Immature pleomorphic lymphoid cells.
- Mitotic figures are seen.
- Tumour giant cells are seen.
- In blood, number of immature lymphoid cell increases and known as ***Leukemia***.

Diagnosis

- Symptoms and lesions
- Histopathological examination

Neoplasms in Cattle and Buffaloes

Tumour or neoplasm is defined as a new growth of cells which proliferate continuously without control, bear a considerable resemblance to the healthy cells from which they arise, have no orderly structural arrangement, serves no useful function and for the present at least, have no clearly understood cause. Tumours are characterized by the following main hallmarks: genome instability, mutation and epigenetic change; sustained proliferation and evasion of growth suppression; evasion of apoptosis; deregulation of energy metabolism; induction of angiogenesis and invasion and metastasis.

There are various etiological factors like hereditary factors, age, pigmentation, hormones (intrinsic factors), extrinsic factors like physical trauma, chronic irritation, chemical carcinogens, ionizing radiation, actinic light rays, metazoan parasites, viruses, etc. These all are involved in the carcinogenesis or development of cancer. In the thirst of modernization and industrialization, man has contributed pollution to the life and ecology of plants, animals and microbes. Increased demand for food and fibre has led to the chemicalization of agriculture and we have reached on such a stage that modern agriculture is dependent on high yielding varieties, which can only be grown under the influence of fertilizers and pesticides. Pesticides are the man-made chemicals which are being used to produce enough cheap food. Majority of these pesticides are beneficial when used for specific purposes, handled properly and applied as per the recommendations of the manufacturer. However, over the years, there has been a mounting fear and concern that indiscriminate and improportionate use of pesticides may lead to their residues in food chain which may exert their harmful effects in human beings and animals. In an ideal pesticide application, the chemical should fall exactly on the target and be degraded completely to harmless compounds but this never occurs and only some part of the pesticide hits the target pests while remaining drifts into the environment. Most of organochlorine pesticides like dieldrin, gamma isomer of benzene hexachloride (BHC), dichloro diphenyl trichloroethane (DDT) and polychlorinated biphenyl (PCB) may cause cancer in liver and lung. Indirectly, a state of immunosuppression for a longer period is helpful in increasing the susceptibility of an animal for malignancy. Since many pesticides are known to cause mutation in chromosomes of man and animals, it is considered that they may also lead to carcinogenicity. Immunity is a result of interactions among various cells of the immune system and tumour cells. The occurrence of spontaneous regression, although extremely rare, and the presence of lymphoid infiltrates in and around tumours indicate that immunological defence mechanisms may interfere with the development and growth of tumours. Tumour cells can be recognized by the immune system because they often bear unique tumour specific antigens. These tumour specific antigens arise from mutations of cellular genes that give rise to abnormal proteins that are expressed on the cell surface or to abnormal expression of genes that would not otherwise be expressed. Tumour cells may also bear non-unique tumour associated antigens that are found in tumour cells as well as in other cells in the body. Some of these are oncofoetal antigens.

A survey was carried out from 1982 to 1995 (14 years) on neoplasms in cattle and buffaloes and the prevalence of different neoplasms was recorded as squamous cell carcinoma (48.4%), fibroma (19.61%), melanoma (6.5%), lymphosarcoma (4.5%) and papilloma (4.2%). The occurrence of neoplasms in different animals were as 62.3% in bullocks, 19.4% in cows, 16% in buffaloes and 2.3% in bulls.

In the present study, the cases of tumours in cattle and buffaloes which had been reported in India during the period 1990-2017 are summarised below:

1. Papilloma and Squamous Cell Carcinoma

Papilloma is a benign tumour from an epithelial surface and involves squamous, transitional or columnar epithelium depending on the tissue of origin. Macroscopically, size is small from few mm to 10 cm in diameter from skin, pedunculated or broad based (urinary bladder). Surface may be smooth or horny. Sometimes finger like projections are seen. Microscopic features are thick layers of epithelium, layer of connective tissue is present and epithelium is irregularly arranged. It had been reported from the oral cavity of a calf in Mathura in 1991 , bovine cutaneous papillomatosis in Tirunelveli in 1992, cutaneous and teat papillomas in cattle in Ludhiana in 2003 , teat papillomas in bovine in Ludhiana in 2004 and papillary transitional cell carcinoma of urinary bladder in a cow in Mysore, Karnataka in 2010 .

Squamous cell carcinoma is a malignant tumour of squamous stratified epithelium which is characterized by macroscopic features like papillary projections or cauliflower like growth, broad base, soft and grey or pink in colour and microscopic features as Stratum germinativum proliferation, concentric layers of keratin forming *'Epithelial pearls'*, presence of mitotic figures seen and thickening of prickle cell layer. This type of tumour had been reported from the eye of a 8 years old Murrah buffalo in Andhra Pradesh in 1991, from bovines in Parbhani, Maharashtra in the year 1992, from 6 years old cow in Durg in 1995, from larynx of 15 years old Ongole cow in Tirupati in the year 2000 , from urethra in a 6 years old adult bullock in Hisar in the year 2000, from gingiva of 7 days old Hariana male calf in Hisar in the year 2001, from neck of 8 years old bullock in Chattisgarh in the year 2002, from the tail of 12 years old bull in Chattisgarh in the year 2002, from lower jaw of a bullock in Karnataka in the year 2010 and from vulva in a cow in IVRI, Izzatnagar in the year 2014. A case of ocular carcinoma was detected in buffalo at Pantnagar.

Horn cancer is commonest neoplasm of cattle in India; however, it may also occur is buffaloes and sheep. This neoplasm was first reported in 1905 from Bombay Veterinary College and since then it has been recorded from every part of the country. Adult cattle of 5-10 years of age mostly suffer from horn cancer. It has been recorded in long horned animals with white coat. The prevalence of horn cancer was found highest in Kankrej (8.24%) followed by Gir (7.33%), Malvi (6.99%), Khillari (2.96) and others (1.11%). Working bullocks are comparatively more susceptible to horn cancer. In a study of 968430 cattle and buffaloes during 1966-70, neoplasm of horn has been recorded in 2652 animals including 2268 cattle and 384 buffaloes. More than 90% of affected animals were in the age group of 5-10 years.

Horn cancer is a squamous cell carcinoma of horn, originating from core epithelium. The disease is characterized by bending and dropping of affected horn, development of cauliflower-like cancerous growth, cachexia, anaemia and death after prolonged illness. Microscopically, it is characterized by the presence of epithelial pearls. The stroma is infiltrated by lymphocytes and polymorphonuclear cells. It had been reported from a 8 years old non-descript buffalo in Namakkal, Tamilnadu in 2000 and from a 12 years old cow in Maharashtra in 2002.

Fibroma and Fibrosarcoma

Fibroma is a benign and fibrosarcoma is malignant tumour of fibrous connective tissue. Macroscopically, they are hard in touch, size varies from tiny nodules to large even several cm in diameter. Microscopic features are that the neoplastic cells make significant amounts of collagen, which separates these cells from each other and presence of interlacing bundles of fibrous connective tissue along with spindle shaped nuclei of the cells. There is increased number of mitotic figures (malignant giant cells) in fibrosarcoma. Fibroma had been reported from the oral cavity of a 12 years old Jersey cow in Bhubaneswar in the year 1990, angiofibroma from the nasal cavity of an adult cow in Ludhiana in the year 1990, neurofibroma from 3 years old HF bull in Ludhiana in the year 1990, from the lower jaw of a crossbred cow in Vijayawada, Andhra Pradesh in 1991, rectal neurofibroma from 6 years old Murrah buffalo in Andhra Pradesh in 1993, from the vagina of 6 years old Jersey crossbred cow in Ludhiana in 1995, from rumen of a 10 years non-descript bullock in Parbhani in 1995, chondrofibroma of udder in a 5 years old crossbred cow in Bhubaneswar in 1996, from point of elbow in a 6 years Sahiwal bullock in Durg in 1997, perianal fibroma in 8 years crossbred cow in Nagpur in 1998, neurofibroma over perineum in 8 years old buffalo in Andhra Pradesh in 2002, unilateral nasal polypoid fibroma in a heifer in West Bengal in 2004, fibroma from the colon of a crossbred cow in Tamilnadu in the year 2016, oral fibrosarcoma in a cow in Puducherry in 2011 and ameloblastic fibrosarcoma in a cow in Kerala in 2012.

Basal Cell Carcinoma

Basal cell carcinoma is a malignant tumour of basal cells of Malpighian layer of epidermis or hair matrix. They are also known as hair cell carcinoma and are not invasive locally with no metastasis. Macroscopically, it may occur singly and has broad base. It is subcutaneous, rounded, encapsulated and firm in consistency. Such skin shows alopecia and ulceration. Microscopic features are presence of pleomorphic cells which are round or cigar shaped with hyperchromatic nuclei. Cells are arranged in columns descended to dermis. Prickle cells are not observed. No hair, mitotic figures are seen. It had been reported from a 7-8 years old bullock in Nagpur in 1990 and from a 14 years old Hariana white bullock in Bhubaneswar in 1996.

Melanocytoma and Malignant Melanoma (Melanosarcoma)

Melanocytoma refers to all benign neoplasms of melanocytes. Dermal melanocytomas are confined to the superficial dermis. Microscopically, the neoplasm is composed of plump fusiform cells arranged in whorls or sheets. There is little stromal collagen between the closely packed neoplastic cells. The neoplastic cells have ovoid, vesicular nuclei with prominent nucleoli. Mitotic activity is low. It had been reported from cattle in Gujarat in the year 2015. Malignant melanoma are malignant counterparts of melanocytoma. Grossly, melanoma is recognized by its deep black colour. Their main characteristic is the great pleomorphism and variation in the pattern of growth and degree of pigmentation of neoplastic cells. The shape of the cells varies from round to polygonal forms(bizarre-odd, unusual) including elongated, fusiform to stellate cells. Spindle-shaped cells dominate and are demarcated by thin fibrous trabeculae. The cytoplasm tends to be basophilic. The nucleoli are large and prominent. The basement membrane is lost. Mitotic activity is high. It had been reported from a 8 years old Jersey cow in Palampur in 1990, from two and a half years old Ongole bull in Andhra Pradesh in 1990, from bovines in Madras in 1990 , from nine and a half years old bullock in Jabalpur in 1990, from a 4 years old Hallikar bullock in Anantapur, Andhra Pradesh in 1994, from a 14 years Deoni bullock in Bidar in 1995, from a 4 years crossbred Jersey cow in Andhra Pradesh in 1995, from a 5 years non-descript bullock in Andhra Pradesh in 1996, from the mammary gland of 4 years old Nagpuri buffalo in Akola, Maharashtra in 1997, from a 3 years old non-descript dark-skinned bull in Andhra Pradesh in 1998 and from a 7 years non-descript cow in Guntur, Andhra Pradesh in 2001.

Myxoma and Myxosarcoma

Myxoma is tumour of fibrous tissue capable of producing mucin and anaplasia. These are observed mostly on subcutaneous, subserous and submucous surfaces. Macroscopically, rounded, bunch of grapes like structures are seen. They are slimy in touch due to mucin content. Microscopic features are presence of spindle shaped cells lying in basophilic mucinous matrix with pleomorphism and presence of several mitotic figures with infiltration of inflammatory cells. The nuclei tends to be round or stellate and the intercellular fibrils are bluish (H&E stain). Myxosarcoma had been reported from the nasal cavity of a 6 years old crossbred Jersey cow in Bhubaneswar in 1993 and from the nasal cavity of Kankrej bullock in Gujarat in 2015. Myxoma had been reported from a 3 years old non-descript cow in Izzatnagar in 2000 and odontogenic myxoma had been reported from a cow in Haryana in 2015.

Histiocytoma

Common sites of histiocytoma are face, pinnae, neck, distal extremities and scrotum. Grossly, the neoplasm appears as a solitary or multiple, raised 1-3 cm alopecic plaque or mass, often with ulceration. So it is also called as button tumour. Microscopically, they are composed of nodular infiltrates or round to polygonal cells arranged in cords or sheets. The infiltrate destroys most adnexal structures. Older neoplasms contain infiltrates of lymphocytes and have areas of coagulative necrosis. It had been reported from a buffalo in 2008 at IVRI, Izzatnagar.

Sweat Gland Adenoma

Sweat gland adenoma is benign tumour of sweat glands of skin of face. Macroscopically, solid nodules are seen which are small in size, hard to touch and grey in colour. Microscopic features are presence of columnar or cuboidal cells arranged in glandular fashion. Acini may have lumen or are solid. Cells have acidophilic and faintly granular cytoplasm. Nucleus is round or oval. If secretion is accumulated, then it can be cyst adenocarcinoma or cyst adenoma. It had been reported from a Murrah buffalo in Chhatisgarh in 2004.

Lipoma and liposarcoma

Lipoma is a tumour of fat cells and seen in subcutaneous, subserosa, mesentery or submucosa. Lipoma is common in old aged animals while liposarcoma, the malignant tumour of fat cells is very rare. Macroscopically, size varies from small nodule (1-2 mm diameter) to large big mass (several cm diameter).They are mostly spherical and lobulated. On section, cut surface is oily and yellow in colour. Microscopic features are presence of polyhedral cells which may have a large fat globule or several small ones with marginal nucleus. Connective tissue divides the mass into lobules. In malignancy, anaplastic cells have little fat. Lipoma had been reported from the abdomen of a 10 years old Murrah buffalo in Tamilnadu in 1990, from duodenum of a 7 years old Jersey cow in Palampur in 1990 and from vagina of a 6 years old crossbred Jersey cow in Madras in 1991.

Trichoepithelioma

It is a benign epithelial tumour developing from basal cells in the hair follicles on skin. Macroscopically, there can be hyperpigmentation on the chest, thigh, perianal region, tail and ear tips. Microscopically, there is increased thickness of dermis and presence of numerous hair follicles. Surrounding this, sebaceous glands are also seen with abundant fibrous tissue formation. It had been reported from a 11 months crossbred cattle in Nagpur in 1991.

Adenoma and Adenocarcinoma

Adenoma is benign and adenocarcinoma is malignant tumour of glandular epithelium. They may arise from any gland of the body. Macroscopically, adenomas are nodular and encapsulated and clearly demarcated from surrounded tissues by its pink colour, polypoid in shape and may occlude gland or lumen of hollow organ. Microscopic features are single layer of columnar or cuboidal epithelial cells in case of adenomas and such cells show papillary projections in adenocarcinoma. Presence of pleomorphic cells, mitotic figures, small nucleus with fine chromatin and fine nucleoli is there and such cells are grouped into masses and invasive to basement membrane. Cystadenoma had been reported from the colon of a 7 years old Kankrej bullock in Gujarat in 1995, fibroadenoma of mammary gland in a Mehsana buffalo in Gujarat in 2015, adenocarcinoma from the salivary gland of a 8 years old non-descript bullock in Andhra Pradesh in 2001and ethmoidal adenocarcinoma in a buffalo in Tamilnadu in 2015.

Mesothelioma

Mesothelioma is a tumour of mesothelial lining cells of serous cavities especially of peritoneum and pleura. Such tumours are found in thorax and abdomen. Macroscopically, they are pink in colour, hard, multiple, nodular and scattered in cavity. Microscopic features are presence of collection of cells resembling epithelial cells and these cells have acidophilic granular cytoplasm and large vesicular nucleus and there are numerous blood vessels in tumour. It had been reported from a 17 years old bullock in Bidar in 1993 and from a 10 years old crossbred cow in Palampur in 1993.

Dental Neoplasms

(a) **Odontomas:** They are hamartomas of enamel origin and contain fully differentiated dentin and enamel. (A hamartoma is a benign tumour-like nodule composed of an overgrowth of mature tissue in which the elements show disordered arrangement and proportion in comparison to normal). It had been reported from ruminants in Bidar in 1998and bovine dental tumours in Gujarat in 2017.

(b) **Ameloblastoma:** This is a generic name used for the epithelial neoplasms of enamel organ origin. It can occur anywhere in the dental tissue. It can be either superficial or deep. It is locally invasive, and results in destruction of alveolar bone. Microscopically, ameloblastoma includes inter branching sheets of epithelial cells, intense keratinization and the presence of extracellular hyaline bodies. These hyaline bodies often stained for amyloid. It had been reported from a crossbred Holstein

Friesian bull in Srinagar in 2006, from bovine in Nagpur in 2014 and from a buffalo in Hisar, Haryana in 2017.

(c) **Adamantinoma:** Adamantinomas are the tumours arising from enamel organ. Macroscopically, it arises from alveolar border of maxilla or mandible and soft nodules occur which are round or lobulated. Microscopic features are presence of dense fibrous stroma having epithelial neoplastic ameloblasts which are arranged in cyst or solid masses. Columnar epithelial cells with a giant basophilic cytoplasm are seen. Cells are arranged in the form of a cyst which may contain acidophilic debris. It had been reported from a 6 years old Ongole bull in Andhra Pradesh in 2000.

Ethmoidal Neoplasms

These are tumours arising from the mucosa lining the ethmoid bone. Grossly, the tumour fills up the nasal cavity and the paranasal sinuses and destroys turbinates. There is congestion and marked oedema of the ethmoturbinates, which are covered with copious mucous. It is fleshy, grey-white and presents a varying degree of necrosis. Microscopically, the tumour consists of irregular clusters of anaplastic cells with prominent mitotic figures along with neutrophilic infiltration and stromal fibrosis. Tumour giant cells with multiple nuclei are present. Areas of necrosis and haemorrhage are also observed. It had been reported in crossbred cows in Ranchi in 1990.

Hepatocellular Carcinoma

Hepatocellular carcinoma is a malignant tumour of hepatic cells. Macroscopically, they are single, projected as brownish or greenish nodule and are round or ovoid. Microscopic features are hepatic cells arranged in columns. They are large and polyhedral with acidophilic granular cytoplasm. Nucleus is very large, central and pale staining. Numerous mitotic figures are present. Tumour giant cells are seen and divided by connective tissue stroma. It had been reported from an Indian water buffalo in Ludhiana in 2011.

Cholangiocellular Carcinoma

These are malignant neoplasms of biliary epithelium which usually originate from the intra-hepatic ducts. Macroscopically, they are small in size, multiple, round and encapsulated. They are yellowish white in colour. Microscopic features are acini lined by columnar cells containing mucin There are cyst like spaces filled with neoplastic cells. Nucleus is located at the base of cells. Cells are surrounded by collagenous stroma. It had been reported from a 17 years old crossbred bullock in Akola, Maharashtra in 1997, from buffalo in Jabalpur in 2004, from a buffalo in Kerala in 2011 and from Kankrej bullock in Gujarat in 2015.

Haemangioma

It is a benign tumour of blood vessels. Macroscopically, they are usually single, vary in size from few mm to several cm in diameter. They are dark red in colour and bleeding is severe on rupture or injury. Microscopic features are presence of many single cell lined capillaries and their lumen is filled with newly formed endothelial cells. It had been reported from a 6 years old crossbred Jersey cow at tip of teat in Thrissur in 2001 and from a cattle in Meerut in 2014.

Lymphoma and Lymphosarcoma

Multiple neoplastic growths are seen, which are moderately firm, pale, yellow in colour and appeared as masses of firm lard with greasy look. Histopathological features include neoplastic lymphoid cells in sheets encircled in delicate strands of fibrous tissues. Tumour cells can show invasion even in muscle fibres causing degeneration and necrosis. Neoplastic cells have large deep staining nucleus with scanty cytoplasm. Mitotic figures are frequent. Lymphoma had been reported from a buffalo in Chennai in 2005. Lymphosarcoma had been reported from a 7 years old non-descript buffalo in Andhra Pradesh in 1990, from a 10 years old crossbred bullock in Akola, Maharashtra in 1995 and renal lymphosarcoma from a 18 years old crossbred bullock in Akola, Maharashtra in 1997.

Thymoma

It is primary neoplasm of thymic epithelial cells and is accompanied by varying proportions of non-neoplastic lymphocytes (thymocytes). They grow slowly. They are usually encapsulated, nodular, firm masses with soft and cystic areas, located in the cranial mediastinum. They are cytologically dissimilar with small lymphocytes and are round to spindle-shaped epithelial cells present singly or in clumps. Variable number of mast cells, plasma cells, eosinophils, neutrophils and macrophages may be present. Microscopically, connective tissue trabeculae of variable thickness subdivide the mass into lobules composed of solid sheets and cords of round to spindle-shaped epithelial cells. Variable numbers of mainly small lymphocytes are present accompanied by a smaller number of medium and large lymphocytes. The cystic structures are lined by epithelial cells, which may be ciliated. It had been reported from a 12 years old Deoni bullock in Bidar, Karnataka in 1995.

Leiomyoma and Leiomyosarcoma

Leiomyoma is a benign tumour of smooth muscle found in different organs like uterus, vagina, stomach, intestines, urinary bladder, oesophagus etc. Leiomyosarcoma is malignant neoplasm of smooth muscles. Macroscopically, they are small sized tumours with broad base, firm, lobulated and pink in colour. Microscopic features are muscle bundles arranged in all directions and planes and these are separated by fibrous tissue with blood vessels. Nucleus becomes cigar shaped and contains filamentous chromatin. In leiomyosarcoma, there is presence of anaplastic cells with shorter chromatin. Mitotic figures are common. Such tumours are invasive to adjacent tissues. Leiomyoma had been reported from the oesophagus of a 10 years old non-descript bullock in Parbhani, Maharashtra in 1995, from the rectum of a 7 years old Mehsana buffalo in Gujarat in 1998 and from rectum of a 5 years old non-descript buffalo in Vijaywada in 1998. Leiomyosarcoma had been reported from the neck of a 7 years old buffalo in Ludhiana in 1990 and from the cervical region in crossbred cow in Gujarat in 2016.

Myofibroblastic Tumour

It is tumour of myofibroblasts with plasma cells, lymphocytes and eosinophils. It is also called as inflammatory fibrosarcoma, inflammatory pseudotumour and plasma cell granuloma. It is circumscribed and not encapsulated. Grossly, it is seen as white tan mass with whorled fleshy or myxoid cut surface. It may have focal haemorrhage, necrosis or calcification. Microscopically, myofibroblastic and fibroblastic spindle cells are seen with inflammatory infiltrate of lymphocytes, plasma cells, eosinophils, histiocytes. Malignant behaviour is associated with highly atypical polygonal cells with oval nuclei, prominent nucleoli, Reed-Sternberg like cells and atypical mitotic figures. It had been reported from the nasal cavity of a cow in Ludhiana in 2016.

Urinary Bladder Neoplasms

Neoplasms of the lower urinary tract occur mainly in the urinary bladder. Lower urinary tract neoplasms usually cause mucosal ulceration resulting in clinical signs of dysuria, haematuria or obstruction. Urinary bladder neoplasms can block the ureters, causing obstruction of ureteral urine flow, increased ureteral pressure and hydronephrosis. It had been reported from cattle at IVRI, Izzatnagar in the year 2014. A study was done on expression of certain cancer biomarkers in urinary bladder tumours of cattle and buffaloes at IVRI, Izzatnagar in the year 2014.

Granulosa Cell Tumour

Granulosa cell tumour arises from the ovary mesenchyma. Macroscopically, they are single, very large even up to 20 cm in diameter. They are yellow in colour, rounded, lobulated and projected on the surface of ovary. Microscopic features are tumour cells arranged in columns, clusters or compact alveoli as irregular mass or pseudo glands. In lumen, hyaline acidophilic material is there and several mitotic figures are seen. It had been reported from buffaloes in Nagpur in 2007.

Perivaginal Granuloma

On gross examination, the tumour is solid, thick, highly lobulated, homogenous and brownish grey in colour. The growth is highly vascular with areas of haemorrhages and necrosis. On histopathological examination, there is presence of mass of granulation tissue in the muscular layer of the perivaginal area. It had been reported from a 5 years old non-descript buffalo in Palampur in 1992.

Ganglioneuroma

It is a rare and benign tumour of the autonomic nerve fibres arising from neural crest sympathogonia, which are completely undifferentiated cells of the sympathetic nervous system. However, ganglioneuromas themselves are fully differentiated neuronal tumours that do not contain immature elements. Grossly, these are solid, firm tumours that are typically white in colour. Microscopically, they are composed of ganglion cells, Schwann cells and fibrous tissue. It had been reported from 2-9 years Murrah buffaloes in Ludhiana in 1992.

Neoplasms in sheep and goats

Tumour is a mass of tissue formed as a result of abnormal, excessive, uncoordinated, autonomous and purposeless proliferation of cells. Common feature for virtually all neoplasms is damage to the cellular genome. Tumours develop from a broad variety of tissues. Multifactorial agents such as viruses, mutagenic chemicals, and radiation induce their outgrowth which are referred as extrinsic factors. Along with these several intrinsic factors like age, species, breed, sex and inheritance which influence cancer development. The genetic damage produced by carcinogens is believed to be random, and many mutations may be inconsequential. Cancer can develop when nonlethal mutations occur in a small subset of the genome. These genetic changes in cells which leads to tumour development causes structural changes on the cell membrane surface which is identified by the immune system and will subsequently be destroyed by either para specific or specific immunity or by combination of both. Failure of the immune-surveillance to detect and destroy the neoplastic cells is attributed to the poor development of the immune system or immunosuppression. This immunodeficiency can be related to the present day scenario where the animals are exposed to the adverse climatic changes, increased exposure to pesticides, and fertilizers leading to their residual effects causing immunosuppression and increased incidence of neoplasms in animals in the recent years.

Spontaneous or naturally occurring tumors in small ruminants are rarely reported due to early age slaughtering of these animals. This is partly attributable to the short life expectancy of domestic small ruminants in present intensive system of rearing. The epidemiological data on occurrence of tumor in sheep and goat in India is limited. This review is an attempt to provide details regarding tumours in sheep and goat based on the available records.

Tumours in Goat

Trichoepithelioma

A trichoepithelioma is benign tumour that shows differentiation to all three segments of the hair follicle with incomplete or abortive trichogenesis. A 5year-old mixed breed goat had a soft, off white, ulcerated, glandular mass at junction of left teat and udder. Microscopically, neoplastic mass was composed of islands and nests of neoplastic cells that form variable sized keratin filled cysts and supported by a moderate fibro vascular stroma. Neoplastic cells underwent incomplete trichogenesis. In the center of islands and nests, neoplastic cells showed symmetrical keratinization indicative of infundibular origin.

Cyst Adenoma of Bartholin's gland

A three and half year old non-descript pluriparous goat was presented with enlarged and hard vulval labia. The vulval opening was constricted by the protruding mass. The growth removed from the right and left labia and size of the growths were 5.5X5.0 and 4.5X5.0 cms, respectively and weighed altogether 36.0 gms. The surface of the growth was granulated giving an appearance of cauliflower. The cut surface is pale yellowish in colour and variably sized cysts filled with clear, yellowish fluid were observed. Hematoxylin and eosin stained sections revealed multi cystic structures and acini lined with well differentiated single layer of epithelial cells. Frequently the dilated cystic spaces were occupied by pinkish hyaline mass. The supporting stroma of fibrous connective tissue was diffusely infiltrated with lymphocytes. Such observations are characteristic of Cystadenoma of Bartholin's gland.

Thecoma and metastatic adenocarcinoma

An ovarian thecoma is a benign tumour of stromal/sex-cord (mesenchymal) origin which account for approximately 0.5-1% of all ovarian tumours. Ovarian adenocarcinoma refers to the malignant tumour of the ovarian glandular tissue. Occurrence of ovarian tumours in small ruminants are rarely reported due to early age slaughtering of these animals. Ovarian tumours arise due to excessive proliferation of granulosa and theca cells. The incidence of ovarian tumours is rare among goats. The pathomorphology of a case of composite neoplasm of ovary in a goat comprising of thecoma and metastatic adenocarcinoma was reported. A carcass of eight year old female goat of non-descript breed, died with a history of weakness and emaciation was brought for post-mortem examination. On necropsy, the pelvic cavity revealed presence of a large ovarian growth weighing about 1.5 kg with presence of hemorrhagic and necrotic foci on the surfaces. Lungs, pericardium, pleural cavity showed the presence of many small clusters/bunches of white nodules. Histopathological examination of the ovarian parenchyma showed proliferation of cuboidal epithelial cells with numerous mitotic figures. The solid sheets of neoplastic cells in fibro-vascular stroma with several concentric layers of calcified tissue (psamoma bodies) were evident in the ovarian parenchyma. The regional lymph nodes also revealed metastatic adenocarcinomatous lesions replacing the lymphoid tissue with proliferating cuboidal neoplastic epithelial cells.

Hepatoma

Hepatoma refers to the benign tumour of the hepatic tissue. In a case study in Izatnagar, a male barberi goat of age 2 years was received with a firm nodular growth in the liver and representative tissue piece from the growth, liver, lung, gall bladder and hepatic lymph nodes were collected. In addition, duplicate sections were also stained by Masson's trichrome method for connective tissue demonstration. A single rounded, well encapsulated about 5.5X5.5 cm in size, greyish-white, solid, firm growth elevated from the surface was noticed in the hepatic parenchyma, located near the left border in the diaphragmatic lobe. On cutting the growth revealed variable sized circumscribed compact nodular structures with varying colours. The growth was encircled and separated from normal hepatic parenchyma by thick connective tissue capsule. The band of connective tissue of variable thickness infiltrated into the growth forming pseudolobulation. The neoplastic growth varied from lobule to lobule with absence of central vein, portal triad and radiating hepatic cords. The hepatocytes in the periphery were elongated, compressed and in the center acini formation having abundant cytoplasm and enlarged hyperchromatic nuclei with evidence of mitotic figures. Some of the acini had increased pinkish secretion with fat globules. In other lobules the acini were variable in size and shape, showed proliferation, papillary projection and presence of multinucleated giant cell like structure. The gall bladder, hepatic lymph nodes and lungs did not reveal any abnormality.

Intestinal Adenocarcinoma

Intestinal adenocarcinoma refers to malignant tumour of the glands of the intestine. A four year adult goat died of debility and anorexia. The carcass was weak and grossly, severe enlargement of mesenteric lymph nodes (MLN), edema and thickening of mucosa of ileum was noticed. Serosal surface of ileum was attached to a large nodular/tumourous mass with hard, gritty consistency. Impression smear from mucosa and MLN stained with ZN/acid fast staining and revealed numerous acid fast bacilli indistinguishable from *Mycobacterium avium* subsp. *paratuberculosis*. Microscopically, intestine revealed diffuse infiltration of epithelioid cells, macrophages, lymphocytes and giant cells in lamina propria and MLN suggestive of JD. In addition, the attached tumorous mass on the intestine showed proliferating epithelial cells in the form of acini with numerous mitotic figures, elongated spindle shaped fibroblast and osteocytes proliferation and disruption of basement membrane was observed in serosal and submucosal region of the ileum. The characteristic infiltration of epithelioid and giant cells with numerous acid fast bacilli confirmed it as Johne's disease but lesions of adenocarcinoma in ileum is one of the important finding in this case. The occurrence of paratuberculosis with adenocarcinoma is a rare finding in goats.

Oral Fibrosarcoma

Oral Fibrosarcoma refers to the malignant tumour of the fibrous connective tissue of oral cavity. A four month old female kid was referred with a hard, bulging, bilateral swelling around maxilla and mandible causing marked stenosis of oral cavity. Histopathology revealed anaplastic hyperchromatic cells arranged in whorls with abundant fibrous tissue. Several mitotic figures were also seen in the area.

Epithelial Thymoma

Thymoma refers to the benign tumour of thymus tissue.Epithelial thymoma in a three year old male kid, presented with bilateral swelling at the ventral neck region just behind the larynx since birth. Grossly, oval, greyish white, hard, nodular growth was observed, weighing around 300grams and was bilobed with a thick fibrous cord in between. Histopathologically, the growth was encapsulated by fibrous connective tissue capsule. Below the capsule, the follicles were separated by a thin layer of spindle shaped nucleated epithelio-reticular cells. Within the follicles there were rosette shaped glandular structures giving a false appearance of gland. The rosette appearance was more distinct towards the periphery of the follicle, indicating cortical zone. The glandular structures were lined by tall columnar to cuboidal cells with vesicular nuclei. The cytoplasm was more basophilic. Karyolysis and vacuolations were also seen amongst these cells.

Auricular Myxoma

Myxoma are rare tumours of primitive fibroblasts that produce excessive mucin and occurs in variety of location. Auricular myxoma was reported in a 2 year old non-descript doe, with a history of having a large mass in the right ear since 2 months. Grossly the growth was extensive and hanging from the convex surface of the right auricle. The growth was hard and brown in colour. The excised mass was 10.0 X 9.5 X 8.5 cm in size and it was circular shaped with a rough surface. The growth weighed 580 g and it was firm, slimy and non-encapsulated. Cut surface of the mass was glossy, wet and cystic cavitation were seen. Histopathologically, stellate to fusiform cells distributed in a vacuolated, basophilic, mucinous stroma containing few tiny blood vessels that was partitioned by collagenous connective tissue septae were seen. The individual tumour cell was stellate or fusiform in shape and the cell nucleus was round, ovoid and elongated with multiple nucleoli.

Bilateral Submandibular Salivary Gland Tumour

Salivary gland tumours are rare in animals except in cats. Among small ruminants, very few number of cases have been observed in the sheep. Even these few cases showed unilateral gland involvement. A nine months old Tellicherry goat in Namakkal was presented with bilateral swelling of the jowl region. The growth was non pedunculated and each excised mass measured eight cm in length and four cm in width. These two pink coloured, soft textured masses were apposing each other, but not fused. Fine needle aspirate smears revealed a few individual and more clumps of round to polygonal cells with anisocytosis and a few mitotic figures. Histopathologically, tissue section revealed different shaped and sized secretary acini with proliferating multilayered epithelial cells making papillary projection within the lumen of the acini. Basement membrane of the acini was intact with non-infiltrative borders. The polygonal cells revealed basophilic cytoplasm when stained with haematoxylin-eosin stain.

Tumours in Sheep

Adamantinoma

Adamantinomas are tumours arising from enamel organ. Fibromatous epulis (gingival hypertrophy) and ossifying epulis is fairly common in dogs and rare in other domestic animals. These may be seen as single or multiple solid lesion protruding from the gums. In the present case report in Akola, a one month old lamb had multiple solid firm and pink growth protruding from the gums of lower jaw were observed causing bulging of the lower lip and difficulty in mastication. Focal areas of ulcerations and haemorrhage were also seen. Histopathologically, growth consisted largely of dense fibrillar stroma separating islands of ameloblasts. Fibrous septa separating the islands showed osseous trabeculae. Proliferating cells showed ameloblasts arranged as in the structure of the enamel organ. Ulceration of the mucosa was prominently seen with infiltration of inflammatory cells and granulation tissue.

Pulmonary Adenomatosis

Pulmonary adenomatosis is caused by Jaagsiekte sheep retrovirus- type D oncorna virus characterized by progressive alveolar epithelial metaplasia, resulting into papillary ingrowths and associated fibroplasia of alveolar septa. Primary pulmonary tumours are less frequently reported than metastatic tumours of lungs in domestic animals and rarely recorded in sheep conducted post mortem examination of a severely emaciated carcass of ewe. Lungs revealed patchy to diffuse areas of consolidation and greyish white nodular foci up to 1-2mm in size in the apical, cardiac and diaphragmatic lobes. On microscopic examination, the alveoli were lined by single to more than one layer of cuboidal to low columnar epithelial cells giving adenomatous appearance. Several alveoli revealed papillary projections of the alveolar epithelium into the lumen. Intra bronchiolar papillary processes into the lumen composed of irregular masses of columnar cells were seen in few areas. There was thickening of the inter alveolar septa due to congestion, proliferation of connective tissue and infiltration of mononuclear cells.

A four year old ram of Malpura breed died in the Central Sheep and Wool Research Institute, was subjected to detailed postmortem examination. After recording gross lesions, the representative tissue samples were preserved in 10% formalin and routinely processed to obtain haematoxylin and eosin stained sections for histopathological studies. Mitotic index was prepared by counting mitotic figures in H&E stained sections. Duplicate sections were stained for interphase nucleolar organizer regions and AgNOR dots were counted under oil immersion lens. Mitotic figures were rarely seen with mitotic index being 2.00±1.60. The Silver Staining for Nucleolar organizer regions (AgNOR staining) revealed many fine AgNOR dots distributed in the nuclei and mean value was 16.20±4.48 (dots per nucleus).

In a study the diagnostic efficacy of certain molecular tumour markers was evaluated by immunohistochemistry on formalin-fixed paraffin-embedded sections using specific monoclonal antibodies. Lung tissues from nine spontaneous cases of pulmonary adenomatosis were collected from Avikanagar, Rajasthan. Out of total nine cases, one was found to be metastasized in the mediastinal lymph node and liver. AgNOR staining revealed many small AgNOR dots (mean value 11.64±0.94 per nucleus) and Mean Proliferating Cell Nuclear Antigen (PCNA) index was 73.90±29.39, suggesting proliferative activity of the alveolar epithelial cells. The cells were positive for p53, c-Myc, PCNA and hTERT, showing specific nuclear staining. The proliferating cells showed reduced expression of cadherin. Strong fibronectin presence was seen in the stroma and connective tissue while proliferating alveolar epithelial cells revealed relatively weak pericellular fibronectin expression. The results showed the successful use of the tumour markers in characterizing the neoplastic properties of the alveolar epithelial cells in the ovine pulmonary adenocarcinoma.

In another study 3698 lungs collected from slaughtered sheep in and around Tirupati and examined morphologically. 396 lungs were showed different pneumonic lesions. Among 396 lung lesions 39 (9.85%) were diagnosed as Pulmonary adenocarcinoma. Grossly, all the lungs were congested, increase in size, weight and oedematous. Consistency varied from granular to meaty appearance and many of them revealed nodules ranging from very small to 2.5 cm in diameter and serous exudate on cut surface of lungs.

The pathological alterations were described in spontaneously occurring bronchiolo-alveolar carcinoma (BAC) in a sheep. A total of 35 lung specimens in 10% formalin were received from Avikanagar during the period from September 2004 to February 2005 for pathological examination. A case of BAC, occurring spontaneously (0.57%), in sheep was encountered on histopathological examination. Grossly, the hard nodules were present in lung parenchyma towards periphery of right diaphragmatic lobe. Microscopically, the bronchiolar and alveolar epithelial cells varied in size and shape and were of cuboidal or columnar types. The proliferating cells were multi-layered and attached to the conspicuous basement membrane.

Squamous Cell Carcinoma (Occular Carcinoma)

Squamous Cell Carcinoma refers to the malignant tumour of Stratified squamous epithelium. Incidence of ocular neoplasms are common in cattle and is rarely seen in sheep (Blood *et al.,* 1983). In this case report , a non-descriptive ewe aged four years was presented to the Veterinary hospital, Anantapur for treatment with the history of bulging dorsally in the left eye at the forehead. On examination it was found that the growth extended to the nictitating membrane and conjunctiva of the upper and lower eye lids and the eye ball was completely covered with the neoplastic growth. Ulceration was noticed on skin, conjunctival mucosa. Histopathological examination revealed typical squamous cell carcinoma with cell nests showing infiltrative columns of neoplastic squamous cells with rarefaction of underlying tissue. Extensive fibrosis with infiltrating columns of the neoplastic cells was also noticed.

Synovial Sarcoma (Cystic Papillary Type)

In Avikanagar, Rajasthan, synovial sarcoma was reported in a Rambouiliet ram of about 4 years and 10 months of age, presented with a history of swelling on the left thigh which was found to be vascular. The tumour was capsulated in a thick fibrous capsule with light greyish mass of muscle on the lateral side of the left thigh involving the regional lymph nodes. Microscopic examination of neoplasm revealed the presence of both solid areas of pleomorphic spindle shaped and polyhedral cells and cystic spaces with papilla like projections lined by polyhedral tumour cells. The cystic spaces were encircled by hyalinised muscle cells. The cell lining of the spaces had no regular basement membrane and were haphazard and surrounded by neoplastic cells. The adjacent lymph nodes were entirely replaced by the tumour cells which were mainly cystic and papillary in type with focal cystic spaces containing mucinous exudate. No metastatic lesions were observed in any other organs.

Metastatic Chondrosarcoma

Chondrosarcoma refers to the malignant tumour of cartilaginous tissue. In a case report in Korutla, a four year old ram was presented with tumour mass in the form of a massive hard swelling at the right lateral abdomen region. Grossly the mass was irregular and well demarcated, measured approximately about 40cm in length, 30 cm in width and 25cm in depth, extending from the rib cage to the lateral abdomen up to flank region. The contoured borders were covered by fibrous tissue capsule. On the surface, the tumour was pale yellowish in colour with small cartilaginous multi-lobular structures. Similar hard nodules were also noticed on lungs, diaphragm and liver during post-mortem examination, indicating metastasis of the tumour. Microscopically the tumour consist of lobulated masses of proliferating pleomorphic chondrocytes that were separated with very thin fibrous stroma. The periphery of the lobule contained cluster of closely packed young chondrocytes while the center contained mature chondrocytes. Based on this morphology, a grade II Chondrosarcoma with metastases into the lung, diaphragm and liver was diagnosed.

Haemangioma and Haemangiosarcoma

Haemangioma is the benign tumour of endothelial cells of blood vessels. Haemangiomas arising from the urinary bladder are uncommon entities in sheep. A case report in Puducherry gross and histopathological features of haemangioma were detected in the urinary bladder of a 4 year old male cross bred sheep. Grossly the urinary bladder was severely distended with extensive serosal vascularization and rupture of few blood vessels. Mucosa was moderately thickened and haemorrhagic. The right kidney was moderately enlarged, greyish white in colour and showed multiple areas of necrosis. Histopathology of urinary bladder revealed varying sized blood filled cavernous spaces that were lined by a single layer of endothelial cells. There was no evidence of mitosis. The gross and histopathological features were suggestive of haemangioma of the urinary bladder.

Haemangiosarcoma is a malignant tumour of endothelial cells. In a case report a two year old sheep was presented with a red lump at the fetlock region, in Gudiwada, Krishna District, Andhra Pradesh,. It was soft, foul smelling and bleeding was observed. Histopathological examination revealed vascular spaces lined by elongated endothelial cells with high cellular stroma filled with RBC, necrotic tissue and inflammatory cells. Undifferentiated round, ovoid, and spindle shaped neoplastic cells with pleomorphic, hyperchromatic, large nucleus and scanty cytoplasm was observed.

Neoplasms in equines, swine and camelids

Tumours are state of excessive cellular multiplication occurring as a result of sublethal damage to the genetic material of the cells that results in the uncontrolled proliferation of the cells. These tumours develop from a broad variety of tissues/ cells. Tumours are usually monoclonal in nature and these cells have the ability to subdivide and grow while limiting the proliferation of the adjacent normal cells. The tumours also produce variety of substances which has various adverse effects on body like loss of body weight, anorexia, fever, anemia etc.

In equines of all breeds, groups and all ages, skin tumours are the most common type of tumours. The incidence of tumour in external genital region is also higher. The common malignant neoplasms of the external genitalia of the mare are squamous cell carcinoma, melanoma and squamous papilloma. The skin tumour that are common in equines are sarcoid, squamous cell carcinoma and melanomas. These skin tumours may metastasize and invade other parts of the horse body. The main concern with the tumours growing in the cranial region is that they cause disfigurement of the face and may affect vision, hearing and difficulty in feeding and proper respiration. Tumours that originate from other organs are less common and more difficult to diagnose in early stage. These tumours in the organs and glands of horses become more apparent with the age of the horse.

The epidemiological data on occurrence of tumour in equines in India is limited. A screening was conducted on neoplasms of equines from 1952 to 1973 in southern India, in which 69 horses and one donkey was found to be affected with neoplasms of skin and glands. Another survey conducted at Hisar from 1980-1988 suggested sarcoid as main tumour of horses. In Gujrat, a study of tumours in horses revealed 30% fibroma, 25% squamaous cell carcinoma, 16% fibrosarcoma, 6% papilloma and 6% melanoma. This review is an attempt to provide details regarding tumours in equines based on the available literature.

Incidence of tumours in swine are less common. This can be attributed to the early age slaughter of pigs and therefore do not live long enough to develop tumours. The incidence is extremely rare in pigs with only a few case reports on lymphangioma, rhabdomyoma, multiple acanthoma, fibroma, haemangioma, histiocytoma, sweat gland adenoma, squamous cell carcinoma, mast cell tumour, dermoid choristoma and haemangiomas in the skin and subcutis.

Tumours are not reported often in camels. This may be due to low prevalence of tumours in camels or lack of reported literature. Also there is small population of camels in India and more over camels are considered quite resistant to the diseases in comparison to other animals. Carcinoma of lungs and adenocarcinomas of the forestomach have been reported in Bactrian camels with metastatic lesions in the liver, hepatic lymph nodes, heart, aorta and the lungs. Squamous cell carcinoma frequently occurs in the flank region, side of the hock and behind the sternal pad and most commonly been seen on the dorsal part of the nail of the foot and in interdigital space.

Tumours in Equines

Equine Sarcoid

Equine sarcoid is an aggressive tumour of fibroblasts seen locally in equine skin. Equine sarcoid are most commonly observed tumours in equines, representing approximately 35 % of all equine skin neoplasms and 20% of all neoplasms encountered in equines. These are benign tumours and classified as nodular, fibroblastic, verrucous, occult or malevolent on the basis of their appearance. Sarcoid are not considered as malignant tumours but they are generally invasive and reoccurring in nature. A case of sarcoid was reported in an Indian chestnut gelding, aged above eight years which was having a large roughly spherical, sessile cauliflower like growth on the medial aspect of the left hind limb just above the hock joint measuring about 16cm and weighed 800gms. The surface was dry, horny and ulcerated. Histopathology revealed slightly hyperkeratotic epidermis with moderate acanthosis and large rete pegs. The growth consisted entirely of fibroblastic components with bundles of spindle shaped cells running at different angle and at times producing whorl like pattern. The large numbers of superficial fibroblasts were arranged in perpendicular to the dermo-epidermal junction giving a "picket fence pattern". Collagen was scanty and mitoses were very few. A case of phalangeal sarcoid was reported in a five year old mare with exuberant granulation over first and second phalanges in left rear limb and mild lameness. Physical examination showed a large diffused swelling in the pastern region of left hind limb. The mass was cauliflower like in appearance, pale with small granulations. On palpation, it was rough and firm in texture. The growth was prominent on anterior aspect, ulcerated and traumatized. Histopathology revealed ulceration with lot of inflammatory exudation and necrosis at places in epidermal and dermal components. The pseudo-epitheliomatous hyperplasia with large epithelial pegs traversing into underlying dermal elements were visualized. It showed keratinizing tendency at various places. The dermis component consisted of fibroblasts and collagen fibres arranged in whorled pattern.

Seminoma

Seminoma is a neoplasm derived from the germinal epithelium in the testis reported rarely in horses. These tumours are frequently observed in cryptorchid testes and in aged horses. Although they behave mostly as benign tumours, they have higher incidences of malignancy than other testicular tumours. They may invade abdominal cavity which is manifested by enlarged spermatic cord. An unilateral seminoma was described in a 16 year old stallion with history of progressive left testicular enlargement for more than 3 year. General condition of animal detoriated rapidly and died. Grossly, unilateral tumour involving the left testis and above 40cm in length & 16cm in width & 53cm circumference & weighing 16.5Kg was present. Tumour mass was attached to the spermatic cord extending into abdominal cavity through the left inguinal canal and was observed adherent to the mesentery & intestine. Epididymis and spermatic cord was also involved. The cut surface of growth was greyish white, smooth and homogeneous except where it was intercepted by fibrous septa or, interrupted by well-marked hemorrhagic necrotic area scattered throughout the mass. No metastatic lesions were found in the other region. Histopathologically, tumour was composed of neoplastic cells supported by scanty stromal tissue. Seminiferous tubule's structural details were lost. Cells were spherical and polyhedral with hyper chromatic nuclei which were large, granular and contain one or two prominent nucleoli. Multi nucleated giant cells were present. The cell mass was separated into irregular lobules by fibrous stroma and there were areas of coagulative necrosis along with areas of extensive haemorrhage.

In a case report, a 17 year old Kathiawari stallion maintained as serum donor at Ranipet died of Seminoma (Rajendra *et al.,* 1997). Various haematological parameters were estimated and biochemical parameters were evaluated. It was observed that the total erythrocyte count in the affected horse was very much lower (3.56 million/cmm) and the white blood cell count (12600/cmm) recorded 30% increase. No apparent changes was noticed in the testosterone and magnesium values. The alkaline phosphatase value of 116.4 IU/L observed in the seminoma affected horse was higher than the observed value 93.2 IU/L in the healthy stallion. SGOT and SGPT showed an increase in the cholesterol level. Similarly the LDH activity was significantly increased in the affected horse.

Cavernoma

Cavernoma is a benign tumour consisting of a mass of blood vessels has been reported to occur in animals at different locations in the body, especially in the dermis or subcutaneous tissues. Superficial cavernoma are friable and easily infected if the skin is broken. A case report in Srinagar, Kashmir pertains to an extensive cavernoma of the penile sheath in a horse. A horse aged 4 years had an extensive tumour mass measuring 6"X4" in size between the penis and testicles on the medial side of penis. Histopathology revealed necrosis and multiple spots of calcification. The tumour mass was enclosed by a fibrous capsule consisting of many dilated blood vessels intervening collagen fibers and fibrocytes. Necrosis and fibrosis have been reported in haemangioma due to intravascular thrombosis in addition to infraction. The blood vessels were dilated and covered entirely by endothelial type of cells filled with blood. The histopathology of the tumours can vary due to thrombosis of vascular channel.

Cavernous Haemangioma

Haemangioma are frequently encountered tumours in subcutis and dermis of most of the species of animals. In a report of thrombosed cavernous haemangioma in a mule a circumscribed growth weighing about one kg and 11X6.5cms size was removed from the subcutaneous breast region of a mule aged about 4 years. The cut surface was dark brown. Fine gritty deposits were noted in the tumour mass each surrounded by a thick white capsule ranging in thickness from 0.5 to 1.5 cms. Histopathologically the tumour consisted of widely dilated vascular channels, lined by a single layer of flattened inconspicuous endothelial cells, filled with blood. The intervening fibrous stroma mainly consisted of collagen fibers. Areas of necrosis and areas of calcification in the form of purplish irregular amorphous granules were noted. The fibrous capsule enclosing the tumour mass consisted of collagen fibres with scanty fibrocytes.

Squamous Cell Carcinoma

Squamous Cell Carcinoma refers to the malignant tumour of stratified squamous epithelium. Squamous cell carcinoma accounts for approximately 20% of all equine tumours. The perianal, vulvar and clitoral regions of mare account for 12% of equine SCC cases. The causes of SCC in mare have been suggested to include papilloma, trauma, chronic irritation, melanin deficiency, exposure to sunlight. SCC is a very common malignant neoplasm and has the tendency to develop in the unpigmented area of skin. Squamous cell carcinoma of eye was reported in a 20 year old thoroughbred horse presented with lachrymal discharge, corneal opacity and ulceration in left eye during the year 2007. There was recurrence of the eye lesions and symptoms annually. Small growth was noticed from inner canthus. Slowly growth increased in size with cauliflower appearance and broad base. The growth was soft, pinkish in colour and protrudes through palpebral fissure and appeared to be originated from conjunctiva of the membrane nictitans. Biopsy was collected, fixed in 10% formalin and processed for haematoxylin and eosin staining method for histopathological examination. The tissue section of the biopsy material revealed infiltrating squamous cell cord-like structures with hyperchromatia and vacuolation. At places tissue section revealed necrosis, haemorrhage and infiltration of mononuclear cells.

In a study at Meerut a total of 19 cases studied, out of which squamous cell carcinoma and equine sarcoid were diagnosed in 8 and 4 cases, respectively. The remaining cases were diagnosed as chronic inflammatory lesions, granuloma and necrotizing dermatitis. Ultrastructurally, sarcoid sample revealed presence of fibroblast with pleomorphic nuclei and abundance of RER with dilated cisternae. All these samples were screened for Bovine papilloma virus-1, -2 and -13 and Equus caballus papilloma virus -2, -3 and -4. Seven samples showed positivity for both BPV-1 and -2 while 3 samples for BPV-2 alone. In the squamous cell carcinoma samples, immunohistoch emical expression of connexin 26 was attempted and positivity was observed in 4 of the 6 samples which are considered more invasive and metastatic.

A case of undifferentiated baso squamous cell carcinoma was reported in an adult mare with a history of tumour like growth in vulvar region since last two months. Histopathologically, the growth revealed islands of neoplastic epithelial cells arranged in either masses or cords and characterized by pleomorphic nuclie and mitotic figures along with proliferation of fibrous connective tissue. It was diagnosed as undifferentiated squamous cell carcinoma. Immunohistochemical investigations showed strong immunoreactivity for pancytokeratin in cytoplasm, p53 and proliferating cell nuclear antigen in nuclei of neoplastic epithelial cells. In conclusion, it may be stated that the increased expression of p53 and proliferating cell nuclear antigen in proliferating cells substantiates its potential malignancy.

A study in Hisar, was conducted on a biopsy sample collected from a 9 year old mare brought with vulvar squamous cell carcinoma with a history of a hard tumour- like growth hanging on one side of the vulvar lips, since the last 4 months. Grossly, the mass was ulcerated and hard in consistency. Histopathologically, it revealed pleomorphic neoplastic epithelial cells arranged in cords and islands without keratinized layer in centre. The nuclei were large, vesicular or hyperchromatic. Island of neoplastic cells were surrounded by marked connective tissue proliferation. Mitotic figures and infiltration of leukocytes were also observed at places.

Squamous cell carcinoma of vulva was reported in an 8-year old non-descript mare in Mathura, with the complaint of protrusion of a reddish mass from the vulvar lips for 1 month. Grossly the growth was the size of cricket ball attached at the right ventral vulvar commissure and invading the clitoris. The surface was ulcerated. Tumour weighed about 150gm, and the cut surface showed solid texture inside.

In a case report in Anand, a thirteen year old, Marwari horse was presented with ocular squamous cell carcinoma with history of blindness, corneal opacity and growth on lower eyelid of right side eye since last six months. The growth was smooth, nodular, elongated (4X2cm) and pink in colour. On histopathological examination, section revealed lobules of neoplastic pleomorphic epithelial cells, showing varying degree of squamous differentiation and central accumulation of dense laminated keratin pearls. Neoplastic cells contained round to ovoid nuclei of varying size.

In a case study a total of thirteen tumour biopsy samples from horses were received at Junagadh during the period of 2013 to 2016 from different parts of Saurashtra region. All biopsies were received from the females only. The average age of affected animals was 9 years, however, within the range from 6 to 16 years. Out of 13 biopsies, the squamous cell carcinoma was observed in seven animals while melanocytic neoplasms were observed in four animals and the fibroblastic type of sarcoid were observed in two cases. The squamous cell carcinoma was mostly seen in Khathiyawadi breed. The histological observation of squamous cell carcinoma revealed moderate to highly differentiated cells. Melanocytic neoplasms showed pattern of the malignant dermal melanomatosis in three cases and malignant junctional melanomatosis in one cases.

Tumours in Swine

Fibrosarcoma

Fibrosarcoma is a malignant tumour derived from fibrous connective tissue, may be circumscribed or infiltrating in nature, and characterized by immature, proliferating, undifferentiated and anaplastic spindle cells. It represents a heterogenous group consisting of malignant tumours of fibroblasts and also unclassifiable and mixed mesenchymal cell neoplasms capable of producing collagen. The reported incidence of fibrosarcoma in pigs is 0.14 %. A report describes a rarely encountered case of fibrosarcoma involving the entire left fore limb of a seven months old, cross bred grower pig. The swelling had spread from the shoulder to the coronet, where it was broadest and the toes were almost invisible. The swelling measured 20 x 15 cm in circumference and was very hard in consistency. Grossly, the cut surface of the solid tumorous mass appeared pinkish-grey to white in colour. Histological examination revealed wavy bundles of fibrous connective tissue arranged in irregular pattern. Nuclei were hyperchromatic and spindle to triangular in shape, with large prominent nucleoli. Frequently, tumour giant cells with darkly stained nuclei were found scattered among the proliferating fibrous connective tissue. No inflammatory reaction was present in the tumorous mass.

2.Hepatoma

Hepatoma is the benign tumour of hepatic cells. Primary hepatic tumour is rare among pigs recorded 1.6 hepatic tumours per million in a year among slaughtered pigs and reported only six (4%) out of 139 porcine tumours examined by them. A hepatoma in a pig out of 242 pig carcasses of both sex and different ages was recorded. Grossly, the liver was enlarged and revealed greyish brown nodules ranging from 2.5 to 3 inches in diameter. Microscopically, nodular area revealed loss of normal hepatic structure. Liver parenchyma showed an attempt to form new hepatic cells and cords with proliferation of connective tissue in between. Hepatocytomegaly and hyperchromasia are seen. The hepatic cells had lost their acinar arrangements and are separated by mesenchymal cells. Vacuolar degenerative changes were present.

Tumours in Camel

Squamous Cell Carcinoma

SCC is a malignant tumour of epidermal cells in which the cells show differentiation to keratinocytes. Factors that are associated with the development of a squamous cell carcinoma, including prolonged exposure to ultraviolet light, lack of pigment within the epidermis at the sites of tumour development, and lack of hair or a very sparse hair coat at the affected sites. Macroscopic features are presence of papillary projections or cauliflower like growth, broad base, soft and grey or pink in colour. Microscopically, The affected keratinocytes show loss of polarity, karyomegaly, nuclear hyperchromatism, enlarged and prominent nucleoli, and mitotic figures of basal and suprabasal keratinocytes. Extending into the dermis, with or without an association to the overlying epidermis, are islands, cords, and trabeculae of neoplastic epithelial cells showing a variable degree of squamous differentiation. The amount of keratin, seen as intracytoplasmic, eosinophilic fibrillar material (keratin tonofibres), produced by the neoplastic cells is quite variable; there is extensive keratinization, and in well-differentiated tumours, there is formation of distinct keratin "pearls" (Meuten, 2002). It had been reported from the solar surface of foot of a 10 years old male camel (*Camelus dromedarius*) in Bikaner in the year 1995.

Neoplasms in Pet Animals

Neoplasms (Tumours/ Cancers) have emerged as the leading cause of death among various species of animals, especially in canines. The etiology of tumours is multifactorial. It may be due to intrinsic factors as age, heredity, sex, pigmentation, immunological factors or may be due to extrinsic factors as environmental carcinogens of physical or chemical nature, hormones and oncogenic viruses. Suppression of immunity plays an important role in generation of tumours as many tumour growths can be suppressed in early stages if immune system is strong. Tumourigenesis involves the accretion of unprogrammed genetic and epigenetic changes, which lead to dysregulation of the normal control of cell population. Information on types of tumours, their characteristic features along with their prevalence and distribution helps for early diagnosis, prognosis and appropriate therapy. In dogs, a survey was conducted from (1940 – 1951) at Madras and 325 (13.5%) dogs were found to suffer from venereal tumour. Among various neoplasms diagnosed in dogs in Hisar (Haryana) are venereal neoplasm, papilloma, round cell sarcoma, adenocarcinoma, adenoma and lymphosarcoma. Canine venereal tumour was found more during summer (57.9%) as compared to winter (42.1%). The age group mainly involved was 1-5 years. Sex wise prevalence was 68.5% in females and 31.5% in males. In another survey, the frequency of different neoplasms in dogs was recorded as 42.2% of skin, 20.6% of mammary gland, 23.5% of genitalia and 13.2% of other organs. Tumour suppressor genes have role in the pathogenesis of tumours. Further the genes associated with p^{53} as MDM2, p^{21}, p^{38}, cdk2 also have important role in tumourigenesis and its progression. Studies on neoplasms of pet animals is also having public health significance , since they share same environment and are exposed to many of carcinogens as humans. Recently scientists have discovered dogs have greater than 80 % similarity to humans as compared to mice which have only 67 % similarity to humans. Hence the etiology of cancer, types of cancer and its distribution in dogs may have some relationships with cancer in humans. The information related to the occurrence and types of tumours in pet animals in various regions of India is not much documented. This review assesses the available literature describing pattern, occurrence and types of tumours in dogs and cats in India along with some diagnostic and prognostic approaches.

The skin is one of most common sites of tumours in animals. Most skin tumours of dogs are benign however malignant skin tumours are common in cats. Canine skin neoplasms may be categorized as about 55% mesenchymal, 40% epithelial and 5% melanocytic in origin. In a survey it was observed that most frequently occurring tumours were that of skin (42.2%) followed by mammary gland tumours (20.6%), tumours of genitalia(23.5%) and other organs comprising 13.2% of total cases observed during the period of survey. The most common neoplasms of epidermis in dogs include papilloma, squamous cell carcinoma, basal cell tumour, keratoacanthoma, melanocytoma and melanoma. The adnexal neoplasms include adenomas and adenocarcinomas of sweat gland, apocrine gland, sebaceous gland, perianal gland and ceruminous gland while hair matrix tumour and trichoepithelioma are relatively less commonly found adnexal neoplasms in dogs. The neoplasms of dermis and subcutis are fibroma, fibrosarcoma, mast cell tumours, haemangioma, haemangiosarcoma, haemangiopericytoma, cutaneous histocytoma, lipoma, liposarcoma, myxoma, myxosarcoma, venereal tumours, neurofibroma, and neurofibrosarcoma. The most common skin tumours in dogs are mast cell tumours and histiocytoma. The most common skin tumour types in cats are basal cell tumours, squamous cell carcinoma and fibrosarcomas.

An evaluation of proliferative fraction in canine skin tumours and a correlation between four cell proliferative markers, mitotic index, AgNOR count, Ki-67 indices and PCNA was done. Out of 105 tumours; 42 were skin tumours which comprised of 23 cases of benign and 19 cases of malignant neoplasms. The benign tumours encountered were canine cutaneous histiocytoma, perianal gland adenoma, cavernous hemangioma, mast cell tumour, fibroma and fibromyxoma. Whereas the malignant skin tumours found were basal cell carcinoma, squamous cell carcinoma, fibrosarcoma, myxosarcoma, perianal gland adenocarcinoma, epidermoid carcinoma and liposarcoma. Tumours were found in an average age of 7.27 years. Protein Ki-67 was observed to be very sensitive followed by PCNA in differentiating and determining malignant tumours. AgNOR count and mitotic index differed between malignant and benign tumours but alone they proved to be poor makers in providing support for the histological grading of tumours.

Histomorphology of different canine skin neoplasms was reported from Puducherry region. Out of 50 growths, 41 were diagnosed as cutaneous tumours among them 24 were benign and 17 were malignant. These were further categorized into 16 epithelial, 20 mesenchymal and 5 melanocytic tumours. Among the epithelial tumours, 7 cases of papilloma were recorded. Out of 7, 5 tumours revealed changes characterized by orthokeratosis and proliferation of all layers of stratified epithelium. Two cases revealed tendency towards malignancy. Single squamous cell carcinoma showed parakeratosis, acanthosis and keratinocytes dysplasia. A single case of basal cell carcinoma revealed neoplastic basal cells arranged in inter twining strands forming ribbon like pattern. Two cases of sebaceous adenoma revealed neoplastic sebocytes arranged in clusters and lobules in epidermal- dermal interface to dermis. The sebaceous adenocarcinomas showed lobular accumulation of pleomorphic and hyperchromatic polygonal cells in the dermis with accumulation of intracytoplasmic vacuoles suggestive of lipid rich content. There was a single case of apocrine cystadenocarcinoma. Two cases of ceruminous papillary cystadenocarcinoma revealed proliferation of glandular epithelium, supported by fibrovascular connective tissue stroma and were arranged in papillary pattern with cystic spaces. A solitary case of hepatoid adenoma revealed presence of neoplastic cells as cords and islands which were subdivided into multiple lobules by fibrovascular trabeculae. Small basaloid germinative cells were present at the periphery of the lobules, while the central area revealed large hepatoid type cells. Among mesenchymal tumours, one fibroma and two fibrosarcoma were seen. A single case of fibromyxoma recorded showed myxomatous lobules, each lobule characterized by presence of fusiform to stellate cells. Three cases of lipoma were observed which showed solid sheets of lipocytes arranged as multiple lobules separated by mature fibrovascular tissue. Two variants of haemangioma were found, capillary haemangiomas were characterized by presence of small vascular channels with plump endothelial lining cells. Lumen varied in size and contained little to moderate number of erythrocytes. Cavernous haemangioma was revealed large vascular lumen lined by flattened endothelial cells aligned on thin collagenous septa and fibrous connective tissue stroma was present.

Nine canine skin tumours were studied for cytology and confirmed by histopathology. Ages of dogs with tumours were between 7 to 12 years. Six were female and one was male dog. Characteristic cytological features like plasmacytoid appearance with perinuclear space of Golgi zone (osteosarcoma), swirling pattern of tadpole shaped cells (haemangiopericytoma,) and signet ring cells (mixed mammary gland tumour) were found. Different tumours encountered were squamous cell carcinoma in which the cells were angular and contained basoeosinophilic cytoplasm. Other tumours were sweat gland adenocarcinoma, ceruminous gland adenocarcinoma. Chondroma showed large binucleated cells embedded in basoeosinophilic cartilaginous matrix. Also cytoplasm contained azurophilic granules. Cystic papillary adenoma of mammary gland and malignant mixed mammary tumours were also seen. Fibroleiomyoma with fusiform cells, eosinophilic cytoplasm and basophilic nuclei were seen. Haemangiocytoma cytological smears revealed swirling pattern of spindle cells with centrally placed nuclei.

In a study of cutaneous and subcutaneous tumours of canines, out of 83 tumours, 22.9% were benign and 77.1% were malignant. Most common epithelial tumours were squamous cell carcinoma and simple adenocarcinomas of mammary gland and most common tumours of round cells and mesenchyme were mast cell tumours and fibrosarcomas respectively.

Pancytokeratin is a diagnostic tumour marker for epithelial tumours and there is a limited role of p^{53} gene mutation in oncogenesis of these tumours. A study of canine skin neoplasms in Kolkata Metropolis was conducted in which during the period of one year from 2016 to 2017 total 272 cases were evaluated. Cutaneous mast cell tumour was the most common tumour followed by histiocytoma, TVT, fibrosarcoma and basal cell carcinoma. CMCTs were most commonly encountered in boxer dogs while histiocytoma were found more in Labrador and Golden Retrievers.

Cytological and immunocytochemical study on primary cutaneous transmissible venereal tumours in dogs with lymph node metastasis without genital involvement was conducted. Tumours were found as hard cutaneous nodules on the skin of different dogs. Aspiration cytology of the nodules and lymph nodes revealed large round cells with abundant cytoplasm containing multiple punctate vacuoles. Immunocytological studies revealed the neoplastic cells were positive for vimentin but negative for cytokeratin, desmin, CD3 and CD79a. Cytology can serve as a rapid, economical and non-invasive technique in the diagnosis of round cell tumours.

A study on cytological evaluation of skin tumours for rapid diagnosis and its comparison with histopathology was conducted. Out of 65 cases of canine skin tumours, 14 were confirmed as round cell tumours. 7 out of 14 were TVT among which six were encountered in 3 to 13 years old non-descript dogs and one in 4 years old, Spitz bitch. On cytological examination, there were punctate vacuoles in the cytoplasm. Four were mast cell tumours, in which both single and multiple growths were encountered. Single form was large and ulcerated and multiple forms were characterized by erythematosus vesicular eruptions. Cytological smears revealed purplish staining granules in the cytoplasm. Large blasts like cells without granules were also seen. Some cells had faintly eosinophilic to baso eosinophilic cytoplasmic inclusions. 2 were histocytoma in a 7 year old male Cocker Spaniel and in a 9 months old non-descript male dog. Histopathologically, there was sheet of densely packed round cells. The nuclei were round to oval and slightly bean shaped. Some cells had folded nuclei. One was histiocytic sarcoma in spleen of 11 years old Labrador bitch. The cytological smears revealed high cellularity. Cells were round in shape and exhibited anisocytosis. Nuclei were round to oval, bean shaped, often showing indentation and fold. Giant cells and multinucleated cells were also seen.

In comparative pathology, canine mammary gland tumors have been given special interest because of their similarities with human breast cancer. Among the various tumours of dogs, mammary gland tumours rank second only to skin tumours and are the most common tumours in females accounting for up to 52 % of all the neoplasms. WHO classification of canine and feline mammary tumours has categorized them into three major categories as malignant, benign and unclassified tumours. Consistency may be soft to edematous, to firm and sclerotic and may contain bone and cartilage. They may be solid or may contain a numerous cysts filled with secretions. Mammary tumours are thought to be age dependent, as bitches less than two years of age encounter it rarely, but there is a sharp increase in the incidence after 6 years of age with peak incidence at 8-12 years of age. The incidence of canine mammary tumours varies from 198 to 622.6 cases per 100,000 dogs per year.

An epidemiological study on canine mammary tumours was conducted, in which 100 tumours were collected from 50 dogs. % incidence of CMT during period of investigation from 1997 to 1998 was 1.04 in relation to dog's presence to the College veterinary hospital, Bangalore. Most frequently affected dogs were between 7-10 years old with sharp increase in incidence after age of 5 years. CMT were mainly recorded in females with 8 % cases in male dogs. Intact bitches had frequent incidence of CMT. Majority of tumours were malignant. Thirteen dogs out of 33 dogs with malignant tumours had recurrence. In dogs with metastasis, regional lymph nodes revealed metastatic lesions in four dogs with malignant tumours.

Occurrence and distribution pattern of CMT studied revealed that there was highest occurrence of these tumours in month of September followed by April. Out of the total 407 tumour cases examined, 99 were of canine mammary tumours. Benign type tumours of mammary gland recorded in 64 cases included mixed mammary tumour, papillary adenoma, fibroadenoma, myoepithelioma and mucinous adenoma in decreasing order of incidence. The malignant tumours of mammary gland were found in 35 which included papillary or mucinous adenocarcinoma, malignant mixed mammary tumour, intra- acinar mammary carcinoma solid type, and intraductal carcinoma. German shepherd was most commonly affected breed followed by Spitz, cross bred, Doberman, Labrador, Boxer and other breeds of dogs. The age- wise distribution revealed that highest occurrence was in dogs of age group 4 – 10 years.

In an epidemiological study on canine mammary tumour, out of 109 neoplastic biopsy samples, 51 were canine mammary tumours. Highest incidence of CMT was recorded in the age group of 10-12 years. Incidence of CMT as per sex was such that out of the 51 cases, only one case of mammary gland tumour was observed in a male dog and rest were all in the females. Breed -wise incidence of canine mammary tumours revealed maximum incidence was observed in crossbred, followed by German shepherd, Labrador and Spitz and non- descript dogs. A study of canine neoplasms at Mannuthy showed tumours having their origin from mammary glands 29.51 %. Among 229 neoplastic conditions, 80 dogs had mammary tumours including 75 females and 5 males. The highest incidences were observed in 8- 12 years old age group.

Heavy metals as mercury, cadmium, iron, zinc have a role in tumourigenesis. Role of heavy metals concentrations in carcinogenesis of canine mammary tumours was studied by Lather *et al.,* 2017. The mean values of iron, zinc, mercury and cadmium were significantly higher in tissue and serum of dogs affected by tumours as compared to tumour free animals.

Cancer is appearing as a leading cause of death in animals as in most of the cases, it is diagnosed in terminal stages after neoplastic cells have metastasized in different organs. To identify cancers in early stage there is need of biomarkers, so that it can be detected before clinical symptoms and metastasis is reported. In a study, out of 67 suspected tumour cases, 63 were histopathologically confirmed as tumours with higher occurrence of malignant (50) than benign tumours (13). There was significant difference in different proliferative markers, argyrophilic nucleolar organizer region (AgNOR), proliferative cell nuclear antigen (PCNA) and proliferative cell nuclear protein Ki-67 (Ki-67) indices between benign and malignant tumours except in mitotic index. There was also significant correlation between AgNOR, PCNA and Ki-67 indices with Ki-67 index being highly sensitive than PCNA in differentiating and determining the proliferation rate of malignant and benign tumours. Among proliferative markers Ki-67 was found to be highly sensitive marker for assessing cell proliferation followed by PCNA and AgNOR indices. Mitotic index was found to be a poor marker of cell proliferation.

A Comparative study on the expression pattern of the proliferating cell markers PCNA and Ki67 in canine mammary tumours and analysis of pattern of expression of proliferating cell markers PCNA and Ki67 by immunohistochemistry in different histological subtypes of canine mammary tumours was done. Immunostaining was performed by employing monoclonal antihuman antibodies against PCNA and Ki67. Out of 103 canine mammary tumours 98 were diagnosed as malignant and only 5 were diagnosed as benign tumours. Reactivity to PCNA and Ki67 was localized to nuclei in non-mitotic cells; but in mitotic cells PCNA immunostaining was cytoplasmic and Ki-67 expression was chromosomal. Proliferation indices determined were generally higher for PCNA compared to Ki67. Intensity and distribution of staining was more in the basal layer of tubular and tubulopapillary carcinomas however, in mixed tumours the intensity and numbers of positive cells were more around the myoepithelial cell nests and cartilaginous or bony metaplasia. PCNA and Ki67 indices were significantly higher in malignant tumours compared to benign counterparts. Among various malignant tumours PCNA and Ki67 indices were higher in osteosarcomas, carcinosarcomas and solid carcinomas compared to other types. Also PCNA and Ki67 indices were positively correlated with each other in both benign and malignant tumours. Results showed that high PCNA and Ki67 indices were associated with malignancy and poorly differentiated tumours.

AgNORs count as a diagnostic marker and cell proliferative rate in canine mammary tumours has been studied at Proddatur, AP. Of the 72 cases, 18 cases had tumour categorized as benign and 54 were malignant. The mean AgNOR count for all tumours varied from 2.38 to 8.32 and a significant correlation was found between the increased AgNOR count and histological grade. Results showed that AgNOR index appears as a reliable diagnostic marker for tumours and provides information about the rate of proliferation irrespective of tumour type. AgNORs in malignant cells were irregular in size and shape and dispersed throughout the nucleus whereas benign cells were larger, sharply defined and confined to nucleolus.

Cell proliferation evaluation has been useful for the evaluation of behaviour and potential malignancy of tumours. High AgNOR counts in stage II than in stage I and stage 0 indicate the presence of greater number of proliferating cells and poor differentiation of cells as evidenced by occurrence of multiple dispersed AgNORs in these tumour's cells (Sarli, 2002). Jayachandra, 2010 studied AgNORs in canine malignant mammary tumour for their prognostic value. Difference of AgNOR count found in alive and dead dogs were observed. Mean AgNOR count found in different stages was highest in stage II followed by stage I and least in Stage 0.

Matrilysin can be used as biomarker for cancer diagnosis and prognosis. Twenty serum samples collected from malignant canine mammary tumours were subjected to quantitative determination of MMP7 by indirect ELISA using human MMP7 polyclonal antibodies. The dot blot ELISA studies indicated that on removal of dog mammary tumour, MMP7 could not be detected in serum. In indirect ELISA the absorbance of tumour serum was found to be 9 times higher as compared to normal serum suggesting over expression of MMP7 in tumour serum. It suggested significant release of pro MMP-7 which showed cross reactivity with human MMP7 polyclonal antibody in serum of dog having mammary tumour as compared to normal dog sera. Certain genes as myc, p53, ras, Rb, erb etc. have significance in the regulation of cell cycle and cell division. Myc oncoprotein are responsible for cell proliferation, cell growth and apoptosis, these on deregulation, lead to genesis of wide range of cancers.The results of strong c-Myc immunolabelling pattern in infiltrative ductal carcinoma of human breast resembled to its canine counterpart, suggesting the involvement of similar molecular and pathological processes in the development and progression of tumours. The study also revealed the conservation of the structure of molecule across species as the monoclonal antibody specific for human c- Myc protein showed excellent immunolabelling in canine tissues.

In a study of the c-erbB2 expression pattern in canine mammary tumours, out of 65 confirmed tumours, 11 were benign and 54 were malignant tumours. In immunohistochemical studies, 23 of malignant tumours showed c-erbB2 oncoprotein over expression. Papillary adenocarcinoma, malignant mixed mammary tumour, solid carcinoma, squamous cell carcinoma, infiltrative adenocarcinoma, mucinous carcinoma, intraductal carcinoma in situ and malignant myoepithelioma were found positive for c-erbB2. Tumours of connective tissue origin (6 cases) were immunonegative. It was interpreted that over expression of c-erbB2 oncoprotein is exhibited more by malignanat mammary tumours than benign ones. Further among the malignant mammary tumours, tumours of epithelial origin are frequently involved.

In malignant mammary tumours, compared to benign tumours and further among malignant tumours in poorly differentiated tumours, there is higher PCNA index. The expression pattern of PCNA and Ki-67 in human tumours shows that in mitotic cells, Ki-67 expression is chromosomal and PCNA immunostaining is cytoplasmic while in nonmitotic cells, PCNA and Ki-67 expression are restricted to the nuclei. The similar pattern was observed in canine mammary tumours. Out of 103 canine mammary gland tumours, 98 were diagnosed as malignant and only 5 diagnosed as benign tumours. PCNA and Ki-67 indices were significantly higher in malignant tumours as compared to benign tumours. There was positive correlation in PCNA and Ki-67 indices with each other in both benign and malignant tumours. High PCNA and Ki-67 indices were associated with malignancy and poorly differentiated tumours.

Plasma proteins albumin, globulin and immunoglobins play important role in identification of sub clinical stages in cancer patients. Hypoalbuminaemia is common in cancer patients and infusion of albumin does not improve their condition. Compensation capacity of globulins in cancers can help in making prognosis. Alteration in protein profile is more pronounced in malignant tumours and in advanced stages of tumour progression. Serum protein profiles were investigated for developing globulin compensation index (GCI) in bitches with mammary tumours and alteration was noticed in tumour group.

Single Strand Conformational Polymorphism (SSCP) profile of axon 5 of p53 gene revealed mutations in 3 out of 15 cases of spontaneous canine mammary tumours. Sequencing also revealed mutations in all samples when compared with wild type p53 gene sequences and results of analysis were same for all three. A study was conducted on immunohistochemical reaction to p^{53} protein expression in which among 38 CMT tissues only 10 expressed presence of nuclear reactivity for mutant p^{53} protein. Over-expression of mutant p^{53} protein of high intensity was found in osteochondrosarcomas and carcinosarcomas. The p^{53} gene expression by real time PCR also revealed its over- expression in osteochondrosarcomas and carcinosarcomas. In a clinicopathological study of canine genital tract tumours, the prevalence of benign tumours was more than malignant tumours. Incidence of the tumours showed that most frequently affected site was vagina or vulva followed by penis or prepuce and testes and uterus. The occurrence of leiomyoma was more followed by TVT, seminoma, fibroma, fibrosarcoma and lipoma. Females were affected more than males. A case of vaginal tumour was reported in a 12 years old Pomeranian bitch. Tumours of vagina and vulva were more common than the tumours of the uterus among the tumours of genital origin. Cardiac tumours are uncommon in pet animals. These may arise in heart tissue (primary tumours) or metastasize in the heart from another location (secondary tumours). Primary tumours include hemangiosarcoma, heart base tumours, mesothelioma, rhabdomyosarcoma, fibrosarcoma and lymphosarcoma. A case of malignant mammary gland tumour with metastasis to heart was reported.

Mast Cell Tumour

Mast cell tumours arise from mast cells of connective tissue of skin. It is mainly a tumour of dogs and occasionally also found in cats. Occur in old age majority being between 6-15 years of age. Metachromatic cytoplasmic granules are characteristic of tumour. Mast cell tumour in a nine year old male Chippiparai dog on the skin of the ventral abdomen was \observed high cellularity of round neoplastic cells and anisocytosis in cytological smears as well as large metachromatic granules in the cytoplasm. Histomorphology and cytology of cutaneous mastocytoma was studied. Cytology revealed sheets of mast cells with very high pigmentation. Histopathology of the mass revealed pleomorphism, high cellularity. There was marked infiltration of eosinophils throughout the tumour mass.

Fibroma

Gingival fibromas or epulis are extremely common tumours in dogs. They are found along the gum line. These are categorised into 3 types depending upon histologic type and tumour behaviour, fibromatous epulis, ossifying epulis & acanthomatous epulis. Fibromatous & ossifying epulides are solitary, non- invasive types & can grow to a larger size. Acanthomatous epulides can be invasive into local tissues & may cause destruction of local bone. An ossifying epulis in a 7 year old male Doberman dog in mandibular region. A case of periodontal fibromatous epulis was reported in a 12 year old Basset hound male dog which on histopathological examination revealed fibroblasts with packed collagen and abundant vasculature with occasional lymphocytic infiltration and there was absence of mitotic figures. A study on cytological and histopathological diagnosis of canine epulids in Chennai showed that acanthomatous epulis was commonly prevalent when compared to the fibromatous and ossifying epulis. Acanthomatous epulis was seen in 2 Spitz, one each in German shepherd, Boxer, Dalmatian and non-descript breeds of dogs. There were 5 females and 1 male. Two cases of fibromatous epulis were found in Boxer dogs involving one 5 years old male and a 7.5 years old female. Single case of ossifying epulis was found in a 9 year old male Spitz. Spitz was predominantly affected (33%). Commonly affected age group was between ranges of 2-13 years. Local invasiveness was observed in one acanthomatous epulis showing malignant lesions. A case of acanthomatous ameloblastoma in a 6 year old female Spitz was reported. Vaginal angiofibroma in a seven year old German shepherd bitch was reported.

Lipoma and Liposarcoma

Lipoma and liposarcoma are tumours arising from adipose cells. These are common tumours in most species of domestic animals in the older age group. Lipomas are made up of cells containing either one large fat globule or several small ones. The nucleus is pushed to periphery. Between fat cells, collagen fibres strands are interspersed. There are certain subtypes of lipoma as infiltrating lipoma, angiolipoma, fibrolipoma and myelolipoma. A case of angiolipoma in a 22 year old German shepherd dog was reported. The most common site for lipoma and liposarcoma in dogs is tissue of thorax and abdomen. Liposarcoma in a 7 year old male German shepherd dog was reported. A case of intrasplenic myelolipoma in spleen of a 7 year old male Labardor retriever dog was reported. Histopathologically, multifocal areas of adipose tissue, focally extensive myeloid precursors, and sinusoidal congestion and hemosiderin deposits in macrophages were observed.

Papilloma

Papilloma is papovavirus induced benign tumour of stratified squamous epithelium. Papillomas are more common in males. Middle and old aged dogs are most often affected. In cats' cutaneous papilloma are rare, affect old cats and are usefully solitary. In a case of cutaneous papilloma in a 4 year old Doberman dog, grossly mass was hard in consistency with thorny surface and appeared as cauliflower like growth. Histopathologically, epithelium formed rete- pegs which appeared to form epithelial pearls. A case of multiple cutaneous digital papillomas in a 10 month old mixed breed dog on digits of both fore limbs was reported. A report of oral papilloma in Beagle male puppy of 4 month old with the cauliflower like growths on the frontal region, upper lip and lower jaw region was presented. Another report in an eight month old male non-descript dog was presented in a dog having a pedunculated cauliflower like growth on the left oral commissure of the mouth which on cytological examination revealed benign squamous cells clusters. Microscopically the mass revealed papillary projections and contained multiple layers of prickle cells with fibrovascular connective tissue core as well as hyperkeratosis.

Squamous Cell Carcinoma

Squamous cell carcinoma is firm nodular mass that may be proliferative or erosive and may extend deep into dermis. Sites exposed to solar radiations are more at risk, especially in animals with light pigmentation. These tumours are in areas of chronic inflammation further progressing to actinic keratosis and eventually develop malignant tumours. Dark coloured, large breeds are predisposed to subungual squamous cell carcinoma. In dogs, SCC of nasal planum is extremely aggressive disease, in comparison to cats. Ocular carcinomas are rare in dogs compared to carcinoma in other sites as skin and oral cavity. A case of bilateral ocular carcinoma was reported in a 6.5 years old male mongrel dog with growths on both the eyes. Ocular squamous cell carcinoma in an eight year old mongrel dog was reported. Incidence of squamous cell carcinoma in dogs in Gujarat region was studied. Out of 510 biopsy samples, squamous cell carcinoma was revealed in 22 cases. Highest incidence was recorded in age group of 5 – 12 years. More cases were found in males as compared to females. Out of 22 cases maximum were found on skin followed by oral cavity, eye, prepuce and vagina. Squamous cell carcinoma was reported in a German Shephard male dog at Pantnagar.

Basal Cell Tumours

Basal cell tumours originate from basal layer of epidermis and also from basal cells of hair follicles, sebacious glands, or sweat glands. These are slow growing nodular tumours. They tend to ulcerate. They have a great tendency to infiltrate the surrounding tissue but metastasis seldom occurs. Microscopically cells resemble basal cells of Malpighian layer. Many cells fuse and have a concentric alveolar arrangement. A red coloured hairless mass w6.as noticed at the poll region on the right aspect of the mid line in a 3 year old male Spitz dog. Basal cell carcinoma on the ear of a mongrel bitch histologically revealed cells arranged both in form of elongated cords and in form of solid groups forming nests separated by extensive collagenous stroma. The connective tissue stroma revealed hyalinization and congestion of blood vessels.

Cutaneous Epidermoid Carcinoma

In canines epidermoid carcinoma is of rare occurrence and has been reported as metastatic lesion in lung. A case of cutaneous epidermoid carcinoma was reported in a dog with high indices of AgNOR, PCNA and nuclear protein Ki- 67.

Calcifying Epithelioma

Calcifying epithelioma is a benign cutaneous tumour which originates from the hair matrix cells. Ghost cells or shadow cells are characteristic features of this tumour. It has been reported in both dogs and cats. A case of calcifying epithelioma was reported in 9 years old cross bred dog. Microscopically there was presence of keratin mass concentrically arranged as keratin nest or whorls along with presence of ghost cells. In some areas increased melanin pigmentation was found.

Trichoepithelioma

In trichoepithelioma neoplastic cells are derived from hair matrix cells. These mostly occur in dogs above 5 -8 years of age and are rare in cats. A case of trichoepithelioma in a dog microscopically revealed islands of basal cells with keratinized centres of horn cysts and few rudimentary hair follicles.

Adenoma and Adenocarcinoma

Adenocarcinoma of cornea was reported in a Spitz dog. A case of ocular adenocarcinoma an 8 year old non- descript intact female dog. Metastasis of adenocarcinoma in spleen of an adult Doberman dog as scattered patches in sub capsular and red pulp sinuses was recorded. A case of prostrate adenocarcinoma in a 10 years old intact male Labrador dog on radiography showed enlarged prostate gland. Metastatic growths were found in lungs. Histopathology revealed neoplastic cells forming cords, nests and acini. Pulmonary metastatic neoplasms are common whereas primary lung tumours are rare in dogs. Among the primary pulmonary tumours, bronchio-alveolar tumours are more common than others. Pulmonary adenocarcinoma in a 9 years old Doberman bitch was reported. Diffuse anthracosis was found in lungs on post mortem examination. Histopathology revealed acinar structures with cuboidal cell lining in adenoid pattern and containing mucin in their lumens.A case of bronchioalveolar papillary adenocarcinoma was reported in a 12 years old female Daschund dog. Ciliary body adenoma in a 10 year old Labrador retriever dog with tumour mass inside the eye globe was observed. Histologically, moderately differentiated cuboidal to columnar cells arranged in tubular pattern, grouped in small islands were revealed. Tracheal adenocarcinoma in a 5 year old male non- descript dog was observed

Osteosarcoma

Osteosarcoma is a mesenchymal malignant tumour originating from osteoblasts. Osteosarcoma in a 7 years old male Pomeranian dog involving nasal, ethmoid, maxilla and palatine bones was reported. Mandibular and maxillary osteosarcomas are fourth most common non- odontogenic tumours of oral cavity in dogs. Axial osteosarcoma in a male Labrador dog with a swelling beneath left eye was reported.

Melanoma and Melanocarcinoma

Melanoma and melanocarcinoma are tumours of melanoblasts and are of neuro-ectodermal origin. Grossly, melanoma is brown, black or of grey colored. Microscopically, clumps of brownish - black pigment granules may be present either with the melanoblasts or in macrophages. Malignancy is indicated by lack of pigment. Melanomas arise mainly from skin and are rarely present in eyes, brain and spinal cord. A case of melanoma was reported in the buccal cavity of a 2 year old dog with a pedunculated grey colored mass in oral cavity.

Mesothelial Tumours

These tumours arise from mesothelial lining cells of serous cavities. These are rare among animals. Primary mesothelial tumours in dogs occur in the pleura, pericardium, peritoneum and the tunica vaginalis of the scrotum. Long term contact with asbestos may be a risk factor for mesothelioma. Pesticides were considered a factor that increases risk of mesothelioma. An unusual case of mesothelioma was reported in a 5 year old female Spitz dog. Malignant biphasic mesothelioma in 1.5 year old non- descript dog was reported. Metastases were observed in lung, liver, kidney, mesenteric, renal and mediastinal lymph nodes. Histologically tumour was composed of both epitheloid and sarcomatoid cells. Immunohistochemically, epitheloid cells were positive for cytokeratin and sarcomatoid cells were positive vimentin. A case of mixed mesenchymal skin tumour was reported in a 7 years old Labrador dog. Microscopically, large, clear vacuolar lipocytes replacing cytoplasm to periphery with pleomorphic nuclei were visible. Also a myxoid variant of scattered stellate cells with foamy macrophages were observed. A case of synovial sarcoma with metastases to lungs was reported in a 10 year old non- descript dog in the stifle joint. On post-mortem examination it revealed white coloured pebble like masses scattered in lung parenchyma. Cytologically, cells were arranged in win throwing pattern which is characteristic feature of synovial sarcoma. Binucleation and nuclear fragmentation was observed. Cytoplasmic vacuoles with mucinous granules were noticed. A case of mesothelioma was reported in a 12 year old female cat.

Spirocercosis

Only a few cases have been reported in form of affections of oesophagus and aorta as fibrosarcoma, fibrochondrosarcoma, osteosarcoma, granulolmatosis and aneurysm of aorta.A case of osseous metaplasia by *Spirocerca lupi* was reported in an adult male dog carcass found as circular nodules in submucosa of oesophagus also aneurysm of aorta was noticed. Few live larvae were present inside the lumen of aorta. Histologically, osseous tissue formation at the centre of lesions in aorta was found surrounded by bands of fibrous connective tissue. Oesophageal submucosa revealed remnants of parasites at the centre surrounded by fibrous connective tissue bands and zone of inflammation. Based on necropsy findings during 1999-2004, eighteen cases of *Spirocerca* were reported in dogs in Mumbai.

Multiple Primary Tumours

Multiple primary tumours are tumours either of different kind in the same or in the different organ systems, or tumours of same kind in different organs. These tumours are generally of different histological origin. A case of multiple tumours was reported in an 11 year old Rampur hound bitch with tumours at skin of thigh region and mammary gland. Histopathologically skin tumour was diagnosed as fibroma and mammary gland tumour was diagnosed as complex adenocarcinoma.

Transmissible Venereal Yumour (TVT)

Transmissible venereal tumour (TVT) is the only known contagious tumour of dogs which gets transmitted from one dog to another during coitus or by licking or coming in contact of the affected dog. Studies suggest that TVT cells do not arise from dog's own cells rather tumour cells from an affected dog might grab the mitochondria of other dogs by fusing with their cells leading to mitochondrial DNA recombination in host cells or there may be some other mechanism. It is of uncertain histogenesis. It may be reticuloendothelial in origin. Some studies suggest tumour cell genes in TVT are different from those of host's cells. It occurs in younger dogs between 1-6 years of age and is more common in females. Lymphocytes may cause cell mediated tumour cell lysis which leads to spontaneous regression of the tumour. A case of TVT was reported in a bitch with metastasis in lymph nodes, spleen and liver. A retrospective study on canine TVT from 1981 to 1984 was conducted and it was observed that the ages of male and female dogs affected ranged from 2 to 9 years and 2.5 to 12 years respectively. Among all cases 65 were mongrel dogs, 26 were Alsatian, 23 were Alsatian crosses, 5 were Doberman and 1 was Apso. A study on occurrence of TVT, 216 case reports from 1987 to 1990 were reviewed. Out of 216 dogs, 57.9% were presented in the spring and summer season followed by 42.1 % during autumn and winter season. Lymphokine activated killer cells (LAK) are capable of lysing a wide variety of autogenic, allogenic and xenogenic tumour cells including that of TVT but there is a need to evaluate their efficacy for their large scale use. Transmissible venereal tumour cells were large, oval or round shaped neoplastic cell with indistinct outline having round or oval nuclei which was very large in relation to the size of the cell. A study on differential diagnosis of canine cutaneous histiocytoma and TVT by AgNOR and PCNA was conducted by Nair *et al.,* (2006) in which they observed that in both types of tumours multiple fine dots within nuclei were noticed. In cutaneous histiocytoma, PCNA positive cells took brick red colour in the nuclei and the reaction was found stronger than that observed in TVT. These findings correlated with that of Pawaiya et al, (2003) who reported higher AgNOR count in CCH than CTVT. Ocular metastasis of TVT in a five-year old German shepherd dog was reported. A study on the prevalence and pathological studies of TVT was conducted in dogs. Out of 161 cases, 41 were diagnosed as TVT. The prevalence was more in young female dogs of age group 2- 11 years. Non- descript dogs were more affected compared to pure breeds.

Ovarian Granulosa Cell Tumours

Ovarian granulosa cell tumours are tumours of granulosa cells or theca cells or of the luteal cells of the ovary. These result in nymphomania and sterility. A case of ovarian granulosa cell tumour was reported in a three year old Doberman bitch. Among various tumours, the incidence of granulosa cell tumours is about 22.85%.The incidence of ovarian neoplasms increase with increase in age and in absence of pregnancy. A case of ovarian haemangiosarcoma was reported in a 10 year old non- descript female dog. Grossly the ovary appeared as tennis ball like, firm and reddish in colour. The cut sections showed multilobulated chambers filled with blood clot, showing honeycomb pattern of fibrous trabeculae separating blood filled cavities.

Testicular Tumours

Sertoli cell tumour arises from sertoli cells of seminiferous tubules and is most common tumour in cryptorchid testes. Tumour is round in shape, firm in consistency. There may be presence of haemorrhages and necrosis. Microscopically, cells are round or polyhedral with central nuclei. Tumour cells produce oestrogen due to which dog shows gynaecomastia. A case of bilateral inguinal cryptorchidism with sertoli cell tumour was reported in an 8 years old Alsatian dog with enlarged and hard cryptorchid testes. ABiochemical analysis revealed increased BUN and oestradiol levels. A case of malignant sertoli cell tumour was reported in a four and half year old GSD. Increase in SGOT and total protein value was noticed which was possibly due to *in- situ* effect of hyperoestrogenism. The presence of substantial fibrous tissue proliferation around seminiferous tubules with indication of hyalinization in right testis was there. The presence of metaplasia and metastasis in left testis confirmed the malignant nature of tumour. Some areas within seminiferous tubules revealed small pockets of eosinophilic secretions, surrounded by abnormal sertoli cells resembling to Call-Exner like bodies which are commonly found in granulosa cell tumour. reported a case of sertoli cell tumour in a five year old male mongrel dog. Mixed germ cell and sex cord stromal tumour was reported in a 7 year old male Spitz dog. Histologically, tumour composed of neoplastic germ cells and sex cord stromal cells arranged in tubular and sheet like pattern. Neoplastic germ cells were large, round to polygonal with vacuolated cytoplasm. Neoplastic sertoli cells were irregular to spindle shaped with elongated or oval nucleus.

Tumours of Haemopoietic Cells

Leukaemia is a neoplastic disease involving one or more types of cells of the haematopoietic tissues. TLC may be extremely high with abnormal or undifferentiated cells in the blood. In canine leukaemia, lymphoma is the most common form of Lymphoproliferative neoplasia. It occurs in dogs of 5 years of age and above. It is characterized by bilateral lymphadenopathy. Dogs also suffer from acute and chronic lymphocytic leukaemia. Feline leukaemia represents about one third of all neoplasms of cats, most being lymphoma. They are caused by C- type oncornavirus, feline leukaemia virus. Lymphoma and lymphocytic leukaemias are common, accounting for 80-90% of all feline haemopoietic neoplasms. Lymphomas involving multiple organs are called multicentric lymphomas. Diffused lymphocytic lymphoma in a 7 year old female Rottweiler dog affecting prescapular, popliteal and submandibular lymph nodes was reported. Leukemic leukemia was reported in a 2 year old Doberman dog. On DLC, eosinophils, basophils and neutrophils were nil and 97% lymphocytes were found. Chronic myelogenous leukemia is myeloproliferation of stem cells leading to overproduction of cells of granulocytic series. Myelogenous leukemia is uncommon in dogs. Diagnosis can be done by blood picture showing normocytic normochromic anaemia, neutrophilia & vacuolations of cytoplasm of myeloid cells. These findings can be confirmed by bone –marrow examination. Chronic myelogenous leukemia in a 10 year old Pomeranian dog was reported. A lymphoma was observed around the bulbar gland of penis in a castrated male dog with complaint of pain, difficulty in urination and blood in the urine for last six weeks. The excised tumour mass was elliptical in shape, pinkish coloured and soft in consistency enclosed within a fibrous tissue capsule. The neoplastic cells appeared to be lymphocytes and some immature form of lymphoid cells. A case of multicentric lymphoma was reported in a nine – year old Saint Bernard dog which on post mortem examination revealed splenomegaly with diffuse enlargement and multiple, pale foci disseminated in the parenchyma. A case of multicentric lymphoblastic lymphoma in a 9 year old female Labrador retriever dog was reported. Cases of cutaneous lymphoma in dogs were studied and it was recorded that 6 cases of lymphoma among which 4 were epitheliotropic lymphoma and 2 were non- epitheliotropic lymphoma. Cytologically, medium to large sized lymphocytes were found in smears. Immunohistochemical differentiation for T- cell and B-cell origin was done by the CD3 and CD79a marker.

Heart Base Tumours

Heart base tumours (chemodectoma) form a group of tumours which have been specially noted because of their location. These are slow growing neuroendocrine neoplasms. These may be found as carotid body tumours or aortic body tumours. They generally secrete catecholamines and serotonin. These usually affect older dogs. Heart base tumours are neoplastic proliferation of neuroepithelial cells in aortic bodies mainly in the adventitia of aortic arch. A case of aortic body tumour was reported in a 7 years old Doberman bitch. Chemodectoma was reported in a 13 year old male non- descript dog. A single large sized mass was noticed near the base of heart involving major blood vessels. Grossly, it was multi-lobulated, red to greyish in colour with spongy consistency. Microscopically, it revealed multiple lobules of neoplastic cells separated by connective tissue stroma in a classical neuroendocrine pattern.

Haemangiosarcoma

Hemangiosarcomas are highly malignant tumours of blood vessels and are the most common cardiac tumours of dogs. A case of multiple haemangiosarcoma was reported in a dog affecting heart, liver, spleen, lungs, intestine and kidneys observed as nodular masses infiltrating intravascular spaces. Grossly, scattered, multifocal dark reddish coloured nodules were observed in left auricular endocardium and also in other organs. Histopathologically, oval to polyhedral endothelial cells were observed.

Leiomyoma

Leiomyoma are the benign tumours of smooth muscles. These are the most common smooth muscle neoplasms of the female dog's reproductive tract and account for 85-90 percent of uterine tumours in canines. A case of scrotal fibroleiomyoma was reported in a 7 years old male Alsatian dog. Leiomyoma was reported involving the urogenital tract of 10 years old cross bred bitch. A case of multiple leiomyoma of genitalia with concurrent pyometra in a twelve year old intact female Spitz dog was reported. 35 tumour masses were surgically excised among which 33 were vaginal, one was cervical and one uterine tumour.

Rhabdoma and Rhabdomyosarcoma

Rhabdoma and rhabdomyosarcoma are tumours of striated muscles. They appear as globular masses in 4 year old male mongrel dog with a large pedunculated swelling on left hind limb.

Hepatic and Biliary Tract Neoplasms

Detailed clinicopathological studies of hepatic and biliary tract neoplasms in dogs were undertaken. Cholangiocarcinomas are rare in dogs. These are malignant liver tumours arising from neoplastic cells of bile duct. Different elements are produced as cystic, papillary & tubular elements which are lined by cuboidal or columnar cells as in normal biliary epithelium. A case of cholangiocarcinoma was reported in a 3 years old non- descript dog with history of inappetance, vomiting, diarrhoea, bilateral abdominal distension and progressive weakness. Ascites fluid examination suggested liver damage. Animal died and at necropsy, multiple nodular growths over entire liver surface were found. Histopathology of liver revealed that neoplastic hepatic cells were arranged in microacinar pattern and at some places, ductule formation was present. Papillary cystic cholangio cellular carcinoma was seen in a 10 year old male Spitz dog with metastasis in the bronchial lymph node. A case of spindle cell carcinoma of mammary gland was recorded in a 10 year old Great Dane bitch with metastasis to liver.

Neoplasms in Poultry

A tumour is a purposeless, uncontrollable growth of the cells that has no useful function and has random arrangement. The factors which cause cancer can be extrinsic or intrinsic. Intrinsic factors are heredity, age, pigmentation, sex and tumour immunity. Extrinsic factors are chemicals, radiant energy, chronic irritation, hormones, parasites and oncogenic viruses. The tumour does not occur in any animal until and unless the immune system is immunocompromised. Malignant transformations can be due to complex genetic modifications. Some of them can result in the expression of proteins that are taken as non-self or foreign by the immune system. This is the concept of immune surveillance. In some animals growth of neoplasm is very fast that leads to early death. In others, tumour growth is slow and the animal may survive for several years. When malignant tumour is clinically manifested, it takes 6 months to 1 year to cause death. There are many systems or functions in the body which works together to fight with neoplastic cells. These are non-specific lysis and phagocytosis of tumour cells by polymorphonuclear cells, lysis of neoplastic cells by natural killer cells, antibodies against tumour antigens restraining tumour growth, etc. Tumour cells develop certain biochemical alterations on their surface (protein change) that makes the **"tumour antigens"**. These tumour antigens may evoke immune response in body by humoral or cell mediated mechanism which may inhibit the tumour cell growth. There can be escape of neoplastic cells from immunological destruction by delayed immunostimulation, antigenic modulation, antigenic overload, general immunodeficiency, specific immunodeficiency and by humoral antibodies which binds with tumour antigens and blocks the effect of more potent anti-neoplastic action by entry of another source.

Neoplastic diseases of poultry fall into two broad classes, namely: those with an infectious etiology and those which are non-infectious. Those of the former category are of the greater economic importance because the viruses that cause these diseases are widely prevalent in commercial stock and the mesenchymal neoplasms that they cause affect relatively young birds. These infections and diseases can be enzootic and epizootic. Neoplasms of a non-infectious etiology occur mostly in birds older than the usual lifespan of commercial birds. Such tumours are often of epithelial cell origin, with ovarian tumours being common in hens over two years of age. Even so, tumours of the magnum region of the oviduct, adenomas and adenocarcinomas, of non-infectious etiology, can occur in commercial laying hens at the end of the first laying season. However, the non-infectious neoplasms are generally sporadic and not of great economic significance.

The cases of Poultry tumours which had occurred in India are summarised below

Squamous Cell Carcinoma

Squamous cell carcinoma is a malignant tumour of squamous stratified epithelium which is characterized by macroscopic features like papillary projections or cauliflower like growth, broad base, soft and grey or pink in colour and microscopic features as stratum germinativum proliferation, concentric layers of keratin forming ***'Epithelial pearls'***, presence of mitotic figures and thickening of prickle cell layer. This tumour had been reported from the lung of 46 weeks old desi hen in Parbhani, Maharashtra in the year 1996.

Fibroma

Fibroma is a benign tumour of fibrous connective tissue. Macroscopically, they are hard in touch, size varies from tiny nodules to large even upto several cm in diameter. Microscopic features are that the neoplastic cells make significant amounts of collagen, which separates these cells from each other and presence of interlacing bundles of fibrous connective tissue along with spindle shaped nuclei of the cells. Tumour had been reported from a two and a half years old desi chicken in Mannuthy, Kerala in the year 1994.

Adenocarcinoma

Adenocarcinoma is a malignant tumour of glandular epithelium which is characterized by its pink colour, polypoid in shape and may occlude gland or lumen of hollow organ. Microscopic features are single layer of columnar or cuboidal epithelial cells showing papillary projections and pleomorphic cells, presence of mitotic figures, small nucleus with fine chromatin and fine nucleoli and such cells are grouped into masses and invasive to basement membrane. This tumour had been reported from the ovary of the 20 weeks old White Leghorn layer bird in Bhubaneswar in the year 1997. This type of tumour had also been reported from Japanese quails in Tirupati in the year 2003. Ovarian adenocarcinoma had been reported from a turkey in Kerala in the year 2012. Oviduct infundibular adenocarcinoma had also occurred in a layer chicken in Namakkal, Tamilnadu in the year 2014.

Myxoma

Myxoma is tumour of fibrous tissue capable of producing mucin and anaplasia. These are observed mostly on subcutaneous, sub serous and submucous surfaces. Macroscopically, rounded, bunch of grapes like structures are seen. They are slimy in touch due to mucin content. Microscopic features are presence of spindle shaped cells lying in basophilic mucinous matrix with pleomorphism and presence of several mitotic figures with infiltration of inflammatory cells. This type of tumour had been reported from a nine weeks old chicken in Chennai in the year 2002.

Mesothelioma

Mesothelioma is a tumour of mesothelial lining cells of serous cavities specially of peritoneum and pleura. Such tumours are found in thorax and abdomen. Macroscopically, they are pink in colour, hard, multiple, nodular and scattered in cavity. Microscopic features are presence of collection of cells resembling epithelial cells and these cells have acidophilic granular cytoplasm and large vesicular nucleus and there are numerous blood vessels in tumour. This type of tumour had been reported as a concurrent occurrence with coligranuloma and nodular taeniasis in a poultry flock in Kerala in the year 2013.

Seminoma

Seminoma is a malignant tumour of epithelium of seminiferous tubules of testes. Macroscopically, they are white or grey in colour, lobulated as bulging from testes and areas of necrosis may be seen. Microscopic features are epithelial cells arranged as sheets or islands separated by thin strands of fibrous tissue. Cells are round, large, uniform in size with acidophilic and granular cytoplasm. Mitotic figures are numerous. This tumour had been reported concurrently with leydig cell tumour from a Giriraja chicken in Mizoram in the year 2016.

Leydig Cell Tumour

Also called as **"Interstitial cell tumour"**, these are the testicular neoplasms which are almost always benign. Grossly, the neoplasm is spherical, of yellowish brown to orange colour and well demarcated. Microscopically, cells of the neoplasms can be large, round, polyhedral or spindle shaped. The cells have abundant cytoplasm, which is often finely vacuolated and has brown pigment. Although haemorrhage, necrosis and cyst formation are common; leydig cell adenomas are non-invasive. This tumour had been reported concurrently with seminoma from a Giriraja chicken in Mizoram in the year 2016.

Granulosa Cell Tumour

Granulosa cell tumour arises from the ovary mesenchyma. Granulosa cell tumour is usually observed in association with Avian leucosis complex caused by retro virus. Macroscopically, they are single, very large even up to 20 cm in diameter. They are yellow in colour, rounded, lobulated and projected on the surface of ovary. Microscopic features are tumour cells arranged in columns, clusters or compact alveoli as irregular mass or pseudo glands. In lumen, hyaline acidophilic material and several mitotic figures are seen. This type of tumour had been reported from a Guinea fowl in Kerala in the year 2011. Immunohistochemical and pathological studies had been done on granulosa cell tumour in Guinea fowl (*Numida meleagris*) in Tirupati, Andhra Pradesh in the year 2016. In these studies, the impression smears from the affected organs were made and stained with Leishman's stain. Representative tissue specimens were collected in 10% formalin and processed for routine histopathology. The tissue sections were taken on APES-coated slides for immunohistochemistry. Immunohistochemistry was carried out using primary antibodies for alpha inhibin and CA125 markers according to the standard protocol. Gross examination revealed emaciated carcass with distended abdomen which on opening revealed accumulation of straw coloured fluid. Large greyish white, multinodular masses with few cystic areas were observed attached to the ovary. Few masses were pedunculated. Cytological smears revealed presence of eosinophilic, polyhedral cells with prominent nucleoli and intracytoplasmic vacuoles with tendency to form follicle like structures. Along with these cells, pleomorphic lymphocytes, plasma cells and lymphoblasts with nucleoli were observed. Histopathologically, the ovarian mass revealed the infiltration of the eosinophilic polyhedral cells forming the rosettes separated by the connective tissue stroma. In few areas, the acinar structures showed the presence of eosinophilic material in the lumen resembling Call Exner bodies- a pathognomic histopathological lesion of granulosa cell tumour. Along with neoplastic granulosa cells, the ovarian tissue also revealed the presence of pleomorphic lymphoblasts, lymphocytes and plasma cells in between the parenchyma. Immunohistochemical staining showed strong positive immunolabelling with alpha inhibin, a specific biomarker for granulosa cell tumour and negative reaction with CA-125, confirming this case as negative for ovarian adenocarcinoma.

Haemangioma

It is a benign tumour of blood vessels. Macroscopically, they are usually single, vary in size from few mm to several cms in diameter. They are dark red in colour and bleeding is severe on rupture or injury. Microscopic features are many single cell lined capillaries are usually seen and their lumen is filled with newly formed endothelial cells.

This type of tumour had been reported from the liver of a seventy-two weeks old Rhode Island Red cock in Parbhani in the year 1995 and also had occurred in a white Pekin duck in IVRI,Izzatnagar in the year 2016.

Myeloid Leucosis

Myeloid leucosis or myelocytomatosis is a neoplastic disease caused by Avian leucosis/ sarcoma group viruses of retroviridae family. Macroscopically, nodules are slightly soft, grey to white coloured and of varied size on peritoneum, inner surface of ribs, liver, mucosal surface of trachea and on the head of femur bones. Microscopic features are marked proliferation of myelocytes and presence of a large, vesicular and eccentrically placed nucleus and cytoplasm is tightly packed with eosinophilic (pink) granules. This type of tumour had been reported from broiler breeder chickens in Mumbai in the year 2013.

Marek's Disease

Marek's disease (MD) is a lympho-proliferative disease of chicken caused by Alphaherpes virus of Herpesviridae family. It is characterized by mononuclear cellular infiltrates in peripheral nerve and various visceral organs, eyes, skin and central nervous system. Neural involvement, leading to paralysis, is the most visible symptom and the names of polyneuritis, fowl paralysis, range paralysis and neurolymphomatosis are commonly applied. In classical Marek's disease, the characteristic gross lesion is enlargement of one or more peripheral nerves. Affected nerves are up to 2-3 times the normal thickness. The normal striated and white glistening appearance is lost, and the nerve may appear greyish and sometimes oedematous. Acute Marek's disease is characterized by diffuse lymphomatous involvement and enlargement of the liver, gonads, spleen, kidneys, lungs, proventriculus and heart. In younger birds, liver enlargement is moderate, but in adult birds the liver is greatly enlarged, which is similar to that in lymphoid leucosis. Microscopically, three types of lesions are seen in peripheral nerves. In the first, there is cellular infiltration of the nerves with mature lymphocytes. In the second, which is the most common, there is separation of the nerve fibres associated with edema followed by less cellular infiltration. These cells are lymphocytes and plasma cells. Infiltration with neutrophils and myelocytes may also occur. In the third type of the lesion, the nerves are infiltrated with lymphoblasts showing numerous mitoses. In this condition, which may be an advanced and progressive stage of the second type, all evidence of the nerve tissue is lost and it has the appearance of a neoplasm. In the central nervous system, perivascular cuffing with lymphocytes is noticed. The most common lesions in visceral organs are lymphoid tumours and the lymphoma consists of a mixture of malignant T-cells and reactive, bursa dependent lymphocytes(B cells), T cells and macrophages. On the skin, there is gross enlargement of feather follicles, appearing as nodular elevations. Skin becomes rough and tough. There is patchy infiltration of lymphoblasts, plasma cells and a few histiocytes. Presence of infrequent pyroninophilic lymphoblasts is the differentiating feature in Marek's disease unlike lymphoid leucosis.

Pathological and serological studies had been done on natural outbreaks of acute(visceral) Marek's disease in chickens in Gujarat in the year 1993. Marek's disease had occurred in vaccinated layer flocks in Haryana in the year 2003. It had also been reported from the commercial chickens in Aizawl, Mizoram in the year 2005. An outbreak had also occurred in vaccinated poultry(White Leghorn) flocks in and around Namakkal region of Tamil Nadu in the year 2010. Marek's disease had also been reported from the desi chickens in Mumbai in the year 2014. It had also occurred in a duck in Nagpur in the year 2014.

Lymphoid Leucosis

Lymphoid leucosis (LL) or big liver disease is the commonest neoplasm caused by the Avian Leucosis Sarcoma Virus (ALSV). It is characterised usually by enlargement of the liver by infiltrating lymphoblasts. LL appears between 14th and 30th week of age. Incidence is usually highest at about sexual maturity. Grossly visible tumours almost always involve liver, spleen and bursa of Fabricius. These include, in addition to liver and spleen, kidney, lung, gonad, heart, bone marrow and mesentery. Tumours are soft, smooth and glistening. Growth may be nodular, granular (miliary), diffuse or combination of these forms. In the nodular form, lymphoid tumours (0.5 mm-5 cm in diameter), usually spherical, may occur singly or in large numbers. The granular or military form consists of numerous small nodules (less than 2 mm in diameter) uniformly distributed throughout the parenchyma. In the diffuse form, the organ is uniformly enlarged and usually very friable. Microscopically, the lesions consist of diffuse areas or coalescing foci of extravascular lymphoid cells. The cytoplasm of most tumour cells contains a large amount of RNA, indicating that the cells are immature and rapidly dividing. The main cell is a lymphoblast; they have B cell markers and carry surface IgM. Lymphoid leucosis is sporadic in occurrence and reported from many parts of the country. One or few cases can be seen in older birds during investigation of routine mortality at the time of post-mortem examination.

Hepatocellular Carcinoma

Hepatocellular carcinoma is a malignant tumour of hepatic cells. Macroscopically, they are single, projected as brownish or greenish nodule and are round or ovoid in shape. Microscopic features are hepatic cells arranged in columns. They are large and polyhedral with acidophilic granular cytoplasm. Nucleus is very large, central and pale staining. Numerous mitotic figures are present. Tumour giant cells are seen and divided by connective tissue stroma. It had been reported from ducks in Khanapara, Guwahati in the year 2008. This tumour had also been reported from a turkey in Jaipur in the year 2011 and concurrently with haemangioma from a layer chicken in Mizoram in the year 2016. Hepatocellular carcinoma may also occur due to aflatoxicosis in older birds.

Cholangiocellular Carcinoma

These are malignant neoplasms of biliary epithelium which usually originate from the intra-hepatic ducts. Macroscopically, they are small in size, multiple, round and encapsulated. They are yellowish white in colour. Microscopic features are acini lined by columnar cells containing mucin. There are cyst like spaces filled with neoplastic cells. Nucleus is located at the base of cells. Cells are surrounded by collagenous stroma. This type of tumour had been reported from an adult layer bird of over 24 weeks of age in Ludhiana in the year 2005.

Nephroblastoma

These neoplasms are of embryonal origin and originate from metanephric blastema. These are common renal neoplasms of pigs and chickens in which they are usually seen at slaughter. At post-mortem, these can be solitary or multiple masses which usually reach a great size. They are usually soft to rubbery and grey with foci of haemorrhage. On cut surface, they are often lobulated. Microscopic features vary, but are morphologically similar to the developmental stages of embryonic kidneys. Characteristically, loose myxomatous tissue predominates. Scattered in this tissue are primitive tubules lined by elongated, deeply stained cells and structures that resemble primitive glomeruli. Nephroblastomas also have such mesenchymal components as cartilage, bone, skeletal muscle and adipose tissue. It had been reported from a copper pheasant at IVRI, Izzatnagar in the year 2007.

Neoplasms in Wild and Zoo Animals

Neoplasm or tumor occurs as an unexplained, clinically silent mass in tissue. Thorough clinical examination and logical procedures helps in the diagnosis of the neoplasm. Tissue biopsy is of utmost importance to classify whether a tumor is benign or malignant. Carcinogenesis involves both the genetic and epigenetic alterations. Genetic involves changes with the DNA and epigenetics involve alterations without changes in the DNA. When a cancer adopts a new gene expression pattern resulting from an epigenetic mechanism, it and its progeny can switch back to the previous gene expression pattern. This preserves the nature that can enhance cancerous growth.Neoplasia involves an intrinsic genetic abnormality in somatic cells that give rise to autonomous growth. Cells rapidly grow and expand onto the adjacent tissue. Progressive development of the cancer is characterized by the evolution of successive clones of cells, each coming closer with the advancement of the stage and the cells proliferate, stopping only with the death of the host. There is a strong geographic difference in tumor rates and types of tumor and these differences may result from environmental factors. Neoplasms due to chemical carcinogens are more common in animals exposed to industrial areas and areas with heavy chemical contamination in the environment leading to immunodeficiency in animals that make them more prone to the occurrence of cancers.

In the neoplastic cells abnormal genes favor proliferation over differentiation. Most of these tumors arise by genetic mutation or due to rearrangement of genes. The abnormal gene may produce mRNA that directs the ribosomes to start overproduction of abnormal gene product. Excess gene product then might produce enzymatic and other reaction to produce cellular manifestations. Initiating change can be due to chemicals or radiations or due to viral cancer genes into host DNA that mimic the normal growth controlling genes. Tumors are frequently encountered and reported in case of domesticated and companion animals but this also affects the one dwelling in captivity in zoological parks, zoo's and the one living freely in the forest areas, commonly called as the wild animals. Neoplasms in case of wild animals have reports from zoo/ zoological parks encountered during general examination of the animal due to presence of swelling which may sometimes affects the normal physiology of the animals otherwise the tumors are generally encountered during the necropsy procedure. Wild animals are grouped according to various orders they belong. Enlisted below are the cases and reports of neoplastic conditions in wild animals over a period of around fifty years.

Artiodactlyla

Animals belonging to this order are called even toed animals as they either have two or four toes on their feet. This order includes many families and some of them are:suidae(wild boar, pigmy hog), tragulidae(mouse deer), cervidae(hangul, barking deer, hog deer, chital , sambhar, barasingha and musk deer) and bovidae (antelopes, gazelles, black buck, blue bull or nilgai, chinkara, goral, yak).Cases of tumors encountered in artiodactyla order over the period are described as reported in the available literature.An adult female hog deer was found with persistent vaginal bleeding and died due to the ailment. Later a tumor was found attached with the wall of the uterus and oviduct. It was diagnosed as adenocarcinoma of uterus. Epithelial tumor of the mucosa of the ethmoid was found in sangai, chital, sika deer and blackbuck in Biological Park, Orrisa. Animals developed swelling in the frontal nasal region and developed epistaxis. Symptoms included unilateral and bilateral blindness and exopthalamos. They were later histologically diagnosed to be adenocarcinoma, squamous cell carcinoma and anaplastic carcinoma.

A chital was brought to IVRI for treatment with the history of impairement in foreleg. Its shoulder joint was swollen after the death of the animal deskinning and defleshing revealed a spongy large swelling involving distal half of radius and ulna. It was reported from the forest division Pilibhit. A 6 year oldserow had multiple cartilaginous exostoses on six ribs. The shaft of the ribs and the area were white in color. The gross and the microscopic lesion revealed it to be osteochondroma. Carcinoma of mucosa of ethmoid was reported in deer in Zoological Garden, Thrissur. Embyonalnephroma in water buck at New Delhi, National zoological park. Fibrosarcoma in hog deer and muzzle mix cell carcinoma was reported in chital from Zoological Garden, Bhilai. A chital from Biological Park, Patna suffered from Cholangiocarcinoma, on Post mortem liver revealed grayish white area, sinusoid were dilated and filled with red blood cells. Another chital from Jim Corbett Park suffered from carcinoma of liver. Gnu in Zoological Park, Andhra Pradesh was diagnosed with histiocytic cell carcinoma of cervical region. Biological Park, Orissa reported tumors from various animals in its captivity which includes lymphosarcoma in Gaur, reticulum cell sarcoma and mesothelioma in mediastinal lymph node and liver in different Nilgai and epithelial tumor of ethmoid in Black Buck.

Leiomyoma in abomasum-duodenal junction and fibroma were reported in a Sambhar and another case of fibroma in vagina of chital, also reported adenocarcinoma of liver in mouse deer and adenoma at vulva of barking deer from Zoological Garden, Assam. Squamus cell carcinoma was reported from a Yak, from West Bengal. A solitary growth was noticed in lower right cheek.

Initially, it was soft but later ulcerated with sticky material. Histopathology confirmed the diagnosis, keratin layers forming pearls were observed. A case of endometrial carcinoma was reported in a spotted deer from Thrissur Zoo, necropsy revealed enlargement of the uterus, left uterine horns showed multiple nodules. Histopathology revealed spindle shaped cells with indistinct borders. Cases which were only maintained in zoo records includes uterine tumor in a chousingha was from Zoological garden, Mumbai. Carcinoma of lung in a wild boar and another of unspecified origin from Sambhar was reported from Zoological garden, Thrissur. Zoo record, 1999, reported a case of tumorous growth at the base of antlers in a Blackbuck from, Bhilai. Zoological Garden, Assam in Zoo Annual Report 1978-1980, presented a case of squamous cell carcinoma in a pigmy hog. Carcinoma of lung in a bluebull and carcinoma of ocular and nasal region in Sambar was presented at Zoological Park, Tirupati.

Carnivora

The order includes the flesh eating mammals, this includes families such as; felidae (lion, tiger, jaguar, leopard, cheetah), ursidae (Himalayan bear, sloth bear), canidae (wolves, jackals, hynae), viveridae (civets, bear cat) herpestidae (mongoose).

Felidae (Lion/ Tiger/ Leopards/ Jaguars)

Neoplasms are most commonly encountered in case of wild felids. A male Tiger at National Park, Delhi, 1979 was reported to be affected from bleeding from mouth and deterioration in physical condition. On necropsy enlarged and swollen reddish posterior part of tongue was found. Histologically, it revealed to be a squamous cell carcinoma (Arora and Parihar, 1990). Lioness at zoological garden Lucknow on necropsy revealed thick growths attached to peritoneum and omentum.Tiger from National Park Ranthambore was diagnosed for mesothelioma recovered from thoracic cavity; another from Zoological Garden, Thrissur had cavernous hemangioma of lung and liver. At National Park, Delhi squamous cell carcinoma was diagnosed in a Tiger and Zoological Garden, Kolkatta reported sebaceous gland carcinoma. Reports of Carcinoma of sweat gland and sweat gland carcinoma in lower eyelid were also reported from the same national park. Kidney hemangioma was reported in Tiger at Kanha National Park, Madhya Pradesh.

Biological Park, Orissa reported numerous cases of tumors in Tigers which includes; Intrahepatic bile duct carcinoma about 2 litres of straw coloured fluid was collected from the peritoneal cavity and liver was enlarged and had multinodular cauliflower like growth, cases of Malignant melanoma of skin, mesothelioma, epidermoid carcinoma was also reported. A case of fibroma in the hind limb of a lionwas reported. The growth was hard and extended into the subcutaneous tissue so it was excised, it was confirmed on histology to be a fibroma and showed interlaced bundles.

Adenocarcinoma of mammary gland in a Tigress was reported from Zoological Garden, Assam. Squamous cell carcinoma of lungs was reported in an Indian Leopard. Animal had respiratory distress and on necropsy one lung was hard and had multiple nodular growths while other was normal, the case was confirmed histologically. Histiocytoma in leopard was reported from Nandankannan Zoo, Orissa. The animal developed a fluctuating swelling at ventral cervical region. Histopathology showed closely packed cells indistinctly grouped by thin fibrous tissue, vacuolar cytoplasm indicating it to be a histiocytoma. Tumors in different Lions were reported such as Adenocarcinoma of intestine, Squamous cell carcinoma, epidermoid carcinoma of gingival, Adenoma of lung, from Zoological Garden, Thrissur. Zoological Garden,Thrissur reported few more cases in Lions which included Epidermoid cysts, Renal carcinoma in which left and right kidney both showed multiple grayish white nodules, pericardial sac and lungs were also affected, multilobular cystic growth. Zoological Garden, Anand reported squamous cell carcinoma. African lion from Zoological Garden, Jaipur reported Bileduct Cystadenoma. Zoological Park, Kanpur reported Bronchiogenic carcinoma of lungs. A case of lipomatosis was diagnosed in a lion from IVRI. Capillary hemangioma in a Lion was reported from Zoological Park, Chennai. A case of lipomatosis in spleen of a Cheetah was reported from Zoological Park, Delhi. National Park, Rajasthan reported fibroma of tongue in a Leopard. In Zoological Garden, Kerela there were two reports of tumor from Leopards, leiomyoma of uterus and hemangioendothelioma. Jaguars from Zoological Garden, Kerela were diagnosed with cystadenocarcinoma of ovary and leiomyoma of uterus and other from Zoological Garden, West Bengal was diagnosed with squamous cell carcinoma.

In Zoological Park, Chennai Leopard suffered from fibrosarcoma of eye. Fibrosarcoma in a Lioness was reported at IVRI, nodular growth on the internal aspect of lower lip was seen. Grossly lung revealed whitish grey fleshy lesions of varying sizes. Histopathology confirmed the diagnosis. A leopard from SV Zoological Park, Tirupati was brought for postmortem examination. The carcass was dull, pale mucous membrane. On necropsy free blood and lemon sized blood clot was found in the abdominal cavity. Histologically, all the lymph nodes and spleen revealed broad sheets of lymphoblast and anaplastic changes and confirmed it to be a case of lymphosarcoma.

A survey was carried out at Zoological Park, Tirupati to estimate the case of tumors in wild felids and they reported tumors in lions, tigers and leopards. Tumors in different lions of different ages were reported to be as gastrointestinal adenocarcinoma, adenocarcinoma, hepatocarcinoma, fibrosarcoma, hemangiosarcoma, cholangiocellular carcinoma, chondrosarcoma, cavernous hemangioma, mesothelioma, lymphosarcoma, leiomyosarcoma, uterine adenocarcinoma, granulosa cell tumor, squamos cell carcinoma, fibrohemangio adenocarcinoma, cholangiocellular carcinoma. In tigers there were case of hemangiosarcoma, cholangiohepatocellular carcinoma and a case of lymphosarcoma in leopard.

Cholangiocellular carcinoma in a leopard was reported from Nagpur, the leopard was anorectic and emaciated and died later. On necropsy there was generalized icterus, multiple pea sized metastatic granule throughout the mesentery, lungs showed area of metastasis. A white tiger at VanVihar, Bhopal developed a growth on lower eyelid, the mass was excised and histology revealed it to be a Squamous cell carcinoma; however it reoccurred and the animal was put on chemotherapy but the Tiger died. On necropsy it was found that nodules of varying sized were present at lungs, spleen, liver, and pancreas.

Extra skeletal chondrosarcoma in a lion was reported from Tirupati, a growth was noticed on the lower side of the abdomen near the sternal area, cut section appeared grayish white in appearance and minimum blood loss. Proliferated pleomorphic cartilage cells with hyaline matrix were also seen. A leopard in Sanjay Gandhi National Park was died due to respiratory distress; on necropsy it was found that lungs were severely congested and consolidated. Uterus showed multiple nodules of varying sizes, and the nodules were hard to cut. Microscopically, uterus showed swirling pattern of smooth muscles in a circular fashion indicating a leiomyoma. In an another case of Leiomyoma from Anand on necropsy the leopard revealed hard consistency of liver and a lemon sized tumorous growth attached to the cornua of uterus and was firm. On histology growth revealed interlacing bundles of smooth muscles fibres confirming the case.

Mammary tumor in a Tiger was reported from Zoological Garden, Pune. Zoological Park Kanpur recorded a case of carcinoma of lung. Metastatic growth of bones at various regions was recorded in a tiger at Lucknow. Another report was from IVRI were a tiger was diagnosed with squamous cell carcinoma of lungs. Zoo record (1999-2000), from Zoological Garden, Kerla reported a case of adenocarcinoma of liver and squamous cell carcinoma in two lions. Lymphosarcoma in a clouded leopard was reported from Assam. Kanpur Zoo reported bone tumor in a leopard. Zoological Park Kanpur presented a case of squamous cell carcinoma in a leopard cat. A case of tumorous growth in eye of a leopard cat was mentioned in Zoological Garden, Thrissur. A golden cat from Biological Park, Orissa was diagnosed to have suffered from squamous cell carcinoma of lungs. Intestinal tumor in a Leopard from Zoological Garden, Kerla was also recorded.

Ursidae (bear family)

Zoological Garden, Kerela reported hemangioma of testes and squamos cell carcinoma of lips, gums in two blackbear and hemagioendothelioma of mesentery and organs in a sloth bear. Case of Adenocarcinoma of mammary gland andcholangiocellular carcinoma in a sloth bear was reported from Zoological Park, Delhi. Cholangiocellular carcinoma was reported in a sloth bear from Mannuthy, there was generalized icterus; subcutaneous tissue was dry and deep yellow. A case of Squamous cell carcinoma was reported in brown bear and fibrosarcoma of armpit and liposarcoma of vulvar lips in sloth bear from Zoological Garden, Kerla. Intestinal carcinoma in a sloth bear was reported from Zoological Park, Kanpur. Dachigam National Park, Kashmir, reported mixed hepatocellular and cholangiocarcinoma in a Himalayan brown bear, the animal showed progressive emaciation and respiratory distress and on necropsy revealed hepatomegally with yellowish white to grey nodular growth. A case of metastatic hepatocellular carcinoma in a Himalayan black bear was reported from MC Zoological Park Chhatbir Zoo, Punjab. On necropsy gross lesions were observed in liver, kidney, heart, lung and spleen, microscopically liver showed variable sized multiple tumorous foci surrounded by fibrous tissue stroma.

Death of male sloth bear was reported due to liver cancer at Zoological Park, Mysore. It had long standing recurring skin disease causing alopecia and itching around the ankle and elbow joints. Post-mortem examination showed cancer of liver virtually occupying whole liver parenchyma and metastasis to left kidney. Neoplastic metastatic lesion was reported in a Himalayan bear from Kanpur. Hepatic tumor in a Himalayan black bear was reported from Jharkhand. VanpraniUdyan, Bhopal reported a case of fibroma in mandible region in sloth bear.

Viveridaea

A bear cat was diagnosed to be affected from Adenocarcinoma in lymph node, lungs, liver, spleen, from Zoological Garden, Assam. Zoological Garden, Thrissur, reported case of intestinal tumor in a Palm civet. A civet in Delhi was diagnosed with alveolar cell carcinoma.

Canidaea

Zoological Garden, Gujarat reported cutaneous melanoma in a Jackal. A case of carcinoma of pancreas was reported in Civet. Ayurvedic medical centre, Thrissur, reported granulosa cell tumor in ovary of a civet. Adenocarcinoma of prostate gland in a Jackal was reported from Zoological Garden, West Bengal. Cauliflower like growth throughout the parenchyma was noticed, rounded, polyhedral cells were observed with hyperchromatic nucleus.

Primata

This order includes monkeys, langurs, orangutan, chimpanzee, gorilla, lemurs and marmoset. Frequency of tumor that was encountered was from reproductive system, digestive system, respiratory system. Adenocarcinoma of uterus was reported in Lion tailed Macaque. Fibroma of cervix in monkey reported from Zoological Garden, Assam. There has been report of seminoma, adenoma, adenocarcinoma in stomach of monkey from Zoological Garden, Assam. Golden langur in Zoological Park, Delhi was diagnosed with uterine tumor. There was a report of bronchiogenic carcinoma in monkey from Zoological Park, Kanpur. A case of Gastric carcinoma was reported from monkey in Zoological Garden, Tirupati. Lipoma from poll to ears in a rhesus monkey was presented from Zoological Garden, Madras. Some cases of neoplasms were mentioned in records of the zoos which include, A golden langur at Assam was diagnosed with uterine tumor another similar case was presented from Hyderabad. A case of intestinal tumor was recorded in a Bonnet Macaque from Kerala.

Proboscidea

This includes mammals having trunks, only one family Elephantidae which includes the Asiatic and the African elephants. Percentage of occurrence of tumor is less in elephants as compared to other animals. Elephants owe this nature of resistance for neoplasm to the multiple copies of gene Tp53 in them. They have 40 copies of this tumor suppressor gene as compared to only two copies in humans. However, there are some reports of neoplasm in elephants. A female Elephant from a private owner had a nodular growth under the thigh region from the last 8 years and has grown in size. Histopathological diagnosis confirmed it to be a fibrolipoma. A case of fibrosarcoma was reported in Elephant from biological park Orissa. Fibroma in trunk of Indian elephant was reported from Jabalpur. It started as a small firm growth which later increased in size. The growth was excised with electrosurgery, and confirmed histopathologically.

Perissodactyla

The order includes mammals having odd number of toes i.e., either one or three toes on each foot. The order includes family Rhinocerotidae, includes the One Horn Rhinoceros and Equidae family which includes Zebras, Wild Ass and Horses. There have been very few cases of tumors in rhinoceros and other wild animals of the family. Female Rhinoceros at Kolkata had a tumorous growth on the uterus of the animal, a hard tissue of around 2 kg was found attached to the uterus. Adenoma of stomach in a rhinoceros from zoological park Assam was reported. Squamous cell carcinoma of horn was reported in rhinoceros at zoological garden Kolkatta. A case of Squamous cell carcinoma was reported in lumbar region of a Rhinoceros from Zoological Garden, Mumbai.

Aves

Cases of neoplasm in birds are mostly reported from the one in zoological park or garden and less from the one living in the free range, therefore the cases are more commonly reported from the zoo record of various zoological parks and gardens. The class aves consist of many different orders and include: Galliformes (pheasants), Anseriformes (water fowls), Psittaciformes (parakeets), Gruiformes (crane) and many more.

Galliformes

Renal cell carcinoma in Lady Amherst pheasant was reported and necropsy revealed embedded margin of neoplastic growth. Neoplastic growth was bulged and fluid filled with blood incavity was present. A case of bronchiogenic carcinoma was recorded in pea fowls. Pulmonary neoplasm was reported in a pea hen with diffuse white encephaloid growth, finger like growth extending into lung parenchyma and another in a pin tail with growth confined in thoracic cavity, tumor surrounded the thyroid gland and classified to be carcinoid with adenopapillary pattern. Also a case of lymphoid leucosis in a Jungle fowl was also reported. A case of adenocarcinoma in a jungle grey fowl was recorded in Delhi.

In Zoological Garden, Mysore, death of female green pheasant due to cancer of the left ovary was reported. By post-mortem examination cancerous growth of the left ovary with adhesion to the visceral organs was notice. Case reports of Carcinoma of kidney in a green peafowl and carcinoma of kidney in silver pheasant. Papilloma in head region of a silver Chinese pheasant from West Bengal and papilloma of esophagus in a white peacock was reported from Bihar.

Anseriformes

Biological Park, Orissa reported cases of tumors in birds such as; Muscovy duck suffered from cholangiocellular carcinoma, mesothelioma, hemangioma, bronchiogenic carcinoma. Bronchiogenic carcinoma in a crested pochard and a case of mesothelioma in a comb duck, and a case of Aortic body tumor in a Brahmy duck was also reported from Biological Park, Orissa. Cutaneous capillary haemangioma was reported in a white Pekin duck from IVRI, CARI. The tumor was ulcerated and localized in the axilla of left hind limb. Histologically it was identified that the dermis was thickened and variable sized blood filled vascular lamina was seen; it was later confirmed to be a capillary hemangioma and considered rare. In a study of incidence and pathology of duck mortality in Assam a total of 1723 duck carcasses were collected and was studied and 7.48% cases of hepatic carcinoma was present, microscopically both hepatocellular and cholangiocellular carcinoma was observed. Tumor in abdomen of a spotbill duck was reported from Biological Park, Orissa. Zoological Park, Andhra Pradesh, recorded cases of carcinoma of liver in a teal and grey-leg goose. Zoological Garden, Assam recorded many such cases of neoplasms in avian species, papilloma of lung and tumor on abdomen of a goose was recorded. Liver tumor in a goose and uterine tumour in a Brahmy Duck was recorded. Liver cancer in a Common Teal and Zoological Garden and State Museum Kerla reported many cases of neoplasms which also included a case of lung tumor in a teal and a case of liver tumor was recorded in a Garganey.

Gruiformes

A sarus crane suffered from digestive disorders was diagnosed as hepatoma and mesothelioma of liver (Rao *et al.,* 1974). A moorhen was diagnosed with the intestinal tumour characterized by presence of anaplastic cells having pleomorphism, hyperchromasia, and presence of several mitotic figures (Zoo record, 2000-2001).

Phoenicopteriformes

A flamingo from zoological Garden, Lucknow reported hepatocarcinoma. Abdominal tumor in a flamingo was recorded from Zoological Garden, Gujarat.

Columbiformes

Pigeon from private owner at Jabalpur was diagnosed with hemangiopericytoma. It is a type of soft tissue sarcoma that originates in the pericytes in the wall of the capillaries. It is a meningeal tumor with special aggressive behavior, has a oval nuclei and a scant cytoplasm. There is a dense intercellular reticulin staining. Tumor cells can be pericytic, myxoid and fibroblastic. Hemangiopericytoma needs to be differentiated from benign hemangioma because of their high incidence of recurrence and metastases.

Psittaciformes

A case of pulmonary hemangioma was reported in a parrot from Madras Zoo. On Post mortem grayish white foci were seen in parenchyma of lungs distorted remnants of tertiary bronchi and proliferating parabronchial epithelium showing cellular pleomorphism was noticed. Internal papillomatosis with pancreatic ductular carcinoma was reported in a blue-winged macaw from Chennai. The bird had progressive deteriorative conditions. On necropsy cauliflower like warty growth was noticed in the glottis and the upper esophagus. A male lory was brought for necropsy with history of chronic wasting and sulfur colored droppings. Grossly, multifocal variable sized grey white area was seen on liver surface. Histopathology revealed cystic dilated bile ducts indicating cholangiocellular cyst adenoma. A case of Cancerous growth in intestine of a lover bird was reported from Zoological Garden, Mumbai also a case of tumor of ovary in a love bird was recorded. In Delhi, papilloma in a parrot was reported.

Pelecaniformes

An adult male heron from Guindly National Park, Chennai was presented for necropsy. It was dehydrated carcass and pale mucous membranes. It was observed that the liver was enlarged and friable. Kidneys were grey brown to tan in colour and with diffuse white areas. There were roundworms in the intestine. Histopathology revealed variable sized nodules around blood vessels and neoplastic lymphocytes. A case of lung tumor was observed in an Ibis white.

Reptilia

The class reptilian consists of many different orders comprising of various animals which includes squamta (snakes, lizards) testudine (turtles, tortoise) crocodilian (crocodiles). Most often the cases of neoplasm are encountered in snakes and few reports from other orders is recorded, and the occurrence of neoplasm is as follows.

Squamata

A cobra at Zoological Garden, Kerla suffered from nephroma. Monitor lizard one from Mini Zoo, Kerla was diagnosed with adenocarcinoma of liver and other from zoological park, Delhi was diagnosed with squamous cell carcinoma in legs. A monitor lizard from Herpetology crocodile bank was reported with reticular cell sarcoma of buccal commissure. Adenocarcinoma in liver was reported a monitor lizard from Mini Zoo, Kerla. squamous cell carcinoma in kidney of a python from Zoological Garden, Lucknow. Duvernoy's (Parotid) gland adenoma was reported in Indian Water snake. Snake rescue team Nagpur presented a water snake with hemorrhagic swelling at mouth part. When it was incised revealed multilobular structure, histopathologically there was tubuloacinar structure lined by single or multilayered epithelium. An interesting case of Thyroid adenoma and intestinal leiomyoma was reported from a dead water monitor. A sample of thyroid and intestine was sent from Chennai Snake Park Trust. Thyroid revealed cells of variable sizes containing proteinaceous material. Intestinal nodular growth was seen in the muscular layer of the intestine, the cells had a homogenous population of smooth muscle cells. Zoological Garden, Kerla reported cases of tumor in wild reptiles including kidney tumor in a monitor lizard and intestinal tumor in a rat snake.

Testudines

Hematoma in capture sea turtle was reported from CFMRI regional centre, Mandapam, a female marine loggerhead turtle had an abnormal swelling on dorsal side of neck and had little inclination to swim.

Rodentia

There have been reports of tumor in Porcupine and Squirrels too, though a very few cases have been reported. Zoological Garden, Kerla reported carcinoma of mammary gland and malignant mesothelioma in a porcupine).

Diagnosis

The case of neoplasm is not identified in wild animals until and unless it enlarges in size and causes problems either in locomotion or in sight of animals and sometimes may include anorexia and behavioral changes. Finding a tumor in wild animals or captive animals is a chance event during post mortem procedures as sometimes they are present but produces no signs and symptoms and go unnoticed. Diagnosis can be made upon clinical examination of the animal whether swelling is present, difficulty in locomotion and / or anorexia. As neoplasms in wild animals are commonly noticed in post mortem a cautious examination of the carcass should be done. Confirmation of the neoplastic condition can only be done on histopathological examination.

Public Health and Safety

Several studies suggest that animal viruses are known to cause cancer; the etiologic role of these exposures in human cancer remains speculative. Animal oncoviruses generally are species specific and do not infect or replicate easily in humans. Epidemiologic studies to date have provided little evidence that animal viruses cause human cancer. The infectious agent may present and react differently depending on a host of factors including geography, seasonal variation and climate, population density, and herd immunity. Animal harbor many of the oncogene and some of them which are most studied includes rodent (Abl, Int1/Wnt1, Int2, Notch1, Pim1/2, Runx, Tpl2), fowl (Erb-b, Fos, Myc, Src), feline (Myc), and fish (cyc). However, some animal viruses have been found experimentally to replicate in *in-vitro* human cells. Furthermore, the use of potentially carcinogenic disinfectant agents or cleaning compounds must be taken into account as related etiologic exposures that might partially or fully explain a positive association between their exposures and cancer in wild and zoo animals. There is no such evidence of occurrence of neoplasm from animals to humans, certainly there are other occupational risk associated with handling of captive and wild animals which includes bite, scratches, allergies and other hazard related with the protocol and general safety; so a due care must be taken whenever approaching a wild animal, as these may not directly serve as a source of transmission of neoplasm but they might surely act as reservoir for other zoonotic diseases.

Neoplasms in laboratory animals

Animal studies are helpful to understand the complexities of the fundamental processes involved in tumourigenesis in humans and animals. Researchers use animals to study neoplasms for a variety of reasons including their shorter lifespan, more rapid generation times as compared to humans. Disease progression is faster hence quick results can be achieved using them. Every animal cannot serve as a laboratory animals and the selection of the animals is based on criteria including: size, availability, species and sensitivity (https://www.scribd.com). Conducting cancer studies in all animals in the clinical setting is challenging and less controllable in terms of outlaying variables hence few specific laboratory animals are used more frequently than others as rats, mice and rabbits. In these animals, tumours are induced to form via direct exposure to known carcinogen or they are bred to harbor specific genetic mutations leading to susceptibility for tumour development. Preclinical cancer studies including spontaneous origin of tumours or induction in hosts can be conducted in these laboratory animals. Most of the cancer studies use chemically induced tumours or may use transgenic models. Research areas where these animals have been used include hypertension, cardiac surgery, infectious diseases, metabolic disorders, ophthalmology, delayed hypersensitivity, immune responses, and anaphylactic shock. Commonly used in research related to toxicity, cancers, genetics, immunology and nutrition. Murine models are used more frequently than others. These are easily available and have simpler genetics further genetically identical mice simplifies studies by minimizing the confusions which arise in experiments on mixed populations.

As these animals are used as models for various studies their health status should be constantly monitored as there have been many reports of neoplasms in laboratory animals due to toxicity of chemicals which are used in day to day human life. Laboratory animal's model particularly the murine model of mammary cancer provided better understanding into alterations of molecular mechanisms that lead to cancer. These models are used to explore the factors involved in tumourigenesis, malignant transformation, invasion and metastasis and to examine the response to treatment. The reports on incidence of spontaneously occurring tumours in laboratory animals are few probably because these animals have a short life span to collect data on tumour occurrences. The available reports on the incidence of occurrence of neoplasms in laboratory animals are as follows.

Rabbit

Hepatocellular tumours are uncommon in laboratory animals except some strains of mice. A case of granulose cell tumor of ovary in rabbit was reported. A female rabbit around 2.5 years of age was culled from its breeding stock for biological experiments. On palpation a large mass in the abdominal cavity was felt. On postmortem examination the body was devoid of subcutaneous fat and had a circumscribed growth in left ovary and completely filled the abdominal cavity. Histologically, growth was well encapsulated from which strands of coarsely vascularized connective tissue entered substance of neoplasm. Neoplastic cells were elongated, irregular, hyperchromatic and resembled undifferentiated cells of ovarian mesenchymal cells.

A case of lymphosarcoma in rabbit was reported from Division of Fur Animal Breeding, (CSWRI) Garsa (H.P.). Eight cases showing the lesions of lymphosarcoma were observed. Among these rabbits 7 were of Angora breed (3 males, 4 females) and one grey giant female rabbit. No genetic correlation was found since no such occurrence was seen in their sire lines. Grossly, enlarged liver, spleen and kidneys were observed. Kidneys were discolored and showed raised areas below the capsules affecting usually the cortex. Mesenteric lymph nodes were enlarged and edematous, cranial cavity also revealed varying degree of meningo-encephalitis. Microscopically, mesenteric lymph node showed infiltration of malignant lymphoblasts, kidney also showed massive infiltration of interstitium by neoplastic histiocytes, lymphoblasts.

A rare case of hepatocellular carcinoma in an Angora rabbit was reported. It was also found to be metastasized to lungs. On postmortem examination, a cauliflower like grayish colored growth was seen on the liver and multiple grey coloured nodules of various sizes were seen in lungs. On histopathological examination, anaplastic cells were revealed in liver. Pleomorphic cells were found along with mitotic figures. In lungs, multinucleated giant cells were seen in neoplastic tissue. Vacuolations was found in some cells. Hepatocellular carcinoma was reported in a two and half years old male New Zealand white rabbit. On the cut section of liver, multifocal yellowish growths was noticed. In lungs also whitish nodules were observed. On histopathological examination of liver, anisokaryosis was revealed in nucleus of neoplastic cells along with presence of multiple nucleoli. In lungs, neoplastic mass was encapsulated with thin layer of fibrous tissue.

Hepatocellular carcinoma was observed in a 2 years and 10 months old white giant rabbit. Nodules were observed in liver lacking encapsulation. Pleiomorphic cells were observed, some cells contained multiple nucleus, in few areas, cells appeared as syncytial mass. Intrahepatic metastases were also observed. In lungs, neoplastic cells were embedded in parenchyma. Cytoplasm of neoplastic cells contained coarse granular eosinophilic material. Few mitotic figures were present.

Adenocarcinoma of uterus is one of the most common tumors in rabbits. Metastatic uterine adenocarcinoma was found in a five years old female Angora rabbit. At necropsy multiple ovoid, cauliflower – like tumors mass were seen on uterine horns. Histopathogically, there was haphazard proliferation of anaplastic cells. Neoplastic cells formed loose sheets and at some places were cystic in appearance. Mitotic figures were frequent. It was suggested as mixed, papillary – tubular adenocarcinoma. It produced metastasis into lung parenchyma and intestinal serosa. In another case of tumor in rabbit, a female rabbit was operated for mammary tumor. Tumor was characterized by multilayering of mammary acini with disorder in the layer. No evidence of capsular invasion or metastasis and the basement membrane was intact. A case of bronchogenic adenocarcinoma of lung with pulmonary metastasis was reported in a two years old female rabbit. At post- mortem examination, multiple grey- white nodules in lungs were observed. Cytology of impression smears from lungs and pre- scapular lymph node showed anisocytosis, anisokaryosis, vacuolations and hyperchromasia in epithelial cells. The metastatic foci depicting acini of alveolar epithelial cells replacing the lymphoid tissue were observed in the tissue sections of the pre-scapular lymph node.

Nephroblastoma (embryonal nephroma) was observed in a male German Angora rabbit. In rat mammary gland tumors were induced byadministration of N-methyl N-Nitroso Urea to study the environmental effect on induction of tumour and the histopathological changes in the induced tumour. The expression pattern of tumour marker-PCNA was also studied. Rabbits are induced ovulators and are in estrus much of the times; the persistent estrogenic stimulus may be the cause for development of ovarian tumors in rabbits. A case of spontaneous occurrence of luteoma and uterine adenocarcinoma in the reproductive tract of a two and half years old Dutch breed rabbit was observed.

Rat and Mice

A case of spontaneous lymphoid leukemia was reported from IVRI in mice. Generally, the natural incidences of such cases are very low. Families of such mice with relatively increased incidence of disease have been developed by selective inbreeding. In the albino mice gross lesions were noticed and processed. In the study of 3553 mice, 12 mice of which 5 were males and 7 females were autopsied during 1972 and 1973 and revealed changes related with leukemia.

Grossly both the lobes of the thymus were enlarged and filled the thoracic cavity. Spleen, liver, kidney, heart were enlarged with grayish white nodules. Lungs and kidney revealed reticular cell hyperplasia. Of the 12 positive cases of the leukemia, 7 showed localized thymic lymphosarcoma and 5 cases showed disseminated lymphosarcoma manifesting multiple lymphosarcomas in thymus, spleen, liver, lungs, heart and kidney.

A case of fibroma in a white mouse was recorded. The mouse had a lump on right ventrolateral aspect of body extending from fore to hind limb. The case was surgically treated and the tumor mass was extirpated. Histopathology of the mass was done to confirm the diagnosis. The tissue was replaced by fibro collagenous tissue and was suggestive of intermuscular fibroma. A chronic study was conducted in a group of rats over a period of 165 days to assess the effect of carbon tetrachloride. The rats were divided in a group of 4 depending upon the treatment received. The experiment revealed presence of preneoplastic and neoplastic conditions in the liver of the rats. A case of fibroma in white mouse was reported from Udgir district Maharashtra. Grossly, a large subcutaneous lump was noticed on left ventrolateral aspect of the neck region. The mass was grayish red in color and firm and weighed around 150 gm. Histopathology was conducted and revealed collagen fibres and abundant fibroblasts. A case of tumor in a mouse was reported from Small animal facility, National Institute of Immunology, New Delhi. The 1 ½ year old female BALB/C mouse revealed solid movable mass on the right side. FNAC was conducted and later the mass was removed along with the entire left ovary. FNAC showed erythrocytes with few PMNC's stromal cells, hematogenous cells, epithelial cells and fibroblasts, polyhedral cells were noticed. A case of sweat gland adenocarcinoma was reported in a Sprague Dawley rat. It is a rare condition in case of rats with high incidence of metastasis. The affected rat showed swelling in the abdominal region, was oval and firm. Tumor was lobulated reddish brown with tendency of bleeding. Histopathologically, variable sized acinar structures lined by single to multilayer cuboidal cells and heaping of neoplastic epithelial cells.

A case of follicular cell adenoma and C-cell carcinoma was observed in a male aged Wistar rat. The animal appeared normal and was devoid of any gross lesion. Necropsy revealed enlargement of the thyroid gland. Right lobe was larger than the left lobe. Right lobe revealed varying sized follicles. Some of the follicles were smaller, some were larger, irregular. Colloid in these follicles was more basophilic. C cells showed marked anaplasia. A case report of cavernous hemangioma in liver of a Wistar rat was recorded. The abdominal cavity of the rat was enlarged. Grossly it was reddish brown in color. Histopathology revealed large blood filled spaces communicating each other, vacuolar degeneration of hepatocytes. Histiocytic sarcoma in spleen of a Wistar rat was reported from Gujarat. Histiocytic sarcoma is an uncommon tumor in case of rats. On necropsy pea size fleshy soft mass was observed. Histopathologically, the mass was incompletely encapsulated by thin fibrous capsule. Two cases of spontaneous cutaneous hemangiosarcoma in Swiss mice were reported. A study was conducted to assess the complete picture of pathomorphological and biological behavior of gastric squamous cell carcinoma in terms of their typing, grading, multi-nodularity. Further their correlation with AgNOR count to revalidate the ability of this count in assessing the proliferative aggressiveness of NMU induced gastric squamous cell carcinoma in rats was also studied.

Renal mesenchymal tumor in rat is also known as stromal nephroma, interstitial cell tumor of kidney, mixed malignant tumor of kidney and malignant mesenchymal cell tumor. It is a tumor of nonepithelial origin and spontaneous cases are rare. Immunohistochemistry and histopathology of renal mesenchymal tumour in a 15 week old male Wistar rat were studied. A case of scirrhous carcinoma of the mammary gland was reported in rat and its metastasis was seen in to the lungs. Scirrhous carcinoma is essentially an adenocarcinoma that stimulates the formation of abundant collagen in the surrounding connective tissue. Histopathology was done to confirm the diagnosis. A case of deciduoma in female Wistar rats was reported from Gujarat. Bilateral deciduoma is a proliferative reaction that mimics the decidual implantation site in a non-gravid uterus. A female rat with mass on thoracic region was diagnosed with mammary tumor. The tumors are generally fibroadenoma and occur after rats stop ovulating. Clinically in this case swelling of the left thoracic mammary gland was noticed.

The development of skin cancer in rodents on topical exposure to chemical carcinogens has been widely used to define the stages of carcinogenesis. Dermal application of dimethylbenzanthracine (DMBA) fortnightly over the hind back of Wister rats could cause skin–papilloma, papillary carcinoma and squamous cell carcinoma with metastasis in lungs, sebaceous gland carcinoma, sweat gland adenocarcinoma and connective tissue tumors such as fibrosarcoma, hemangiopericytoma, dermal neuro-fibroma were encountered. A case of mammary adenocarcinoma in a 12 week old female Wistar rat was reported. Pathology of LA7 cell induced tumors was studied in 50 female Sprague Dawley rats of about 30 days of age. Zymbal's gland or auditory sebaceous gland is located anteroventral to the external auditory meatus. A case of zymbal gland carcinoma with complication of leukemia was reported. A three year old female rat was presented in madras veterinary college with the history of progressive swelling on the ventral abdomen since 6 months. On examination the growth was hard and extended from xiphoid to inguinal region. Histopathology confirmed the mass to be a fibroadenoma.

Hamsters

An experiment was conducted to know the protective effect of withaferin A on tumor formation in 7,12-dimethylbenzaanthracene induced oral carcinogenesis in Syrian golden hamsters. The animal was assessed for the presence of tumor in the animal. The animals that were administered with dimethylbenzanthracine alone showed 100 percent incidence of tumor. A study was conducted on preliminary antitumor peptide therapy in bovine papilloma induced virus experiments taking hamsters as modal animal. The experiment was conducted to assess the effect of anti tumour WCS peptide in BPV 1 and 2 virus induced hamster dermal fibroma. Gross and microscopic lesions in the early peptide treatment showed that the growth was arrested while in the well grown tumors the effect was not much appreciable. In a study of cancer in hamster as a model animal, betel quid ingredients were tested separately and in various combinations for carcinogenicity using hamster cheek as the experimental site. Untreated controls and standard carcinogen DMBA treated controls were also maintained. A total of 317 golden hamsters were used for the experiments. They were killed in 2 groups 6-12 month age and another of 13-24 months age. Untreated controlled animals were free of malignancy. In the test animals various betel quid ingredient were under test and induced both oral and gastric lesions ranging from massive atypia and precancerous lesions to frank carcinomas.

Guinea pig

In general, neoplastic conditions are extremely rare in guinea pigs. A case of granulosa cell tumour was reported in a guinea pig. Histopathologically, cells had scanty cytoplasm. The nucleus was vesicular and hyperchromatic. Ovarian tumours are rare in Guinea pigs. Malignant ovarian teratoma was found in an aged Guinea pig. On post- mortem examination, enlarged large ovary was found. Histologically, in ovary replacement of normal tissue by embryonic neurogenic tissue was observed.

12

Necropsy

- General Consideration
- Post-mortem examination of large animals
- Post-mortem examination of poultry
- Steps in post-mortem examination
- Writing of post-mortem report
- Collection, preservation and dispatch of specimens for laboratory diagnosis

General Consideration

Necropsy is examination of animal after death also known as post mortem examination. It helps in diagnosis of diseases and their control. It is said that ***"Necropsy is a message of wisdom from dead to living"***. Necropsy include systemic examination of dead animal, recording of pathological lesions, their interpretation to make diagnosis of disease. Sometimes it is difficult to arrive any conclusion merely based on gross examination of dead animal. Then one should seek the help of laboratory examinations such as Histopathology, Microbiology, Immunology and Toxicology for confirmation.

Necropsy examination is an integral part of disease investigation. Therefore, veterinarian must have the knowledge of the techniques of post-mortem examination, recording of lesions, collection of proper material for laboratory and most importantly their correlation to arrive at conclusive diagnosis. The technique of post-mortem examination is as under:

Post-mortem examination of large animal

- Place animal on left side (Ruminants) (Fig. 12.1).

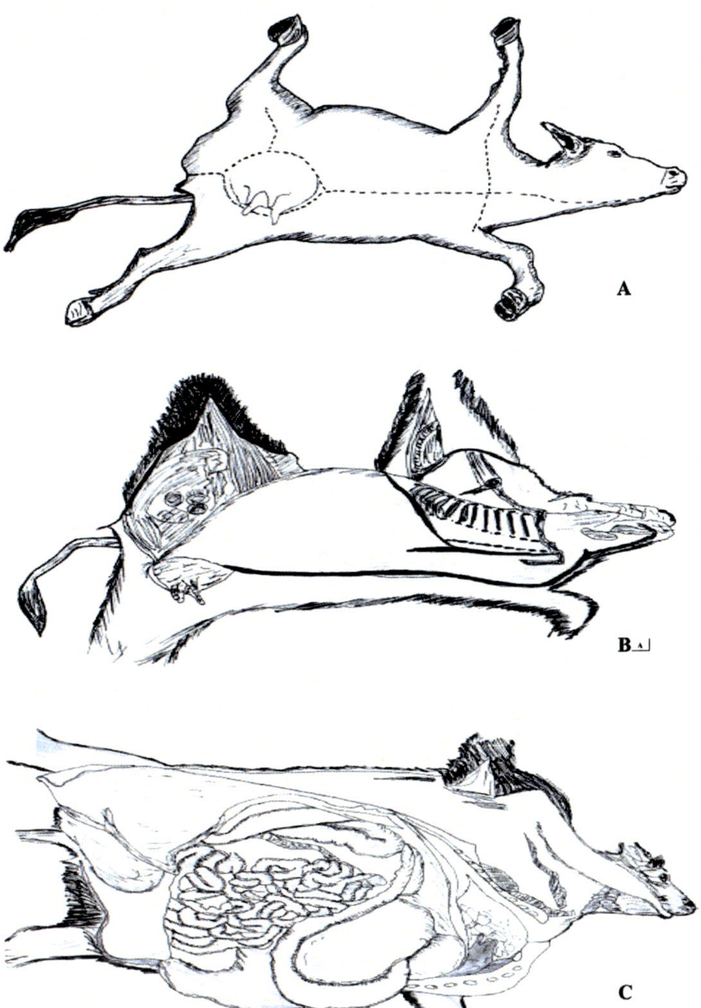

Fig. 12.1: Diagram showing post-mortem examination of ruminant **(A)** position of cow and the marking for incision **(B)** after removal of skin and **(C)** after exposure of abdominal cavity

- Place horse on right side and dog on vertebral column (Figs. 12.2 & 12.3).

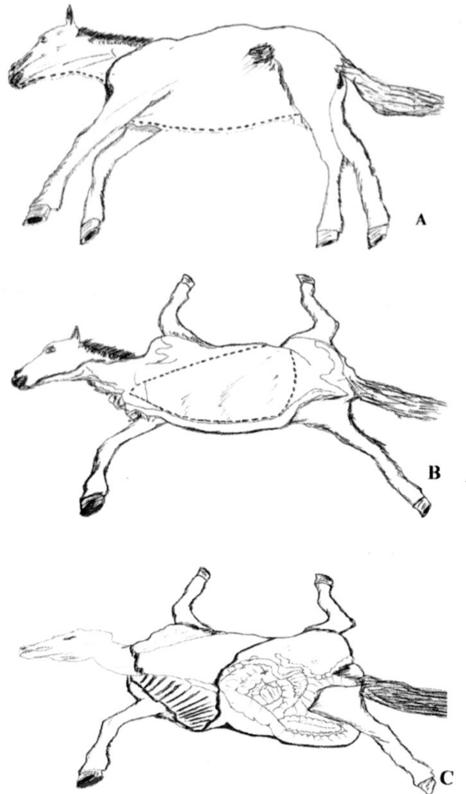

Fig. 12.2: Diagram showing post-mortem examination of horse **(A)** position of horse and marking for incision **(B)** after removal of skin and **(C)** after exposure of abdominal cavity

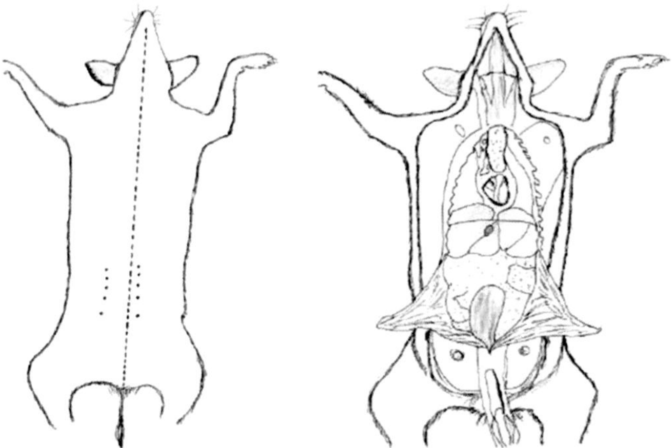

Fig. 12.3: Post mortem examination of dog **(A)** Incision and exposure of abdominal cavity

- Make midventral incision with knife from chin to anus.
- Surround the prepuce, scrotum/mammary gland.
- Remove skin dorsoventrally. Remove skin at face, neck, thorax and abdomen.
- Cut the muscles and fascia in between scapula and body; remove fore legs.
- Raise hind legs, cut the coxo femoral ligament.
- Examine s/c tissue, muscles, superficial lymph nodes- pre scapular, pre femoral supra mammary, etc.
- Open abdominal cavity by cutting muscles and peritoneum
- Open thoracic cavity by cutting xiphoid cartilage at sternum; lift ribs and press them to break at joints with vertebral column.
- Examine the visceral organs in both cavities:

Thorax : Heart, Lungs, Trachea, Oesophagus, Mediastinal lymph nodes, Diaphragm

Abdominal cavity:

Ruminants : Rumen, Reticulum, Omasum, Abomasum

Other animals : Stomach

In all animals : Liver, Pancreas, Intestines, Mesenteric lymph nodes, Spleen, Kidneys, Ureter

Pelvic cavity : Urinary bladder, uterus

Post-mortem examination (poultry, fig. 12.4 to 12.22)

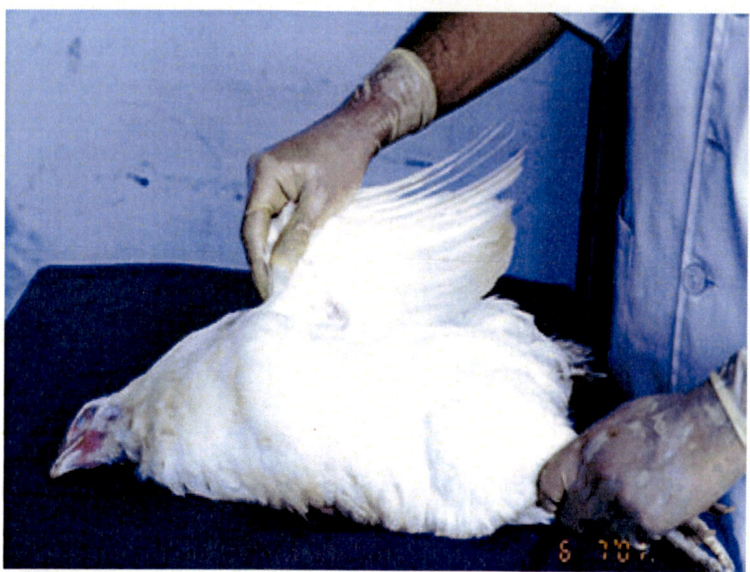

Fig. 12.4: Post mortem examination of poultry- External examination

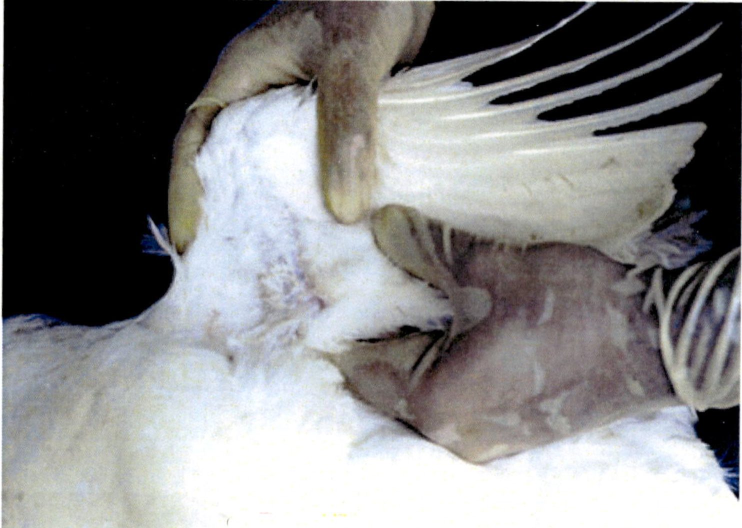

Fig. 12.5: Post mortem examination of poultry- External examination

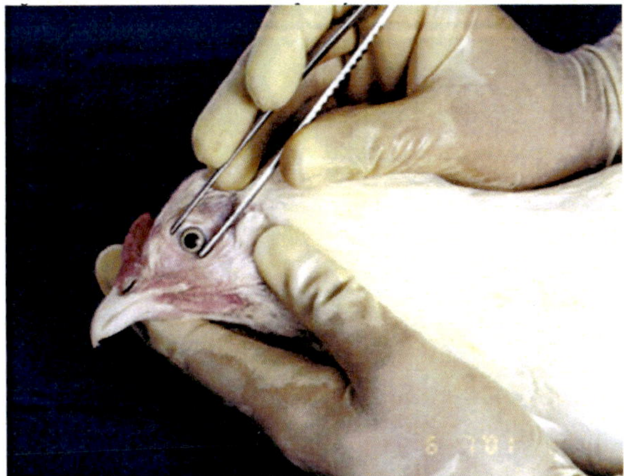

Fig. 12.6: Post mortem examination of poultry- Examination of eye

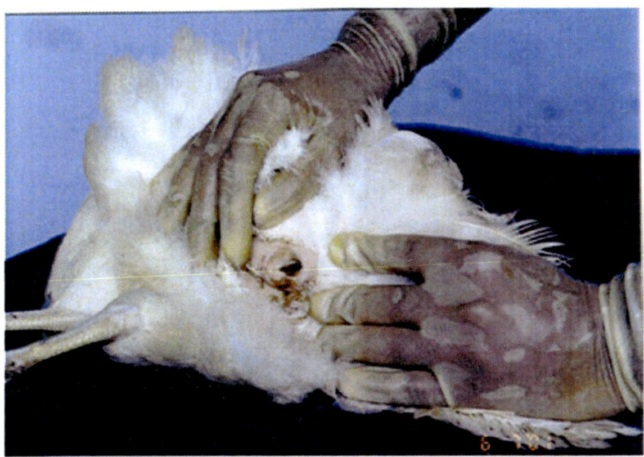

Fig. 12.7: Post mortem examination of poultry- Examination of vent

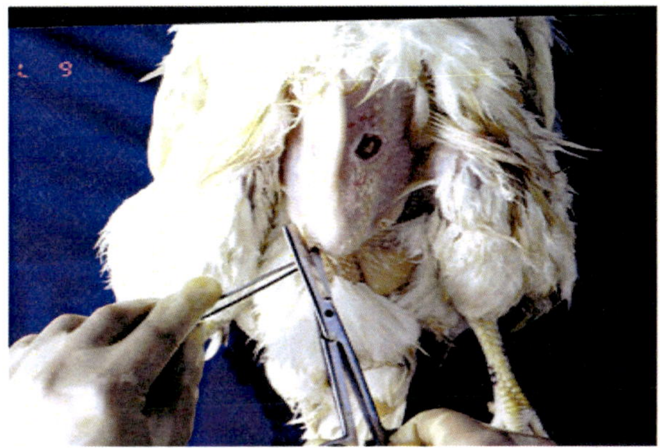

Fig. 12.8: Post mortem examination of poultry- Removal of skin

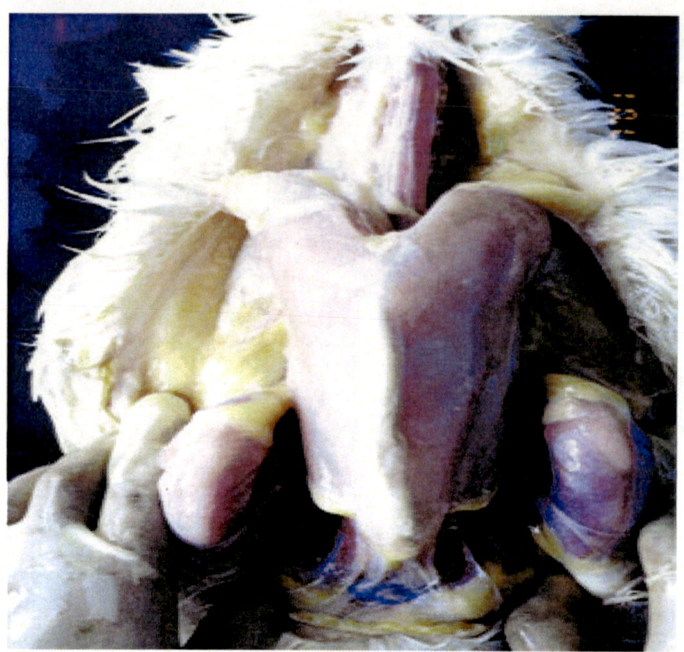

Fig. 12.9: Post mortem examination of poultry- Coxo-femoral joint break

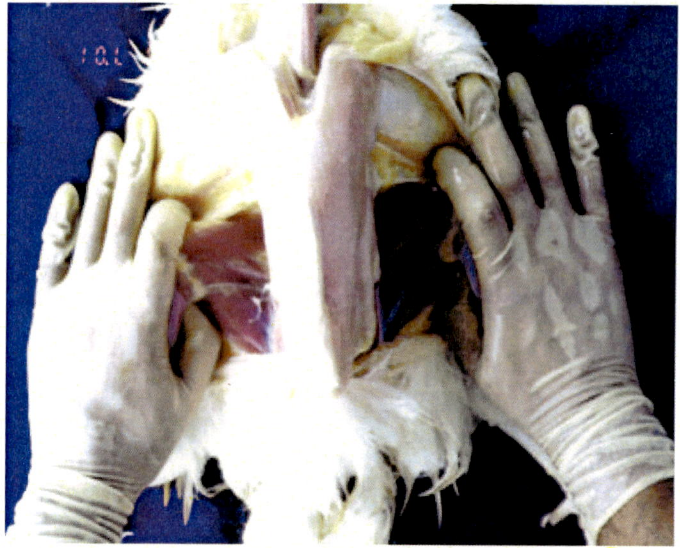

Fig. 12.10: Post mortem examination of poultry- Exposure of muscles for examination

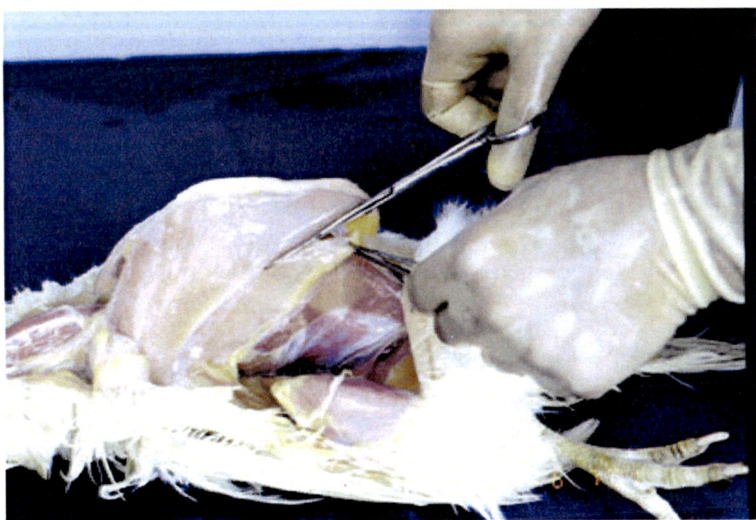

Fig. 12.11: Post mortem examination of poultry- Removal of breast muscles

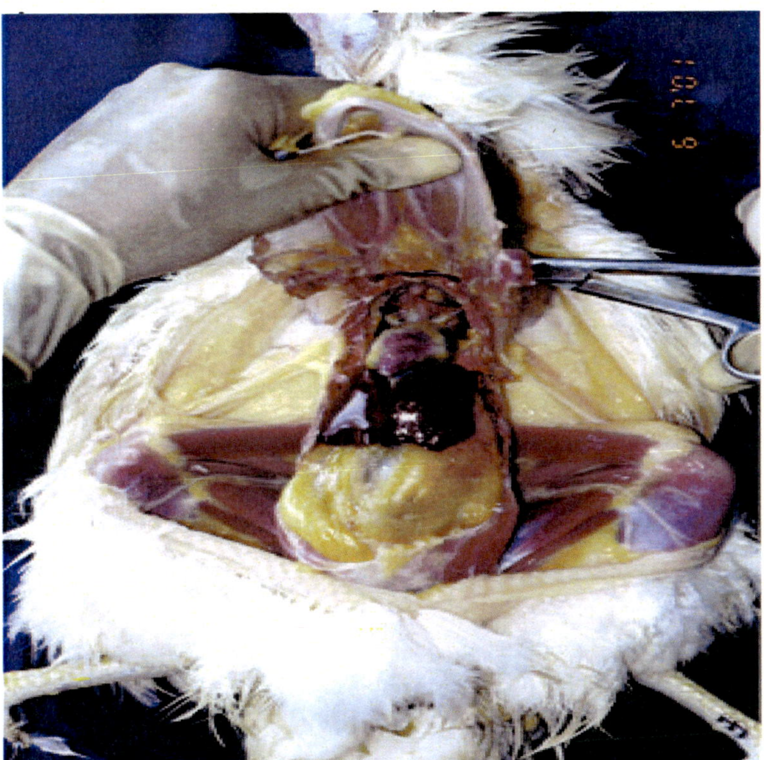

Fig. 12.12: Post mortem examination of poultry- Cutting of neck bones

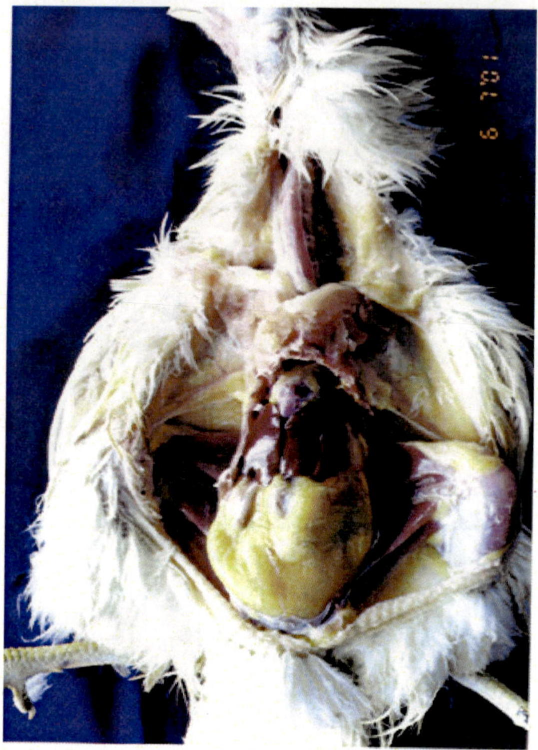

Fig. 12.13: Post mortem examination of poultry- Exposure of internal organs

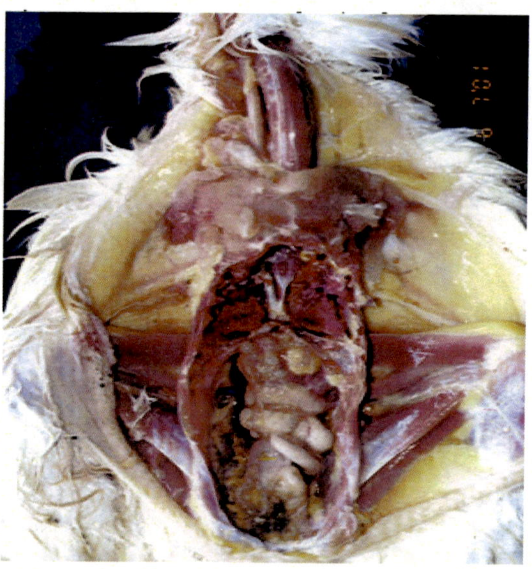

Fig. 12.14: Post mortem examination of poultry- Exposure of kidneys, ovary, oviduct after removal of digestive tract

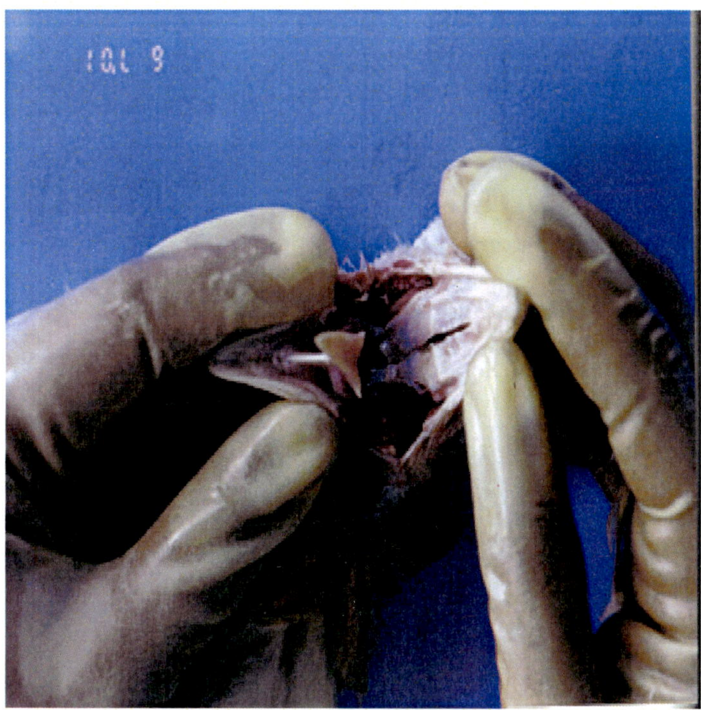

Fig. 12.15: Post mortem examination of poultry-Examination of mouth cavity

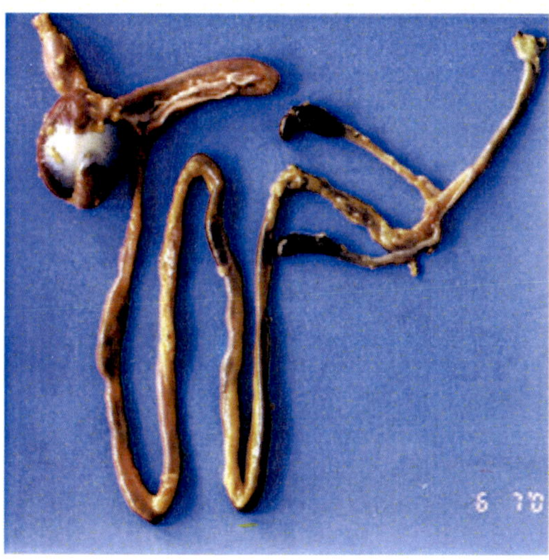

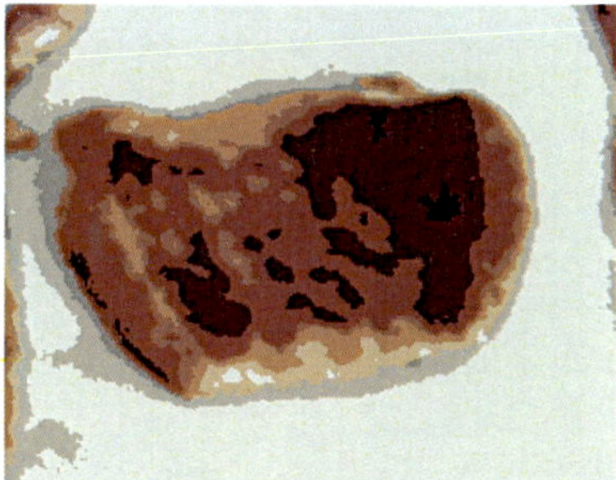

Fig. 12.16: Post mortem examination of poultry- Examination of intestine, caecum, proventriculous

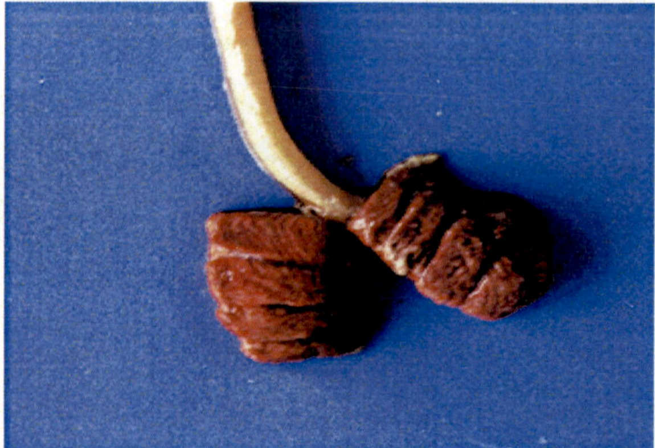

Fig. 12.17: Post mortem examination of poultry- Examination of lungs, trachea and bronchi

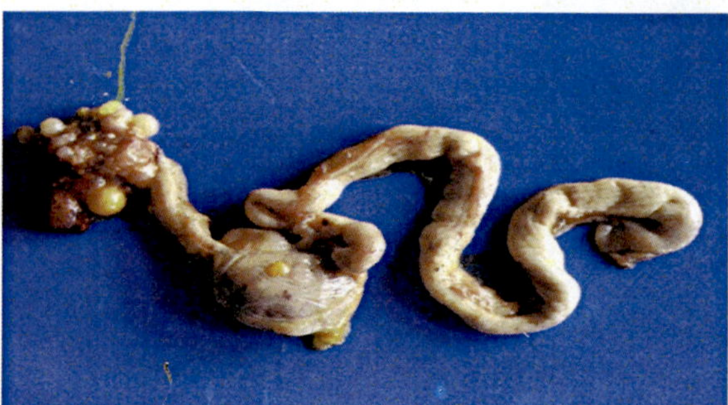

Fig. 12.18 Post mortem examination of poultry- Examination of female reproductive tract

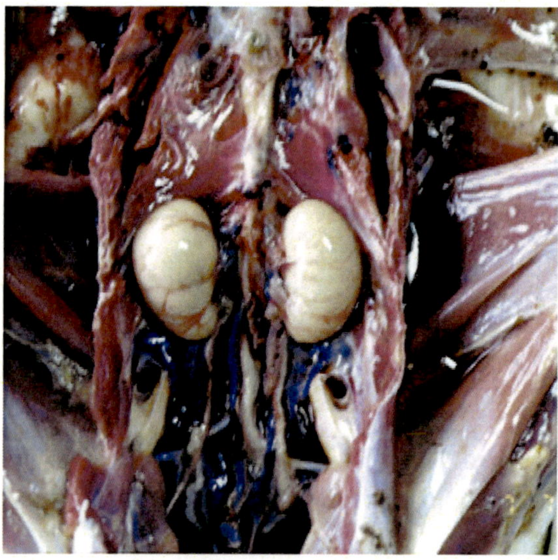

Fig. 13.19: Post mortem examination of poultry- Examination of testes

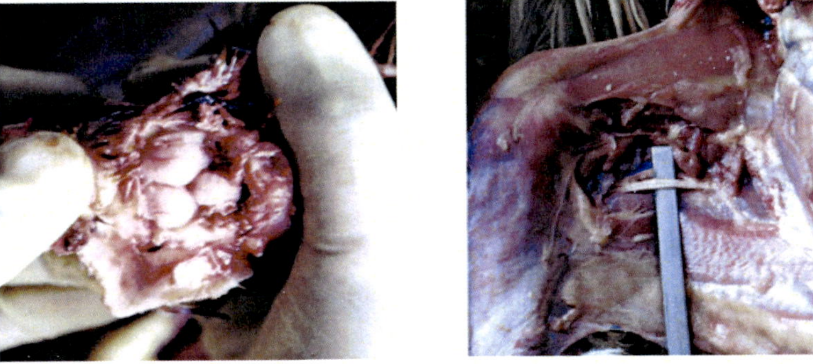

Fig. 12.20: Post mortem examination of poultry- Examination of nervous system

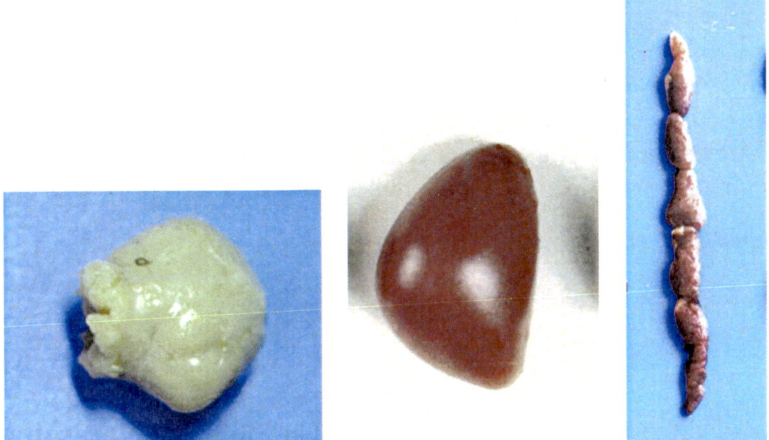

Fig. 12.21: Post mortem examination of poultry- Examination of immune system

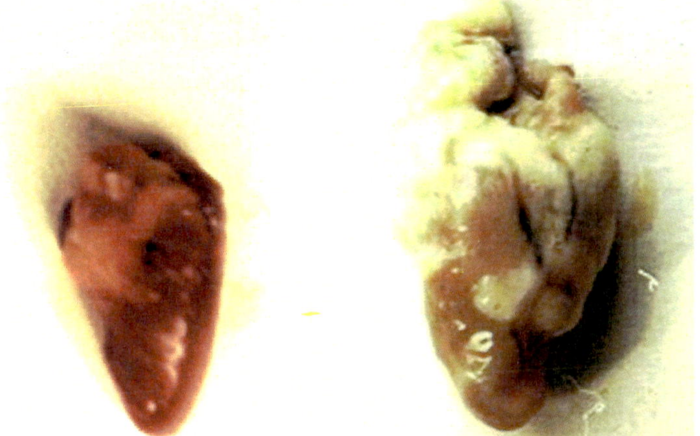

Fig.12.22: Post mortem examination of poultry- Examination of Heart

- Dip the dead bird in antiseptic solution or in water; to avoid feather contamination.
- Keep the bird on post-mortem table at vertebral column and look for any lesion or parasite on skin.
- Examine the eyes, face and vent.
- Remove skin through a cut with knife and with the help of fingers. Expose thymus, trachea, esophagus in neck.
- Break the coxofemoral joint by lifting the legs. Examine the chest and thigh muscles.
- Cut on lateral side of chest muscles. Lift the chest muscle dorsally and break bones at joints with thorax. Cut bones at both sides and remove muscles, bones to expose thorax, abdomen.
- Examine different organs.
- Cut proventriculus and pull the organs of digestive tract out. Separate liver, spleen, intestines, caecum, proventriculus, gizzard, etc.
- Expose bursa just beneath the cloaca.
- Cut beak at joint, examine mouth cavity and expose esophagus and trachea.
- Remove skin of head and make a square cut on skull to expose brain.
- Take a forceps and place in between thigh muscles, remove fascia and expose the sciatic nerve.
- Separate each organ, examine them for the presence of lesion.

Steps in post-mortem examination

Post-mortem examination should be conducted only after receiving of a formal request from the owner of animal having details of anamnesis and date and time of death. Without formal written request, one should not do post-mortem examination of animal. The post-mortem record includes the aspects of animal identification, illness, therapeutic and preventive measures adopted and date and time of death. This information provided by the owner or person requesting post-mortem, which helps in post-mortem examination and recording of lesions to make a conclusive diagnosis.

Various steps in post-mortem examination are as under:

1. External examination

Animal should be examined externally before opening the body for the presence of lesions on body surface. Eyes, ear, anus, vulva, mouth, nares etc. should be specifically examined for the presence of blood and any other lesion. If the blood is coming out from natural orifices, it should be examined for the presence of anthrax bacilli and such carcasses must not be opened for post-mortem examination. Following points should be taken into consideration while conducting external examination.

- Trauma, wound, fracture, cuts, etc.
- Fungal infection *e.g.* ringworm
- Parasitic infestation *e.g.* mange, lice, ticks
- Side of animal is lying down on earth.
- Discharges from openings.
- Burn, ulcers, erosions etc.

2. Subcutaneous tissue and musculature

Examine the subcutaneous tissue and musculature after removal of skin for the presence of lesions such as:

- Congestion, hemorrhage, oedema, nodule, anemia, icterus.
- Fat deposits
- Necrosis on muscles, hardening, calcification.

3. Abdominal and thoracic cavity

Just after opening the carcass, one should observe the presence of any lesion in abdominal and thoracic cavity and following points must be kept in mind.

- Accumulation of fluid (serus, serosanguinous, blood, pus etc.)
- Fibrinous or fibrous adhesions.
- Parasites
- Abscess, tumor etc.

4. Respiratory system

Organs/tissues to be examined

External nares, nasal passage, larynx, trachea, bronchi, lungs, air sacs (poultry) mediastinal lymph nodes.

Lesions to be observed

- Discharge from external nares.
- Growth (granuloma/polyp) in nasal passage if there is blood mixed nasal discharge.
- *Trachea and Bronchi*- Congestion, hemorrhage, presence of caseous exudate, frothy exudate etc.
- *Lungs*- Congestion, consolidation, nodules, presence of exudate on cut surfaces, oedema, atelectasis, emphysema, hemorrhage, necrosis.
- *Mediastinal lymph nodes*- Oedema, hardening, calcification, congestion, hemorrhage.

5. Cardiovascular system

Organs/tissues to be examined

Heart, aorta, arteries, veins and lymphatics

Lesions to be observed

- Fluid, blood, pus etc. in pericardial sac
- Adhesions, fibrin, fibrosis
- Congestion, hemorrhage, necrotic foci
- Hardening of blood vessel, obstruction, thrombi
- Presence of parasites
- Post-mortem clot/thrombi.

6. Digestive system

Organs/tissue to be examined

Mouth cavity, esophagus, crop, proventriculus, gizzard (poultry), rumen reticulum, omasum, abomasum (ruminants), stomach, intestine (duodenum, jejunum, ileum, caecum, colon, rectum), cloaca, vent (poultry), anus, liver, pancreas, gall bladder, mesenteric lymph nodes etc.

Lesions to be observed

- Erosions, ulcers, vesicles
- Congestion, hemorrhage, oedema

- Necrosis
- Icterus
- Abscess/pus
- Perforation, needles or hard objects in reticulum.
- Intussusception, torsion, volvulus
- Parasites
- Atrophy, hardening, nodules
- Contents, catarrhal, blood mixed, digested/ undigested feed material, thickening of wall of intestines.
- Cut surface of liver for parasites, lesions in bile duct.

7. Cardiovascular system

Organs/tissue to be examined

- Kidneys, ureter, urinary bladder, urethra

Lesions to be observed

- Congestion, hemorrhage, infarction, oedema.
- Necrosis, hardening, nodules
- Deposition of salts, calculi
- Obstruction

8. Genital system

Organs/tissue (female)

- Ovaries, oviduct, uterus, cervix, vagina

Male

- Testicles, Epididymis, penis, prepuce

Lesions to be observed

- Cysts in ovary
- Congestion, hemorrhage, oedema
- Foetus in uterus, pus, fluid

- Necrosis, overgrowth, nodules
- Atrophy, adhesions, granularity

9. Immune system

Organs/tissue to be examined

- Spleen, lymph nodes, bursa and thymus (poultry), bone marrow
- Peyer's patches, GALT, RALT

Lesions to be observed

- Size, shape, atrophy, hardening.
- Oedema, congestion, hemorrhage

10. Nervous system

Organs/tissue to be examined

- Brain, spinal cord, nerves, meninges

Lesions to be observed

- Congestion, haemorrhage, hematoma
- Oedema, swelling
- Abscess
- Hypoplasia

11. Miscellaneous observation

- Adhesions in pleural/peritoneal cavity
- Any other left over information pertinent to post-mortem examination/ diagnosis

12. Post-mortem diagnosis

- Diagnosis should be made on the basis of above findings which involve any system or organ. The most involved organ based diagnosis should be written with suggestion of etiological factors or etiology based diagnosis.

Writing of post-mortem report

Post-mortem report consists of two parts post-mortem record and post-mortem examination as given in the format on next page. The first part *i.e.* post-mortem record is having information related to animal and is supplied by the owner or person requesting post-mortem examination. Actually, it is a part of request form of the case for post-mortem examination. This is necessary for the identification of animal. It should be filled in before conducting post-mortem examination. The proper record will be helpful in establishing accurate diagnosis based on post-mortem examination.

Post-Mortem Record

1. **Species:** Here one should write the species of animal such as bovine, porcine, equine, poultry, etc.
2. **Date:** Date of the post-mortem examination.
3. **Case no.:** The serial number of your post-mortem book. It shows cumulatively how many animals are examined by you in necropsy.
4. **Breed:** Mention the breed of animal, if known or supplied in the request form, such as Murrah buffalo, Jersey cattle, etc.
5. **Age/Born:** Age of animal or its date of birth. In case the exact age is not known then mention young, adult or chick, grower, adult in case of poultry.
6. **Sex:** Sex of animal (male or female).
7. **Identification number/mark:** It must be filled with utmost care; the number (tattoo number or brand number) should be the same as on animal. If the identification number is not available/illegible then write the characteristic mark of animal.
8. **Owner:** Here, the name of owner with complete address must be filled clearly. The address should be complete enough so that the report can reach the owner through post also.
9. **Referred by:** In this column, the name of Veterinary Officer/any other officer who referred the case for post-mortem examination should be written. Sometimes owner himself/herself is interested in post-mortem examination of animal; in such case the name of owner should be written.
10. **History of the case:** This includes the clinical illness of animal, duration of illness, epidemiological data, tentative diagnosis, therapeutic and preventive measures adopted. This is very important and information of this column has an important role in making the diagnosis.
11. **Reported date and time of death:** It should have the exact date and time of death of animal. Sometimes, it is difficult to note the exact time

then one can write morning, noon, evening, midnight etc. to approximate the timings of death of animal. In some large farms, it is very difficult to record information with regard to each individual animal/bird so here one can write "previous night" as time of death.

12. **Date and time of post-mortem examination:** Pathologist conducting post-mortem examination should write here the exact time and date of the post-mortem examination.

The above information is very important to arrive any conclusive diagnosis. The correct information enhances the specificity of post-mortem diagnosis. Some points might be looking like insignificant but one should not overlook them and write as correct as information he/she can gather from the owner's request letter/form.

Post-Mortem Report

Post-Mortem Record

1. Species:
2. Date:
3. Case No.:
4. Breed:
5. Age/Born:
6. Sex:
7. Identification No.:
8. Owner with address:
9. Referred by:
10. History of the case:
11. Reported date & Time of Death:
12. Date and Time of post-mortem examination:

Post-Mortem Examination

1. External appearance
2. Subcutaneous tissue and musculature
3. General observations after opening the carcass

4. Respiratory system
5. Cardiovascular system
6. Digestive system
7. Urinary system
8. Genital system
9. Immune system
10. Nervous system
11. Miscellaneous observations
12. Post-mortem diagnosis

Date: Signature of officer conducting post-mortem

Place:

Post-Mortem Examination

It includes the observations made by the pathologist conducting post-mortem examination. This part of report should be filled in as soon as possible after the post-mortem examination. It is advisable that one should record some points on a small paper or diary during post-mortem examination and fill them in report after the conduct of post-mortem examination.

1. **External appearance:** Record the lesions observed in intact animal before its opening. One should place on record the side of animal lying down, lesions on skin, external parasites, trauma etc.
2. **Subcutaneous tissue and musculature:** The observations made after removal of skin, on subcutaneous tissue and muscle should be included in this column.
3. **General observations after opening the carcass:** It contains the general information or lesions present in abdominal and thoracic cavity such as accumulation of fluid, pus, blood, clot of blood, post-mortem changes such as pseudomelanosis, etc.
4. **Respiratory system:** Record the lesions observed in respiratory system right from external nares, nasal passage, trachea, bronchi and lungs along with mediastinal lymph nodes.
5. **Cardiovascular system:** Record the lesions present in heart, aorta, arteries, veins and lymphatics.

6. **Digestive system:** Record the lesions observed in digestive tract from month cavity, esophagus, crop, proventriculus, gizzard (poultry), rumen, reticulum, omasum abomasum (ruminants), stomach, intestines, rectum, anus, cloaca, vent (poultry), liver, pancreas, gall bladder etc.
7. **Urinary system:** Place on record the lesions present on kidneys, ureter and urethra.
8. **Genital system:** Record the lesions present in ovaries, uterus, oviduct, cervix and vagina in females and testes, penis etc. in males. Be careful in recording lesions in this column as it should match with the sex of animal written in post-mortem record section.
9. **Immune system:** Record the lesions present in spleen, bursa, thymus, lymph nodes, respiratory associated lymphoid tissue (RALT), gut associated lymphoid tissue (GALT) etc. Careful recording of lesions in these organs will be helpful in diagnosis.
10. **Nervous system:** Place on record the lesions present in brain, spinal cord and nerves. Most of the pathologists overlook this system and often not taken pain to examine the brain. It should not be done and every effort should be made to examine and place on record the lesions present in this system.
11. **Miscellaneous observations:** Here one can record any missing observation which has not been covered above.
12. **Post-mortem diagnosis:** This is very important. Based on the history and lesions present in different systems, pathologists by using his experience and conscience conclude the diagnosis. He/she may also write suggestions along with diagnosis or some points to suggest the diagnosis and/or contain the disease in other animals.
13. **Signature of officer conducting post-mortem:** Each and every report must be signed by the officer doing post-mortem examination. Without signature of competent officer, it has no validity.
14. **Place and date:** The person signing the post-mortem report must also write date and place of post-mortem examination.

Collection, preservation and dispatch of specimens for laboratory diagnosis

Tissue samples are collected from dead or live animals for laboratory examination to confirm the tentative diagnosis.

Purpose

- Diagnosis of disease or for identification of new disease.
- Confirmation of tentative diagnosis.
- Prognosis
- To observe the effect of treatment and give directions for future therapy.

Precautions

- Collect the tissues as early as possible after death of animal.
- Representative tissue/sample should be collected.
- Sharp knife should be used for cutting
- Collect the tissues directly in fixative.
- Size of tissue should not be more than 1 cm for histopathology in 10% formalin.
- Hollow organs should be taken on paper to avoid shrinkage.
- Hard organs like liver, kidneys etc. should be collected along with capsule.

Collection of specimens for bacteriological examination

- Collect the tissues under sterile condition.
- Sterilize knife/ scalpel/ spatula on flame or in boiling water.
- Surface sterilized by hot spatula
- Cut with knife and collect sample from inner tissue.
- Body fluids/blood should be collected in sterilized syringe or in Pasteur pipette.
- Specimens should be collected directly in media (liquid media-nutrient broth, peptone water, tetrathionate broth or even in normal saline solution/phosphate buffer saline).
- Seal, pack and transport the collected material to laboratory in ice/under refrigeration conditions.

Bacterial Diseases

Abscesses

- Swab in sterile conditions/pus in vials
- Collect material from margin of abscess

Actinobacillosis/ Actinomycosis

- Tissues from affected parts in 10% formalin.
- Pus in sterile test tube/from edge of lesion
- Slides from Pus for sulfur granules.

Anthrax

- Blood smear from tip of the ear
- Blood for cultural examination
- Muzzle piece for biological test.
- Mark the specimen as "***Anthrax suspect***"

Black Quarter/Black leg

- Smear from swelling
- Affected muscle piece in ice.

Brucellosis

- Serum after 3 weeks of abortion
- Foetal stomach tied off
- Swabs from uterine discharge
- 5 to 10 ml milk in ice

Glanders

- Smear from discharge
- Lung, liver and spleen in 10% formalin
- Serum

Johne's disease

- Bowel washings in sterile bottle
- Smear from rectal mucosa
- Mesenteric lymph node in 10% formol saline

Leptospirosis

- Serum 21 days after abortion
- Milk/urine in vials (1 drop of formalin in 20 ml)
- Liver, kidney tissue in 10% formalin

Listeriosis

- Half brain in ice
- Half brain in 10% formalin

Mastitis

- 10 ml milk in sterile vial in ice

Pasteurellosis

- Heart blood
- Lung, spleen and mediastinal lymph nodes in ice.
- Affected tissues in 10% formalin.

Salmonellosis

- Liver, spleen, kidney and intestine tied off in ice.

Strangles

- Smear, swab of pus in ice.

Erysipelas

- Blood
- Spleen, kidney, liver in ice.

Campylobacteriosis

- Foetal stomach tied off
- Vaginal mucosa in ice.

- Preputial washings
- In pig, intestine and liver in 10% formalin.

Colibacillosis

- Heart blood in sterile vial.
- Tissues from intestine and lymph nodes in 10% formol saline.

Tuberculosis

- Lungs, mediastinal and bronchial lymph nodes in ice and in 10% formalin.

Collection of specimens for virological examination

- Collect tissue under sterilized condition
- Body fluids/ blood in sterilized syringe or in Pasteur pipette
- Tissues in buffered glycerin
    - PBS pH 7.2- 50%
    - Glycerin- 50%
- Avoid samples in glycerin from sensitive viruses *e.g.* Rinderpest, canine distemper
- Seal and mark the specimen bottle and transport to laboratory.

Viral Diseases

Foot and mouth disease

- Tongue epithelium, vesicular fluid, saliva, pancreas in 50% buffered glycerin
- Serum

Hog cholera/ swine fever

- Serum under refrigeration
- Spleen, liver, kidney in 50% glycerin/ice
- Tissues from intestine, mesenteric lymph node and half of the brain stem in 10% formol saline.

Infectious Canine Hepatitis

- Several pieces of liver, gall bladder and kidney in 10% formol saline.

Pox

- Scabs in ice and in 10% formol saline.

Rabies

- Intact head should be soaked in 1% carbolic acid.
- Fracture the skull with hammer.
- Remove skin and bones
- Half brain in 10% formalin
- Half brain in 50% neutral glycerin.
- Tissues from cerebellum and hippocampus in Zenkers fluid for 20 hrs, wash in tape water for 24 hr and keep in 80% ethyl alcohol for Negri bodies.

Ranikhet disease

- Liver, spleen in 50% neutral glycerin
- Proventriculus in 10% formalin
- Brain in ice.

Rotaviral enteritis

- Faecal sample
- Intestinal tissue in 10% formol saline.

Gumboro disease

- Bursa of Fabricious, kidney, muscles in 10% formol saline.
- Bursa, kidney in 50% buffered glycerin.

Systemic diseases

Diarrhoea/Enteritis

- Faecal sample in sterile vial
- Serum
- Tissues of intestine, mesenteric lymph nodes in 10% formol saline.

Abortion/Metritis

- Faetal stomach content tide off or in sterile vials.
- Serum of dam after 21 days of abortion.
- Vaginal discharges in sterile conditions.
- Tissues of placenta, foetal liver, stomach, kidney in 10% formol saline.

Pneumonia

- Nasal discharge/nasal swabs.
- Lung tissue/pieces in sterile vials.
- Lung tissue and mediastinal lymph node in 10% formol saline.

Dermatitis

- Skin scrapings in 10% KOH.
- Skin tissue in 10% formol saline.

Encephalitis

- Cerebrospinal fluid in heparinised vials.
- Brain tissue in 10% formol saline.
- Brain tissue in 50% glycerol.

Nephritis

- Urine sample in sterile vial.
- Kidney tissue in 10% formol saline.

Collection of specimens for toxicological examination

- Stomach/ intestinal contents
- Liver, kidneys, heart blood
- Urine
- In clean glass jars
- In ice/refrigeration without any preservative
- Seal, label, transport to laboratory.
- In veterolegal cases all specimens must be collected in presence of police.

- Type of poison suspected along with detailed history, signs, lesions/ treatment etc. should be written on letter with specimens.

Toxicosis/Poisoning

Heavy metal Poisoning

- Hg, Pb, Bi, Ag
- Liver, kidney, stomach content in ice in separate containers.

Alkaloids

- Liver, stomach contents and brain tissue in ice.

Nitrate

- Fodder
- Stomach contents, blood in ice

Strychnine poisoning

- Stomach contents, intestinal contents, urine, liver, kidney in ice.

Hydrocyanic acid

- Plants
- Stomach contents, blood, liver
- Preserved in 1% solution of mercuric chloride.

Pesticides

- Fatty tissue, liver, stomach contents, blood in ice.
- Subcutaneous, omental, mesenteric fat.

Collection of specimens for immunological examination

- Heart blood in syringe/ Pasteur pipette
- CSF/Synovial fluid /peritonial fluid
- Tissues in formol sublimate or in buffered formalin
- Blood/serum/others should be sent to laboratory under refrigeration conditions.
- Add one drop of 1:10000 merthiolate in 5 ml serum as preservative.

Dispatch of Material

Following points must be kept in mind while dispatching the material to laboratory for diagnosis.

1. Describe the clinical signs, lesions, tentative diagnosis and treatment given to animal in your letter. Also mention the type of test you want with your tentative diagnosis.
2. Write correct address on letter as well as on the parcel preferably with pin code, if the material is sent through post.
3. Mark the parcel 'Biological Material', 'Handle with care', 'Glass material', 'Fragile' etc. in order to avoid damage in parcel. Also mark the side to be kept on upper side with arrows.
4. Seal the container so that it should not leak in transit.
5. Try to send the material as soon as after its collection from animal.
6. Keep one copy of cover letter inside the parcel and send another copy by hand or post in a separate cover.
7. Keep adequate material like thermocol etc. in the parcel which will save the material from outside pressures/jerks.
8. Use dry ice, if available otherwise use ice in sealed containers.

Index

C

D

E

F

G

H

I

N

O

P

U

V

W

X

Y

Z